Food for Life

Also by Tim Spector

Identically Different
The Diet Myth
Spoon-Fed

Food for Life

The New Science of Eating Well

TIM SPECTOR

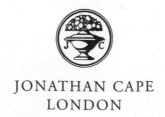

JONATHAN CAPE
LONDON

7 9 10 8 6

Jonathan Cape is part of the Penguin Random House group of companies
whose addresses can be found at global.penguinrandomhouse.com.

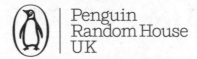

Copyright © Tim Spector 2022

Tim Spector has asserted his right to be identified as the author of this
Work in accordance with the Copyright, Designs and Patents Act 1988

First published by Jonathan Cape in 2022

penguin.co.uk/vintage

A CIP catalogue record for this book is available from the British Library

ISBN 9781787330498 (Hardback)
ISBN 9781787334267 (Trade Paperback)

Typeset in 12/14.75pt Bembo Book MT Pro by Jouve (UK), Milton Keynes
Printed and bound in Great Britain by Clays Ltd, Elcograf S.p.A.

The authorised representative in the EEA is Penguin Random House Ireland,
Morrison Chambers, 32 Nassau Street, Dublin D02 YH68

Penguin Random House is committed to a sustainable future
for our business, our readers and our planet. This book is made
from Forest Stewardship Council® certified paper.

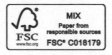

To my children, Sophie and Tom, and planet Earth

Contents

Part Three: Food Tables and Tips

Introduction:
Why care about food?

Writing this book felt like starting my own version of Phileas Fogg's adventure, setting off in his hot air balloon; armed with a map of what the world of nutrition science had in store, and a time frame in which I wanted to complete my journey, but not yet knowing the many twists and turns my voyage would take. My curiosity about food and nutrition was first piqued after a frightening episode at the top of an Italian mountain in 2011. My blood pressure shot up, having been normal two weeks before, and I was left with double vision and an anxious few weeks when I thought I had a brain tumour, multiple sclerosis, or a stroke – none of them good news. Luckily, I fully recovered after a few months, but that incident prompted me, like many people with similar life-defining moments, to start exploring my own health and nutrition. My job as an epidemiologist had been to look at the health of large populations; my own health scare forced me to look from an individual perspective for the first time.

The first phase of my journey led me to the new concept of the gut microbiome. In *The Diet Myth* I outlined the central role of our gut microbes, and in *Spoon-Fed* I introduced personalised nutrition. Both books showed why we have been so misled by bad food advice and generalised guidelines, which hardly anyone follows anyway. Yet the questions I most often get asked by readers are about individual foods and ingredients. Is brown bread always good for me? Is wild rice healthy? Is it OK if I eat full-fat yogurt, or cheese, or soy milk? These questions laid the foundations for the piece that was missing: a more practical and positive guide to nutrition, focusing not so much on the misinformation about food, but drawing on new scientific understanding to discover different food types and individual ingredients, and the many extraordinary things that happen when we eat them.

This book is an eater's guide to food and nutrition. I will show you what we should all know about the food we eat, and how to navigate the mass of information to make good, informed and practical eating choices – for our health and the health of the planet. I will introduce the true complexity of the new science of food, but you won't need a degree in advanced chemistry to decipher it. We will look at individual foods using the latest scientific knowledge about key chemicals, genes, and the role of the trillions of bacteria that live in our guts – collectively known as the microbiome – and discover how they all interact in unique and highly personalised ways. We will also explore the latest technology which allows us all, in theory, to have our genes, gut microbes and blood sugar and fat responses tested with home kits.

Researching this book made me appreciate the fantastic diversity of food and drink available to us and has strengthened my admiration for traditional, artisanal or whole foods, by which I mean those not made with complex processing in giant factories. Most of us have unprecedented choice in what we eat every day with large supermarkets stocking tens of thousands of items. But we are overwhelmed by the choice on offer and find ourselves returning to the same foods for our weekly shop or work lunch.

We have lost our innate relationship with foraging, growing and producing food for health and wellbeing, and need to re-discover food as preventive medicine. We have known for centuries that food and health are closely linked. Hippocrates realised that food should be treated with respect and can be both harmful and beneficial. My research team at King's College London (KCL) and personalised nutrition company ZOE, along with our US collaborators, highlighted during the pandemic the impact our simple food choices have on the likelihood of being severely ill and even dying from Covid-19.[1] Poor diet has been estimated to account for around 50 per cent of common diseases; if everyone ate optimally we could prevent or delay around half of the disease burden of heart disease, arthritis, dementia, cancer, type 2 diabetes, autoimmune diseases and infertility. For the first time in history, there are now 200 million more overweight and obese people in the world than those starving and underweight; over-nutrition is now a real problem. Virtually every common disease has some link with diet, either directly or via the effects of obesity.[2] Our food decisions are the single most important modifiable factor in preventing common diseases and staying healthy. Using food sensibly alongside modern medicine gives us unprecedented potential for good health. Harnessing the power of our microbiome and using evidence-based information, rather than relying on myths, marketing or snake oil, is the key to unlocking this potential.

Countless books have been written about the culinary properties of food and the scientific processes that take place when we cook it. Many other books have been written proposing different diet plans promising to help us lose weight, live longer or even improve our brain power. But we now know that there is no single diet that will work for everyone, just as there is no such thing as a superfood or a toxic food. As we will see – with a few exceptions – no food is simply good or bad. Provided it is a real food, there is no such thing as a bad ingredient. There is also no miracle cure to 'detoxify' our bodies. When it comes to our nutritional health, we should stop looking for a single villain or magic pill. This book aims to do something different. My intention is not to tell you what to eat, though I will share some tips and ideas that I've picked up along the way. Instead, I want to look in detail at the many different foods we can eat, and reveal what the latest science has to tell us about them, to allow you to make your own informed choices.

*

Some of us want to know about food to keep our weight under control, but we have been brainwashed into thinking that counting calories is the best way to do this. Even if calorie counts were accurate (which they rarely are), this would mean that eating equal calories of bread or yogurt, ultra-processed foods or whole foods would have precisely the same effect on metabolism and appetite, or that eating the same meal at breakfast or lunch would have an identical effect.

Unfortunately for the food industry, calorie-control diet companies, and the hundreds of millions of followers of traditional diet plans, none of these statements is true. Calorie counting has been the main obsession in nutrition for decades. Much like counting the macros of fat, protein and carbohydrates, keeping count completely ignores the complexity of our metabolism and the individual and variable response we each have at every meal.

Yet food and ingredient labels continue to rely on outdated notions about the importance of calories, and are made purposefully more complicated than necessary. Take this one:

> Aqua, vegetable oils, fructose, sucrose, dextrose, starch, carotene, E306, E101, nicotinamide, pantothenic acid, biotin, ascorbic acid (E300), palmitic acid, stearic acid, (E570), oleic acid, linoleic acid, malic acid (E296), oxalic acid, salicylic acid, soluble fibre, purines, sodium, potassium, manganese, iron, copper, zinc, phosphorus, chloride, pigments, chlorogenic acid, procyanidins, flavanones, dihydrochalcones, prussic acid, 50 k calories per 100 grams.

You might assume it is a margarine spread, instant noodles, ketchup, or perhaps salad cream. You probably wouldn't guess that it is in fact an ordinary apple.

An apple might seem like a simple food: best known for giving us plenty of vitamins, fibre, making a good pie, and keeping the doctor away. But a food label only tells us so much, and in practice, it tells us very little that is useful. No two apples are the same in their nutritional properties, and no two human beings will respond to eating an apple in exactly the same way. And what about what happens when you cook the apple, or combine it with fat, or ship it around the world in cold storage? As we'll see, there are many different questions we should ask about our foods, rather than obsessing about calorie counts.

Our theoretical apple food label, which you won't find in your local supermarket, also reminds us just how astonishingly complex even the most familiar ingredients can be – and this is just a list of the chemical components we know about. We experience food in colour, with its associated memories, emotions and flavours, but have tended to view food science and nutrition in monochrome. We often associate foods with a single chemical; oranges for vitamin C; bananas for potassium, coffee for caffeine; sardines for omega-3. In fact, most foods contain hundreds of chemicals we still know very little about. The true complexity of food has only recently been revealed with technology called high-resolution mass spectrophotometry, which clearly identifies at least 26,000 different chemicals in the foods we eat; yet modern nutritional databases focus on a mere 150 nutrients – individual chemicals identified in foods that have clinically identified functions in the body – we actually know something about.[3] In the past when we talked about garlic, we would be focusing on the one chemical, allicin, that gives it its pungent flavours, but we would be ignoring the other 4,249 chemicals that we can now identify. As we will see, this new holistic big-data approach to nutrition is in its infancy but will soon reveal the complexity of our foods with even greater precision.

Our concern with individual nutrients, chemicals and minerals has its origins in the aftermath of World War Two, a time of mass starvation, nutritional deficiencies and food rationing. We no longer see scurvy, nutritional blindness and protein deficiencies in most countries, yet this mentality lives on. There are countless articles, interviews, books and products to help us reach the perfect levels of vitamin D, chlorella or magnesium, when most of us aren't deficient in these components at all. This nutrient and vitamin obsession in the last two decades has fuelled a $30 billion industry. The irony is that healthy people who know how to eat well shouldn't need them, even if there was proof that they work.

Many of our problems around the science of food come down to over-simplifying the properties of foods and our responses to them. I want to restore the complexity and the wonder to our food. I want to show you what we now do know about food, but also what we don't yet know.

*

Compared to traditional sciences such as physics or chemistry, nutrition is a very new discipline with degrees in the subject only starting in the 1950s. A lack of funds, support and kudos combined with its youth have meant that there is still so much left to discover, and it is probably the most exciting and fast-moving area of science today. Much of the void in academic independent funding in recent decades has been filled by the food industry.

We can now dispel many outdated myths that have benefitted the food industry: all calories are equal, low-calorie foods are good, high-fat foods are bad, artificial sweeteners are healthy, high levels of processing are harmless, and food and vitamin supplements are as good as real food. Blanket guidelines telling us everyone would be far healthier eating fish rather than meat have not been backed up by science. Salt and coffee, once demonised, are now recognised as quite safe in normal quantities, with recent studies attributing coffee's beneficial effects to some of its plant chemicals that were previously overlooked.[4]

We used to believe that the only bad thing about ultra-processed food was that it contained too much fat, sugar and salt, so if a reformulated version appeared with reduced amounts of these ingredients and lower calories it would be just fine. We have ignored the fact for too long that these ultra-processed foods (UPFs), made up of many chemicals, make us feel hungrier, over-consume, and increase risks of disease and earlier death. Research and associated media coverage are starting to highlight the terrible impact which UPFs are having, especially on our children.[5] The 2021 UK National Food Strategy (Dimbleby) report, which I helped to advise, resulted in recommendations to tax snack foods that are ultra-processed and lacking in nutrients, to help our health and the environment, but this was vetoed by the Government the year after. We are in the midst of a food health crisis, and it is time to take some serious action ourselves.

We need to accept and embrace the complexity of food and our individual reactions to it. We have to ditch the clumsy attempts to give us one-size-fits-all advice about which foods are healthy and stop letting the food industry dictate what we should eat – increasing their profits and our waistlines in the process. This is obvious from the ground-breaking work of my team at KCL and ZOE in large-scale nutrition intervention studies, which give participants food and measure their unique individual response in the largest in-depth nutritional research program in the world, known as the ZOE PREDICT studies. These studies are led by scientists at some of the world's best universities and were made possible by funding from ZOE, the nutrition company I co-founded to help understand this complexity.[6] This individuality is also clear when you look at the varied diets eaten by the longest-lived inhabitants in the so-called blue zones around the world. The diets that support longevity vary widely in carbohydrate, fish, dairy and meat intakes, but what they all have in common is that these people eat hardly any highly processed foods.[7] One of the main reasons we got nutrition so wrong in the past is that we hadn't discovered the missing piece in the puzzle, an essential organ in our bodies – the gut microbiome – which is key to understanding how we each interact with food.

The traditional mechanistic view of nutrition and digestion, which I was taught at medical school and is still prevalent today, urgently needs to be dispelled. We can't continue with the dogma that categorising food by its calories, fat, carbohydrate and protein content, or by a few vitamins, is the best way to produce healthy recommendations.

The revolution may have already started. The team at ZOE surveyed thirteen professors of nutrition at prestigious institutions in the US and UK in 2020 and asked them to rank 105 common foods for health. For half of the foods they had excellent agreement: most fruits and vegetables were ranked consistently highly beneficial to health, while highly processed snack foods, cheap fried foods, processed meats, high-sugar foods and drinks were consistently marked as low. For other common categories such as milk, yogurt, low-fat dairy, lean meats, eggs, dried fruits and artificial sweetened drinks, however, there was virtually no consensus and scores varied widely. Ten years earlier, it is likely there would have been far greater consensus. This tells us that many experts have already changed their minds and are viewing foods differently to the outmoded guidelines and the revolution may have already started.

All the experts agreed that eating plants is healthy; so why don't they agree that all carbohydrates are healthy as this is the main component of plants? Again, the problem is our eagerness to over-simplify. 'Carbohydrates' is an overused umbrella term that scientifically includes all the subtypes of sugar, starch and fibre found in plants. Each of these three carb groups has very different effects on the body, but we foolishly lump them together. Studies and experts are highly divided on whether eating high carbohydrate diets (which also means low fat) are good or bad for you. Most US-led guidelines (which includes the UK) recommend higher carb intakes. But the large PURE study of eighteen populations in five continents (mainly in China and developing countries) showed the *opposite* effect on mortality.[8] Over-simplistic cohort studies show that extremes of carbohydrate consumption (very low or very high) both impact mortality, whereas a middle ground of 50–55 per cent consumption is generally protective.[9] Yet many indigenous populations have adapted to exist on virtually no plants or carbohydrates without obvious ill-effects, such as the Inuit, Sami and the Tsimane in Bolivia, suggesting that in some environments, carbs, unlike fats or protein, are not essential. What we don't know for sure is whether adding plants to traditional Inuit diets would have made them any healthier (though those that move to urban areas are becoming unhealthy and dying early because of processed foods and poor health care).[10] Rather than arguing over the percentage in our diets, we should be looking at the type and quality of the carbohydrate. You only have to look at the beneficial impact of the Mediterranean diet and long-term veganism, where good-quality, whole-food, high-carbohydrate intake go hand in hand with longevity.

Fat recommendations have been similarly over-simplified. Most official guidelines still tell us to limit saturated fat to around 10 per cent of total intake. This is based on outdated epidemiological studies going back fifty years. The latest data generally shows no consistent effects of saturated fat on heart disease, with some recent studies actually showing it may be beneficial.[11] Saturated fat is made up of many different types of fatty acids of different lengths that have different properties, such as how solid they are at different temperatures and their functions in the body. Some highly processed meat products have high saturated fat levels and may be associated with heart disease. But other foods with high levels of saturated fat, such as full-fat dairy, lean meat and dark chocolate, are not associated with any heart problems. Extra virgin olive oil is high in saturated fat but also contains many other types of fats and hundreds of chemicals which make it one of the healthiest foods you can eat. Food is not about individual chemical components ingredients; it is about the whole complex matrix and structure.

*

I've called this book *Food for Life* because I want to look beyond food as a tool for weight loss or gain, and instead think about food for our health in the broadest sense: our individual health, the health of our society and the health of our planet. We didn't have the space to add all of the research and nuances on the common drinks we like without this book becoming a huge tome, so I touch briefly on the main points in the final 'liquids' chapter. There is, however, so much evidence, controversy, history and interest that it probably deserves its own book, so watch this space.

We are all now more aware of the impact of our food choices on climate change, pollution and loss of biodiversity, from deforestation for palm oil, to methane production through farming, to pollution in plastic bottles and packaging. Although most of us are not in charge of the multinational companies responsible for the worst crimes, the single most important way we can contribute to reducing greenhouse gases is not by giving up our car or foreign holiday, but by changing what we eat. Some foods we have taken for granted, like red meats and cow's milk, consume a disproportionate amount of the planet's resources and our demand is driving down prices. The health of the planet obviously affects our human health too, through natural disasters and pandemics due to climate change and growing populations, to air and sea pollution, collateral damage via pesticides/herbicides and antibiotics for farming, as well as reduced food diversity, fresh produce, and localised water scarcity. We now need to factor environmental considerations into our food choices. Once we change our mindset and start thinking about meals as mini daily transactions for our future wealth, we can start investing for ourselves, our loved ones and, if we are clever, maybe even the planet.

*

It would have been impossible to write a book like this when I began working in medicine a generation ago. A vast and exciting new area of food science, which sits somewhere between medicine, nutrition, biology, chemistry and food history, is opening up to us. We now have the tools and motivation to fully understand our own personal relationships with food and why we all respond differently. Food education in schools hasn't changed for the better in the last forty years, and usually revolves around a discussion of calories, body weight, and the ability to make a cupcake or a brownie, and it has totally failed to curb the unacceptable levels of eating disorders and obesity in children of school age. Hopefully this is all about to change.

I hope to help you to look beyond the deliberately deceptive food labels, miracle product media claims, and misleading divisions of foods into calories, carbohydrates, fats and proteins. I also hope to encourage you to try new foods, vary your choice and number of plants and combinations of flavours. This book will make ingredients easier to understand and help you know what to look out for. I have added food tables in Part Three to help you plan your weekly shops. Armed with a greater overview of food facts in this book, I hope that you will become an expert in your own diet and what makes you unique.

PART ONE
Food for Life

1. What is the microbiome?

We all need to know more about our gut health and its impacts on our overall wellbeing.[1] This is not just our occasional episodes of wind, bloating, constipation or acid reflux, but the health of our gut microbiome – the thousands of bacterial species that make up our gut community, 99 per cent of which inhabit our large intestine (or colon). Current estimates suggest there are as many bacterial cells as there are human cells in our bodies (actually it's slightly more bacteria at a ratio of 1:1.3), which really means we are half human, half bug. Many people suffer long term from some gut symptoms, such as IBS, but know nothing about the state of their gut microbes and the role they play in their health. This is all about to change. Using the latest genetic sequencing technology, we can now accurately measure and classify these microbes and assess your microbiome health, and we are beginning to understand their multiple functions by exploring their genes and the chemicals they produce.

Although this technology has reduced in cost twentyfold in the last ten years, it still costs several hundred pounds if performed to a good standard using full shotgun sequencing methods. Luckily my team at KCL and ZOE have come up with a cheap and fun solution that everyone can try to provide a snapshot of their gut health. I should warn you that it involves turning your poo blue. As part of the PREDICT study participants ate muffins coloured with bright blue food dye to make recognition easy and we measured the transit time of food (from eating to toilet bowl): the shorter the transit time the healthier the gut microbiome, and the longer, the worse. The 'blue poop challenge', as it became known, was more successful than we could have imagined, beating the traditional stool test that is still being used by doctors to predict overall gut health.[2] The average time was 29 hours, with some people seeing their blue poo as long as four to five days after eating the muffin. Generally, around 24 hours was healthy (mine are around 18–19 hours) and provide a snapshot as to the state of your gut microbes and ratio of good to bad guys. Shorter transit times were also linked to less type 2 diabetes, better blood sugar control and less internal fat, but too short (less than eight to ten hours) indicates you may have an infection or other health problems. This test was better than just counting the number of times per week you have a bowel movement or the consistency of the stool. Although the test is just correlation and not causation, it clearly shows that a healthy gut is related to having a swifter transit time and not being constipated. You can get the simple blue food dye recipes to test and educate your family and compare notes and results on the website.[3]

The current research focus is on at least 40 trillion bacteria in our guts, but our microbial garden is teeming with other forms of life. Viruses also play a role in our digestion and health and outnumber bacteria by five to one, but we cannot yet measure them accurately. These viruses eat bacteria and are crucial in controlling their numbers when they get out of control and may also be helpful to us. We are also full of natural fungi, of which the best known subtype is yeasts. As well as yeasts used in beer- and bread-making, we also have plenty of candida living happily inside us. Despite misguided attempts by some practitioners to eliminate them, yeasts play a protective role in reducing inflammation and maintaining a good immune defence. Much larger parasites have also long inhabited our guts, especially in people who live in the tropics. They can cause problems sometimes by competing for the same food, but they also help the host by reducing allergies and inflammation. It wasn't thought that Western guts were home to many parasites, but as our detection methods have improved, we are finding more of them. I recently discovered I was one of 25 per cent of adults in the UK and only 4 per cent in the US to have a parasite called 'blastocystis' living permanently inside me. Amazingly, this bug actually keeps me (and other people) thinner and somehow makes me produce less internal fat. I'd love to know which foods to eat to keep this guy happy as they are found in virtually all non-developed populations and probably in all our ancestors.

The individual gut microbes in the microbiome community are best thought of as little chemical factories or pharmacies. The cells in our gut lining can produce only about twenty chemical enzymes to digest our food, while, with collectively 200 times more genes than we have, our microbes produce thousands of chemicals that our own cells cannot. These chemicals start working in the saliva in our mouths, in our stomach and in our small intestine, where most food is absorbed, and then in our large intestine, where they have more time to digest tougher plant fibre. When microbes break down food with their arsenal of chemicals and in turn produce other chemicals, it is known as fermentation.

The latest research tells us to eat a rich variety of plant foods each week (and our work suggests ideally thirty different plants), but there is little discussion of the pros and cons of different foods and ways of cooking or processing them. Much of what we are told about gut health is pretty basic and comes from labels advertising products high in fibre or commercial yogurts that promote certain bacterial strains. Bacteria that are believed to confer a health benefit when consumed live as supplements or added to food are called 'probiotics'. These have become more familiar on our supermarket shelves and are added to all kinds of food including sugary drinks and even chocolate. As you can imagine, not all the claims are substantiated, and some are ridiculous. Often probiotic yogurts have added sugar or artificial sweeteners and dozens of chemicals that would easily reverse any potential benefits. Many so-called probiotic sauerkrauts, for example, are pickled in vinegar to give them a better shelf life and so kill all the microbes. We now know that some strains of healthy bacteria die off quickly and others, such as those in sourdough or wine, are more robust when faced with the harsh changes due to food processing.[4]

As well as fibre, which comes in many different forms and provides a source of food for microbes, we now know of another group of vitally important plant chemicals that only our microbes can utilise: polyphenols. Polyphenols are essentially plant chemicals created to protect against environmental attacks such as harsh weather or specific predators. Foods vary massively in the quantities of polyphenols they contain – with a tenfold difference between different coloured vegetables of the same type, which can also vary if processed or super-heated. In general, plants have more polyphenols if they have grown in a stressful rather than a cushy environment. Plants use these chemicals as defence mechanisms for two reasons. The first is to prevent their fruit being eaten by mammals before their seeds are fertile. The other is to defend themselves against the local environment, such as excess wind or sunshine, as well as fending off microbes and insects. Some plants have been cultivated to dominate world markets simply because they have long shelf-lives and don't get damaged on long transport journeys, with no consideration of taste or polyphenols, such as an iceberg lettuce, which is devoid of both. Until polyphenol content appears on food labels, it pays to be well informed about these chemicals for the sake of your microbes.

In the age of pandemics, we are more aware of the importance of our immune systems than ever before. Some people remained completely immune to Covid-19 and never carried the virus or carried the virus without symptoms, others rapidly succumbed and died, and others suffered with a huge range of symptoms including fatigue and other nerve, skin, lung and gut problems which could last for a few days, months, or years afterwards. Northern Europeans and North Americans suffered most in terms of fatalities for every confirmed case, while developing countries in Africa had confirmed cases but relatively fewer deaths. Some of these differences were due to reporting and younger populations, but lower-income countries experienced lower death rates among elderly residents of nursing homes compared to higher-income countries, suggesting a role of diet and environment.[5]

Our immune function depends to some extent on our genes and the sanitary conditions in which we were raised, which we cannot change ourselves, but there is increasing evidence that diet can also have an effect. Our immune function worsens with age, obesity, and with associated diseases like type 2 diabetes, all of which also affect our gut health. Mice bred in laboratories without gut microbiomes also lack a normal immune system as these two are closely connected. This is what helps us to differentiate between tasty morsel and dangerous intruder; every protein, pathogen and parasite we eat is presented to our immune cells for testing. Whether we react to the peanut protein (such as in peanut allergy) or not, as well as our body's ability to fight and get rid of dangerous microbes and parasites, is what we refer to as 'immunity'. An overreactive immune system can lead to allergy, sensitivity and even autoimmunity (as with coeliac disease), while an unresponsive or sluggish immune system leads to increased risk of illness. It's a fine balance which requires a good, varied diet and a strong, diverse microbiome.

Our microbes also break down fibre to produce chemicals that energise and communicate with our body's immune cells, most of which are in the gut lining. These are the cells that sense when there is an infection and send certain key white blood cells to the site of the infection. They mount an initial T cell attack to neutralise infected cells and stimulate the slower B cell response to produce antibodies, and this provides a memory of the attacking agent so it can act even faster next time, thanks to what are known as memory T and memory B cells.[6]

I like to think of the gut microbiome as a beautiful garden, which has all of the necessary elements to blossom into a diverse and colourful oasis. The food we eat forms the soil for our microbial garden, specifically so-called prebiotic foods; the fibres and other non-digestible food components (including some fatty acids, long sugars like those in breast milk and polyphenols) that act as food for the microbiome, stimulating growth of our existing gut bacteria. The microbes themselves we can think of as seeds, which will only be able to thrive if the soil is ready and rich. A healthy, thriving microbial garden will then have flowers, leaves and lush grass, all releasing oxygen, water vapour and other chemicals into the garden's microclimate. Many of the chemicals are created by our microbes themselves and are known now as 'postbiotics'. A delicate balance exists between pre-, pro- and postbiotics and, as we shall see throughout this book, the food we eat is crucial for the success or failure of our internal garden.

When we have a poor non-diverse or ultra-processed food diet, our immune system suffers and when faced with infections such as Covid-19 either responds too slowly or feebly or is delayed, then overreacts, causing a self-induced 'cytokine storm' – like an anaphy-lactic reaction. We are still learning about Covid-19, but one of our early studies in 2020 from users of the ZOE Covid Study app showed that 8 per cent of people (and one in six children) had a skin rash, which for many looked just like a food allergy symptom. Around one in six people also suffered from nasty diarrhoea and most people with Covid-19 were found to be secreting the virus in their stools and saliva for weeks afterwards. Around one in ten people found it hard to shake off the virus and developed long-term symptoms which in about 2 per cent of people lasted over three months. Many of these people couldn't get rid of the virus from their gut, lungs or nervous system because their immune system wasn't doing its job. I believe diet and gut health are major factors in this immune failure; indeed this has now been shown in published studies.

A 2021 study of over 750,000 ZOE Covid study volunteers who filled out a detailed nutritional survey of their regular diets, revealed some fascinating data – poor diet was related to a slightly increased risk of Covid-19 even after accounting for other risk factors like age, social class, deprivation, other diseases, gender and obesity. A poor diet was even more strongly linked to the severity of the Covid-19 infection and risk of going to hospital. When we looked at the poor diets in detail, we found an obvious lack of foods related to promoting gut health. Covid has served as a wake-up call on how important good food and healthy diets are for our immune systems.

As well as fighting off viruses, our immune system needs to be in good shape to prevent food allergies, which are an unnecessary response to harmless food proteins and have become an epidemic in the young. The immune system is closely involved in monitoring our body for the earliest signs of cancer and destroying early micro-tumours without us ever knowing about them. Just a few years ago a diagnosis of metastatic melanoma or lung cancer was nearly always rapidly fatal. The latest cancer immunotherapy drugs stir up an immune response specifically against the tumour cells. These miracle drugs can now save the lives of over one in three people with advanced metastatic disease without the major side-effects of traditional chemo-therapy. I led an international study, called the PRIMM study, with over 200 patients with metastatic melanoma on immunotherapy, and we saw a powerful effect of their diet on their response to the drug and that doubled their chances of survival after a year.[7] This is all due to the links between food, microbes and the immune system, which may add credibility to the many unproven anecdotes of people taking herbs such as turmeric to help fight cancer. So all this new science suggests we should keep an open mind on the potential links between diet and other diseases.

2. Why do we love food?

Food has shaped the way we have evolved over the last million years. When we started to cook our food, our digestive tracts slowly became shorter as a result of the more easily absorbed cooked foods. Our brains became larger thanks to this increased nutrient intake, with a major part dedicated to our senses, in particular those neuronal areas related to food. As omnivores, we needed a good system to distinguish edible from non-edible foods, and those that were higher risk or those that gave a bigger reward. This is why, from a young age, we are hard-wired to be wary of bitter or sour foods that may be dangerous and programmed to love sweet foods, with energy-dense fatty or savoury foods lying somewhere in between. The smell, texture, colour or shape of a food or plant give us clues as to what chemicals it contains and what it might taste like. Taste is an imprecise term often used interchangeably with flavour, which is a combined food experience. Today, these signals are most clearly seen in infants, even before they are exposed to many foods. But we learn to overcome many of these inherited traits as we age. We all know young children can be fussy eaters, but before the age of two they are still highly receptive to many novel foods, textures and colours presented to them by their parents, enabling them to overcome their initial distaste of bitter vegetables such as broccoli.

Visual appeal

Why did you decide to eat an apple and not a biscuit and then pick that particular piece of fruit rather than the others in the basket? This is where all our senses come in, but what exactly influences our decision? Perhaps the apple was redder and shinier so it looked tastier?

Why do we associate certain colours with tastiness? Millions of years of evolution have told us that brightly coloured fruits have a high chance of containing a high sugar content, rewarding us with sweetness, valuable energy and nutrients. Fruit trees have evolved to exaggerate the growth and appeal of their fruits so that their seeds will be eaten by animals and spread to other sites to produce more trees. Over centuries, farmers have bred the ancestor of the modern apple, the tiny bitter crab apple, into over 7,000 different varieties, which can be ten times the size of the original. So, consciously or unconsciously, we look at colour, size and any signs of damage, mould, worms and ageing to help us choose the best, ripest and freshest fruit. Just the sight (or even the memory) of a red shiny apple can make us salivate and feel hungry, thanks to the large part of our brain dedicated to linking food with taste memories. Producers, shops and advertisers understand this psychology and how to manipulate it to fool us. Many shiny apples we eat are actually months old, picked unripe and stored for months in dark warehouses then sprayed with ethylene to chemically ripen them. Most supermarket apples are cleaned and polished to remove the natural protection, and then sprayed with a wax coating to make them look shiny and still ripe.

Up to half of our brain can be engaged in visualising food compared to a much smaller fraction allocated to taste. Our vision and memory help us anticipate and prime our senses for how the food will likely taste within quite a narrow range so that, most of the time, we are not in for too big a shock. I still remember eating basil ice cream for the first time in Rick Stein's restaurant in the 1980s, thinking it was pistachio. It was initially unpleasant, but now that flavours like green tea ice cream are commonplace my brain can anticipate the tastes and I enjoy them.

We can find it difficult to grasp the concept that objects have no inherent colour. The colour 'orange' didn't exist in our language until the fruit was brought to Europe by the Portuguese and Spanish in the sixteenth century and the word 'naranja' became both an orange and a new colour. A yellow lemon is not really 'yellow', it is just a fruit that reflects light at a certain wavelength perceived differently by receptors in our eyes and converted by the brain into an image of the colour yellow. When margarines were first developed, they were a dull grey colour, and had to be dyed bright yellow; orange and yellow food dyes are still often used to make food more appetising. No foods are routinely dyed blue (except the aforementioned muffins), as we rarely see blue fruit or vegetables in nature and we are programmed to not trust them.

We humans can distinguish colours and tones better than other animals, many of whom only see life in monochrome. We can in fact distinguish an estimated 5 million colours and 340,000 colour tones, which probably helped our ancestors pick the right foods, but the theory is hard to test, as we lack the vocabulary to describe the 11,000th shade of red.

Smell, taste and flavour

We are even more discerning in food flavours. By using our 400 smell receptors, capturing all the thousands of different floating natural chemicals, we can distinguish around a trillion combinations of odours. Our brain cleverly converts these into smell images, which are then stored in a lifelong smell memory bank in a dedicated part of our brains – the prefrontal cortex – which is proportionally much larger than in other animals. This is key to our anticipation of food. Just think of how sensitive we are to the different smells of burnt toast, burnt rubber, burnt fuses or burnt chicken, or how we can recognise hundreds of scents of flowers and plants. As well as detecting minute doses of chemicals, our brain can make different concentrations of the same chemical appear as different flavours. For example, there is an odour chemical which in different amounts can be perceived as a tropical fruit, grapefruit or, at high doses, something very unpleasant. One way to think of smell or flavour is like a pointillist painting, made up of thousands of tiny individual dots of odour, which blend together to form a unified sensation.

We see, smell and anticipate taste in our brain, which informs our salivary glands and our stomach to prepare for a meal. The greater the appetite the more intense the stimulation. Signals pass down from our brain through the long vagus nerve to our second brain – the vast network of nerves and neurons lining the gut – roughly the same size as a cat's brain. Saliva is stimulated even before we pick up that red apple, and like Pavlov's dog, it can be enough just to imagine one. Just the thought of this apple stimulates our digestive system and appetite hormones, which allow acid in the stomach to be released.

The primary role of your mouth is to rapidly decide if you are going to spit or swallow, and it has evolved as a sophisticated defence mechanism against poisons. Your tongue may be extra sensitive to slimy or unusual textures to stop you swallowing a worm or insect that might be in the apple. When you bite into the apple, your brain expects to hear a crunch and if it doesn't it will rapidly downgrade the apple as potentially worth spitting out. The crunchier the sound the higher the edibility rating, even if the flavour is indistinguishable. Many apple varieties are bred for their 'crunch' as much as their flavour, given names like 'Honeycrisp' which make your brain anticipate the crunchy noise. Food manufacturers have also manipulated this desirable quality in crisps and breakfast cereals, and in their packaging and storage choices.

Once the first bite is in the mouth, the taste and odour receptors are triggered, anticipating and reinforcing the flavour of the food. Saliva moistens each mouthful; it contains water, salts, mucus and many enzymes to help release the chemical aromas, and as you chew more of the food's surface area is exposed and its taste develops further. The shape or texture of the apple perceived by the sense of touch can also modify our taste. Soft rounded food shapes or food labels convey greater sweetness than sharp angular ones. When Cadburys smoothed out the edges of the angular square blocks of their bestselling Dairy Milk chocolate without altering the recipe they had complaints from loyal customers saying they had made it creamier and sweeter. If the apple is pre-cut with sharp edges it will taste less sweet than one cut in smooth semicircles. Some of this could be our visual perception and part could be the sensation on the tongue.

Some foods, including apples, have chemicals that provide a key characteristic called astringency. It is neither a taste nor a smell but a tactile sensation of puckering or drying of the mouth and tongue.

You will notice this when eating a slightly tart apple or drinking dry cider, certain wines, black tea or an unripe banana. It is due to certain polyphenol chemicals called tannins which make proteins in our saliva stick together, making the tongue surface seem rougher. A little bit of astringency in a sharp apple or dry cider can be pleasant but can be overpowering if the effect stays in the mouth too long. One reason milk is popular with strong black tea is to block the astringent effects of the tea leaf chemicals so they can't stimulate the tongue proteins.

When we rate the taste and flavour of a food, we are unable to distinguish which of our senses we are relying on. We are fooled by our brain into thinking that sight and taste are the most important. We have five main tastes we can distinguish – sweet, sour, bitter, salty and umami (savoury) – but we may actually have many more, though experts can't agree on their credentials. Although the sight of an apple is often what we think attracts us, the aromas are an underrated guide to freshness. The ancient Greeks believed smell was the basest of the senses. Our brain tricks us into thinking that the sense is coming from our mouth disguised as taste. We also have a communication problem: it is hard for us to describe the thousands of aromatic chemicals floating around inside our heads, which also vary by our culture and language.

There is a common myth that we have super-specialised receptors for different tastes in different areas of our tongues. This tongue map was propagated by a German scientist in 1901 and wildly exaggerated in the 1940s by a Harvard academic, inappropriately named Professor Boring. Receptors (which look like tiny onions) occur all over the tongue, except for a bald patch in the middle, and are not in fact specialised but can detect multiple tastes. Our brains deceive us into thinking they are localised to make the message clearer. My brain still regularly fools me into thinking that I have specialised beer receptors at the back of my tongue, and these are extra sensitive when I'm thirsty on a hot day. Genetic differences in the number and sensitivity of these receptors explain some, but not all, of the taste differences and preferences between people. We also have taste receptors in other parts of our body, including the pancreas which makes insulin, and scattered throughout our intestines, and even in men's testicles, suggesting these receptors may have other mysterious properties.

Our tongues and palates are specially geared up for rapidly detecting bitter tastes as a protective mechanism against poisonous plants. Biting into an unripe plum or a bitter crab apple would make our face pucker up in an instant reaction – just as when babies are given bitter foods. Some people will taste the sourness and bitter flavours of the apple more than others. Some prefer a sharp Granny Smith to a Sweet Gala and some enjoy munching a bitter cider apple that most of us would immediately spit out. If detecting bitterness and sourness is our main defence mechanism against poisoning, why do we often seek them out in small doses? One reason is that humans, unlike most animals, stopped making our own vitamin C about 60 million years ago, so seek out sour plants, apples and citrus that make the vitamin for us. The other is that we have strangely evolved to like the sour taste of the acids produced by fermented foods like yogurt and fermented milks and cheeses. Perhaps we evolved to like foods that were good for our microbes despite the fear of poison.

We have known about bitter taste genes since 1931 when a laboratory prank led a chemist to discover that one in three of his lab staff couldn't detect any bitterness in a chemical called PTC, while one in five people were extremely sensitive and found it very unpleasant. There was a lot of excitement when in 2000 two genes were found (called TR1 and TR2) which appeared to control this response.[1] Most scientists naively believed, like I did, that the key to understanding taste would be to look at the tongue taste receptors and find the few other genes underlying them. But we were wrong and, as so often is the case, biology is much more complicated.

There are big differences between us all in what and how we smell and taste; the 20 per cent of us at the upper range are especially sensitive to bitter taste and are also generally more sensitive to sweetness and detecting odours. These people are known as 'supertasters' and are less likely to drink coffee, red wine, dark chocolate, beer, spicy food and brassicas like broccoli or spinach. Studies of identical twins – who share (for practical purposes) identical genes in every cell of their bodies, and are effectively clones – have shown only modest genetic effects in detecting odours, meaning our environment, upbringing and chance all play a role. When we rated the twins' food preferences, we found that bitter and spicy foods (like alcohol, quinine, garlic) were most genetically influenced, but most of the differences were unexplained. Many of these genetic differences can be overcome by continued exposure to these foods, especially when young.

A simple and fun experiment that you can do at home, with or without assistance, is to place a selection of small bites of different foods on a plate, close your eyes or use a blindfold, fully pinch your nose, then use a fork to place each on your tongue. I did this recently and was surprised at the results. I could not tell a piece of apple from a slice of red pepper, melon, garlic, onion, salami or cheese. Of the ten foods placed on my tongue, the only ones I reliably identified were the sour lemon and spicy chilli. I tested three other friends and got the same results. This brought home to me that the key to taste is not my tongue but my nose.

Follow your nose

Food is made up of thousands of edible chemicals, many of which break down with time, cutting or cooking, into lightweight chemicals called volatiles. We humans can smell these volatiles when we are in proximity of the food. This crucial survival skill helps us to avoid rancid meat or rotten plants. Dogs have a nose specially designed for detecting scents, as seen in their amazing ability to smell the presence of cocaine or Covid virus. This kind of direct smelling method is called 'orthonasal'. But humans are actually pretty good at smelling too. Our heads and noses are specially designed for a different kind of smelling, called 'retronasal' (behind the nose). As we chew the apple, and as we breathe out with our mouth closed, we drive the fruit's odour chemicals backwards and upwards to smell receptors in our nose. Our palate and nasal passage are specifically designed for this purpose. Our anatomy allows very close direct contact between the odour chemicals released in our mouth, which are recognised by the nose receptors, fast-tracked to the olfactory bulb and put together and stored by the brain's clever prefrontal cortex.

Smell is the only sense that has a direct link to the brain — like a superfast broadband connection. This allows us to rapidly construct flavour images from hundreds of chemicals. If you observe how dogs eat, there is little savouring of the subtle flavours. Dogs get most of their pleasure from the anticipation and initial odours rather than from the full mouth gastronomic experience. We credit cats with all kinds of extra powers and sixth senses, but they can't even detect sweet tastes or aromas. Rats have great orthonasal skills and can even detect if food is lacking in some nutrients, such as essential amino acids. However, it is unlikely that they quite have the tasting skills to rival the fictional gourmet chef Remy in one of my favourite films, the 2007 animation *Ratatouille*.

We have all experienced the effects of a heavy cold or sinusitis on dulling our taste. Coronavirus attacks the nerves in the odour receptors, which affects up to a quarter of people with Covid-19 symptoms and, in about 1 per cent, can last over six months. Using data from the ZOE app, my research group was the first to pick up this loss of smell as the best predictor of infection of all the twenty symptoms associated with the virus.[2] We managed to get the UK government to add it to its official lists of symptoms as well as other countries around the world. The long-term effects, which also include distorted taste and smell, are devastating and often lead to depression.

Cigarette smoking and age are major factors in diminishing sensitivity and ability to distinguish smells and taste, which drops off after the age of seventy-five. But we are much more flexible than we think: we can exercise and retain our taste by continuing our exposure to multiple odours which increases the number of nasal nerve fibres.

Losing your sense of smell can be due to early dementia, however, as the brain centres that record food memories become damaged or cut off from the other parts of the brain. Even if the loss of smell is more subtle, it can be a harbinger of death. A 2014 study looked at 3,000 Americans aged fifty-seven to eighty-five and tested them with five classic smells – rose, leather, fish, orange and peppermint – and followed them for five years. Those with problems smelling had a fourfold risk of death. So, for whatever reason, smell and taste are pretty crucial to us humans. We don't yet know the answer, but we are studying whether loss of smell through Covid-19 has any long-term consequences.

Much is still unknown about our taste mechanisms. Different microbe communities live on the distinct areas of the tongue surface and we are just realising that they, along with the microbes in saliva, are involved in taste. Many people notice the reduction in taste that occurs when on antibiotics. Temperature also changes taste. If food is eaten straight from the refrigerator, the sweetness is masked, whereas a warm fizzy drink tastes much sweeter. On a plane journey, food also tastes less sweet because of the decreased pressure reducing the spread of the volatile flavour molecules and the reduced ability of your smell receptors. Airlines select sweeter fruit varieties and saltier dishes to compensate for this – and with all the extra intestinal gases and smelly socks surrounding you on long flights this loss of smell can be a bonus.

Listen to your gut

Most ultra-processed foods (UPFs) contain mixtures of fat, salt and sugar in quantities that have been tested on human volunteers to produce the perfect bliss point which lights up the pleasure centres. The brain, once tricked, then produces feel-good neurochemicals like dopamine which override any signals of fullness from our gut hormones or even our microbes.[3]

These three key flavours – fat, sugar and salt – with the addition of a 'crunchy' mouthfeel, are used to convert cheap, tasteless and nutritionally useless base ingredients into addictive foods.[4] Recent additions of flavour enhancers, artificial sweeteners, sugar alcohols and other new wonder chemicals are designed to increase this brain response and further disrupt our normal feedback loops of satiety. No foods in nature possess this heady, addictive mix, so we lack any evolutionary defence mechanism to stop us gorging on them. As a result, we are becoming fatter but less nourished, which is especially a problem for our children who are now growing up eating UPFs.

The gut–brain axis and the gut–lung axis hold answers to many questions around dietary quality and health, as well as the promise to improve some of the most common and deadly health problems in the modern world. Our sense of smell and how food feels form a huge part of our eating experience but also predict our overall health.

The latest evidence shows that our microbes actually help inform us about what foods we should be eating, even causing us to crave certain foods. Our microbes literally send chemical messages to our brain to encourage us to eat what they need for their survival. Having lots of unhealthy microbes in your gut, therefore, can lead to a vicious cycle whereby you crave foods that help these less friendly bacteria, which in turn drive you to become less healthy. A stark example of this is seen in the difference in microbiome species between vegetarians and meat-eaters. When looking at 'good' and 'bad' microbiome species, we look for those that help reduce inflammation and those that promote it. Inflammation is our body's normal immediate response to trauma, stress or foreign bodies, including food proteins, which starts the healing process. Acute inflammation is a bit like the intense heat of a pizza oven that can be turned on or off. Chronic (meaning long-term) low-grade inflammation is like a smouldering fire that never goes out and stresses the body and is associated with nearly every long-term disease we know of. The meat-eaters tend to have many more pro-inflammatory species living in their guts which are associated with a tendency to crave meat products, whereas those who eat lots of plants have more beneficial microbe strains with less inflammation and often report not feeling the desire to eat animal products. Worryingly, this trend is exaggerated with UPFs, which not only look, smell, taste and feel good to our palates, they also bamboozle our bacteria and make us want more of the same.

3. What foods are really healthy?

Most people reading this book will know that eating plants is generally healthy. On average vegans and vegetarians are healthier and live longer in most countries. We tend to think that eating fish is also healthy (though the evidence is lacking), but when it comes to eating meat opinion is much more divided.

Meat eating has been linked to increased risks of heart disease and cancer mainly, it was believed, because of its saturated fat content. As the saturated fat health story has become less clear, so has the evidence that red meat is always unhealthy. Epidemiological studies consistently find an increased risk of heart disease, cancer and mortality with eating low-quality processed meat – cheap sausages, ham and burgers – often found in ultra-processed foods and ready meals – with a smaller but still significant increase in risk for white meats like chicken. The same risk is not seen with fish consumption, which is why fish is often thought of as a 'safer' animal food choice. The data is always strongest in the US, where people eat enormous quantities of often poor-quality meats, and no associations are seen in Asia where smaller quantities of meat are consumed. The reasons for these differences are still uncertain: they may involve the chemicals such as nitrates or nitrites in processed meats, or the simple fact that the context of the meal is important and the more meat on your plate, the less room there is for a diverse range of plants.

Of all the UK government's 'Eatwell' recommendations, only the directive to eat more than five fruits and vegetables a day had a significant effect on reducing mortality.[1] There are huge numbers of potentially edible plants, of which we only eat a tiny fraction. Are they all good? We need to know more about them and what properties make some better than others, and that is not simply their fibre or calorie content.

Plants as factories

Most of our diet comes from plants even if we don't always recognise them. The spices you add to your stew, the peanuts you nibble as a snack, your cup of coffee in the morning, tofu in your stir fry and pickles in your sandwich, all count towards your daily plant intake; it's not just about spinach and carrots. What do plants have in common? They have all evolved to use energy from the sun to convert nutrients from the soil to produce the sugars they use for energy and growth, a process called photosynthesis, which also generates oxygen. Plants inherited this skill from algae, who in turn inherited it from some clever bacteria about three billion years ago that had mutated to produce a chemical similar to chlorophyll, which is now found in all plants. Because plants don't have legs or wings, they are stuck in the same environment with the same nutrients and seasons. As they need to be able to live off whatever minerals the soil provides, they have evolved as complex chemical factories, with thousands of enzymes able to construct or deconstruct whichever compounds they need. We humans, by contrast, manufacture few chemicals, and use our legs, eyes and nose to obtain the nutrients we need. Our gut microbes, on the other hand, also evolved this amazing chemical production capacity in common with plants, as they have to cope with whatever we decide to feed them.

The thousands of chemicals that plants produce are still largely uncharacterised. It is worth knowing more about these phyto (leaf) chemicals. The overriding aim of a plant is to sustain itself long enough to produce fruits or seeds in order to reproduce and continue its species. Many chemicals ensure that the timing of this seed production event is perfect, but defences are needed to ensure the fruits and seeds are not eaten too early or by the wrong animals. Because leaves are exposed to daylight, protective chemicals, called polyphenols, are needed to prevent sun damage to the cells. Plants must also deter parasites and fungi from living off them, or insects or mammals from eating them. These leaf polyphenols work both as colourful pigments like sunscreen, and act as a defence mechanism for the plant as toxic deterrents. Polyphenols that can be good for us but are poisonous in excess include alkaloids such as the stimulants nicotine and caffeine; coumarin in lavender and clover, which stops blood clotting; cyanide in many fruit seeds, which can be poisonous; psoralens, found in some environmentally stressed parsnips and celery, which cause DNA damage in the skin and are also used as psoriasis treatment; and of course, mushrooms, which contain hundreds of toxins, some of which can be deadly.

The different parts of a plant all have different roles and contain varying mixes of both nutrients and chemicals to protect it. The fast-growing leaves or the tips of the young sprouts need the most protection, and so have the highest concentrations of polyphenols. They also hold the most flavour compounds, which is why we often use these tips as herbs to enhance our food. Sometimes these will be darker or brighter in colour to alert us to their chemical secrets. One of my favourite fruits, which clearly shows the link between polyphenols and survival, is the blood orange, which grows well in Sicily and California. The reason for the vivid dark red flesh is the huge amount of a polyphenol called 'anthocyanin' which the orange produces to survive the temperature swings of a Sicilian winter, with warm days and cool nights.[2]

The phrase 'Eat the Rainbow' has become overused, but it is actually very useful nutritional advice. Eating the rainbow should equate to eating a variety of colourful fresh fruits and vegetables, representing a wide variety of polyphenols. Deep purple aubergines, bright red peppers, vibrant green courgettes and sunshine yellow peaches all contain powerful plant chemicals that contribute to our overall health. We just need to make sure we are eating these colourful foods whole and in their natural form, rather than in a pasteurised smoothie with added colourings and flavourings.

Some endow individual plants with multiple anti-ageing, immune boosting, anti-cancer, or antioxidant properties. More specifically, individual nutrients are attributed problem-solving superpowers, such as magnesium for insomnia and leg cramps. Some nutrients are essential and easily obtained from food, but most are just good marketing tools for the food and supplement industry. The benefit of healthy food is unlikely to be via single nutrients but a combination of the hundreds of chemicals that interact with our gut microbiome. The body has a wonderful 24/7 defence system against disease, ageing and cancer. Our body is constantly repairing itself and fixing small genetic mutations, killing off misbehaving cells or sending out repair signals to build more protein or tiny blood vessels. Studies show that over the age of sixty, most of our bodies contain a multitude of micro-tumours, which never get to become fully blown cancer thanks to our effective immune surveillance systems. But these multiple defences get harder to maintain as we age. The microbiome plays a key role in all of these, and a few nutrients and vitamins in tiny levels are also critical to the many essential chemical reactions we need to thrive.

The vitamin myth

Vitamin C or ascorbic acid provides an interesting illustration of the good and bad sides of vitamin-rich foods. Chilli, cabbage, yellow sweet peppers, kale, broccoli, sprouts and parsley are lesser-known great sources, but we all know that citrus fruits are full of vitamin C. Like many fruits, the ancestors of oranges, grapefruit, lemons and limes were impossibly sour and hard to eat. The Romans used citrus zest or juice to add flavour to food and drink, or as medicines and antidotes to poisons. In the seventeenth and eighteenth centuries around half of enlisted sailors died of scurvy, directly or indirectly – an estimated 2 million men. In 1749, two centuries before vitamin C was discovered, after performing probably the first ever controlled trial, James Lind, a British naval doctor, found that citrus fruits helped prevent scurvy. Twelve scurvy-afflicted sailors were 'volunteered' for the trial, divided into six treatment groups, and given extra rations of the following potential 'cures': dilute sulphuric acid to burn away the 'putrefaction of the guts' (which was widely believed to be the cause); six spoons of vinegar; a quart of cider; half a pint of seawater; spicy barley water; or oranges and lemons. Unsurprisingly, the seawater and acid were not a success, and only the seamen taking the fruit or cider improved. Lind wrote up his findings in 1753, and then promptly left the navy to earn money in private practice and his findings were buried for decades.

Lind's citrus cure was finally officially approved in 1795, leading to British domination of citrus-growing trade routes. All British sailors were given rations of limes (hence 'limeys'). It turned out that limes were not the best source of vitamin C, but they were tough and highly transportable, and the nation's now healthier navy dominated the world for the next hundred years.

Once ascorbic acid (vitamin C) was discovered in 1927, it was promoted as the cure for all our ills and added to as many processed foods as possible. The idea was that if it cured scurvy, extra amounts would have powerful effects on our immune systems, fighting infections, cancer and ageing. A flawed study by Ewan Cameron in 1976 suggested that mega-doses could help terminal cancer.[3] Although no other group could prove this effect, the food industry loved it. They started selling more orange and fruit juice, and then chemical supplements, which were encouraged for the whole population, sometimes in massive doses. The science has finally caught up and meta-analysis of over twenty-nine studies and 11,000 people shows that extra vitamin C does *not* help prevent cancer, obesity or immune conditions. It also doesn't help prevent any new colds or reduce cold symptoms by more than a few hours. A recent large population study using the ZOE app showed that vitamin C supplementation does not help prevent Covid-19 infection but it still enjoys soaring sales as a supplement promising salvation from infections of all kinds.[4,5] Anyone eating a diverse range of fruits and vegetables never has to worry about vitamin C or dubious supplements. As well as having no benefit, taking vitamin supplements can sometimes be harmful. This is because taking isolated nutrients outside of their food matrix is unnatural and can cause serious consequences. Excess vitamin E can cause cancer and too much vitamin A in pregnancy can cause abnormal foetal development.

Vitamin D is another vitamin with celebrity status, and it is added to a wide variety of foods. I was always a big fan, but after spending twenty-five years researching and promoting calcium and vitamin D for bones in my hospital clinics, and writing over thirty related research articles, I have realised the data doesn't add up. It is one of the most studied 'vitamins' and one of the most hyped, having been proposed as a treatment or prevention for over a hundred diseases, with no good evidence to back any of the claims. The final nail in the coffin for me was when I played a minor part in a massive genetic study of fractures in over half a million people. It found there was no effect whatsoever of vitamin D, or milk drinking (and therefore calcium) on the risk of fracture. This data supports summary studies (called meta-analyses) of multiple trials of both vitamin D and calcium supplements, which, when you factor in poor-quality studies, show there is no effect on preventing fracture or falls.[6] Overuse of vitamin D supplements has been linked in several trials to increased falls and fractures, and calcium supplementation in normal doses has been linked in trials and genetic studies to modestly increased risk of heart disease.[7] So unless you are *really* deficient or are caring for someone who spends most of their days indoors, you are much safer getting your vitamin D from fifteen minutes of sunlight per day. In winter, underrated natural sources of vitamin D are oily fish, egg yolks and sunbathed mushrooms (especially shiitake and button), as well as fortified foods. The levels of vitamin D are generally not affected by cooking.

Metabolic stresses, sugar peaks and the food matrix

Even a healthy apple is not just carbohydrate but also contains a small percentage of protein and saturated fat plus tiny amounts of poly- and monounsaturated fats. The pancreas is a small organ next to your liver that sends out enzymes that break down carbohydrates and complex sugars into smaller glucose and fructose molecules that can be absorbed into the bloodstream. It also produces the hormone insulin to help regulate how much and how quickly glucose and protein get to the blood and other organs. Proteins are mainly broken down (digested) here by specialised cutting enzymes allowing the small pieces to be absorbed. Any fats reaching the small intestine start to be broken down by liquid produced in the liver called 'bile salts'. These allow the fat to be dissolved by water and absorbed into the blood and the cholesterol which is the main way fat is absorbed, reused or stored.

Our gut microbes play an important role in getting rid of fat. They produce a chemical enzyme which converts some of this bile liquid into 'active bile salts' which break down the excess fat further, making it harder to be absorbed, so it continues its journey and ends up in the toilet instead of your bloodstream. Depending on which combination of specialised gut microbes you have, your body will vary in how much of both the good and bad fat components get recycled in your bloodstream and how much you excrete. If the fat stays too long in your bloodstream after a meal, some of the smaller particles irritate the blood vessel walls and lead to inflammation which can lead to furred up arteries and signals that increase build-up of fat stores.

So most of the major nutrients in food, such as the sugars, fats and proteins, get absorbed in the middle part of the gut – the small intestine. The rate at which this happens and subsequent changes in the blood which occur are crucial to our health and vary in all of us. This enormous variability is dependent both on the composition and complexity of the food (what we call the matrix) and more importantly on our unique metabolism, which is the basis of the new field of personalised nutrition. My team and I have been studying this intensively on an unparalleled scale for the past five years. Every piece of food has a different rate at which it increases blood sugar after eating depending on the composition and the amount you eat. Those foods with a high score indicate a likely sharp rise in blood sugar after eating, and for the last few years we have relied on a crude average measure called the glycaemic index (GI).

Although short-lived blood sugar peaks after food are a normal response, we now believe that having too many high peaks or large fluctuations with subsequent dips is unhealthy – high peaks and subsequent dips in our blood sugar will make us hungrier and tend to overeat later in the day.[8] Often this depends on the structure (food matrix) and composition of the food, as well as how you eat or chew. Once the food structure has been broken down by chewing, the fats and sugars (glucose) inside the food are released from inside the food cells and absorbed into our bloodstream where they affect our blood fat (commonly known as lipid) and blood glucose levels; in simple terms how much fat and sugar we have in our blood. Some small studies have shown that eating whole foods by chewing them thoroughly results in healthier insulin, blood lipid and glucose responses after eating when compared to consuming foods in a processed form or eating very quickly.[9,10] Chewing is an important way of giving your body more time to react to food arriving. For example, an average apple produces a three times lower blood sugar peak compared to the equivalent unsweetened apple juice. If you ate your apple as mashed-up baby food or as a smoothie, its sugars would be more rapidly accessible because the cell walls containing the starch would be already broken down. This means it would produce a higher glucose peak in the blood, and less would reach the colon. When you digest whole foods such as a sandwich made of sourdough bread with traditional cheddar you expend 50 per cent more energy compared with the same highly processed versions using a white supermarket loaf and plastic cheese.[11]

This matrix effect is also seen with fat levels in nuts which are less accessible when eaten whole than when crushed into a nut powder in processed foods. Changing the matrix of the nuts, from whole almonds to powdered almonds, for example, by crushing and destroying their structure, changes both the blood lipid levels (fat) and energy levels (calories) from the same amount of whole almonds. Like sugar peaks, having high levels of circulating blood fat six hours after a meal is bad for your metabolism and triggers low levels of inflammation as described earlier. Over time this accumulated stress causes permanent changes such as heart disease, type 2 diabetes and weight gain. This shows how different foods, and the different forms in which they are eaten, have crucial health consequences, which aren't reflected in their calories or fat levels.

In the second major report of the ZOE PREDICT nutrition intervention study, published in the journal *Nature Medicine* in 2021, we showed for the first time a link between microbes that were associated with health and the specific foods that changed their frequency.[12] The ZOE PREDICT studies started when I co-founded ZOE. With the help of scientists from Massachusetts General Hospital, King's College London, Stanford Medicine and Harvard T.H. Chan School of Public Health, we wanted to find out how different foods impact each of us individually. We also discovered fifteen good and fifteen bad bugs that were consistent across populations in their links with health and specific foods. We don't understand many of the mechanisms yet, but what is certain is that by interacting with and fermenting our food, microbes can control the rate at which both fat and sugar are absorbed into the body as seen by the spikes in our blood and the way they affect our metabolism. Whatever your starting point, having a diverse range of microbes and a good ratio of good to bad bugs means you can eat the same amount of carbs or fats but have less harmful effects. Keeping the microbes well fed means they produce many chemical metabolites such as butyrate and other short chain fatty acids, key vitamins like vitamin K, biotin, folate B6 (important in pregnancy) and small amounts of B12, as well as having a major role in supporting our immune system.

Foods for a healthy gut

After five years collecting over 11,000 samples from citizen scientists around the world, the American/British Gut Project team produced its first findings. What turned out to be more important for gut health than whether you were a paleo follower, a fruitarian, a vegetarian or even a vegan, was the number of *different* plant species you ate each week.[13] Thirty different plants per week appeared to be optimal. We adjusted for all kinds of possible biases, such as education level, age, social status, smoking, alcohol, constipation, number of children, pets, body weight, diseases, medications, but all the data pointed to the same powerful effect – the diversity of plants you regularly eat.

Why should this be important? We have been brought up to think that if we eat an apple a day it will keep the doctor away, that carrots help your vision, spinach makes you stronger, and broccoli may make you live longer. If you ate only these plants every day, you should be super healthy. Well, not according to our results, at least not for your picky gut microbes. They would prefer you eat apple, broccoli and carrot on one day, but at least twenty-seven other different plants on other days of the week. Of course, plants include seeds, nuts, herbs and spices, which we may eat regularly in small quantities, and might not normally consider when we think about eating plants. Under the old nutritional paradigm of calories, sugars, fats and protein as building blocks, coupled with the simplistic view that plants mainly provide vitamin C and roughage to bulk up the gut, this idea makes no sense at all. But each plant, and sometimes specific bits of plants, has a unique set of chemicals, structure and flavour, and of course a specific role in nourishing our bodies via our microbes. So, it is the diversity of different plants that counts.

After the small intestine stage, most highly processed and refined food we eat has already been absorbed. But what I call 'real' food, which has structure and fibre (like the remains of our apple) enters the large intestine (or colon). At 1–2 metres long the large intestine is actually smaller than the small intestine. At medical school I was taught that this is the boring stage of digestion, designed to retain water and make nice firm stools. But what happens in the colon, and what food reaches it, is crucial to our understanding of food and health. In the large intestine, most of the dozen or so different polyphenols found in our apple are now liberated by microbes either to be used directly or converted to yet more complex polyphenol chemicals. These chemicals (such as quercetin, catechin or chlorogenic acid) help the body fight cancer, depression, diabetes or heart disease. They also help prevent obesity. In an observational study of nearly 2,000 twins we found those that ate large amounts of foods containing polyphenols had a 20 per cent reduction in risk of obesity, even after adjusting for fibre intakes.[14] Fibre intakes were also a major predictor of weight gain or loss over ten years in the same group, showing that polyphenols and fibre improve our health independently.[15]

Some polyphenol chemicals are used by microbes directly as energy like rocket fuel, enabling them to replicate and also create a waste by-product that might actually be an invaluable chemical component for us: short chain fatty acids (SCFAs). These tiny molecules have many functions. When SCFAs reach the human cells lining our gut they supply them with energy, literally keeping them alive and letting them replicate. They are key for sending signals to our immune cells, keeping down inflammation and suppressing allergies. They also act on our brain and gut hormones, suppressing appetite. An example of one such SCFA is butyrate which helps our gut barrier, that separates the contents of our gut from our blood supply, to remain intact and prevent what is known as 'leaky gut'. The thin single-cell gut barrier is delicate and recurring infections, poor diet and high stress can result in it breaking and causing unhelpful gut contents to 'leak' into our circulatory system, causing more inflammation and damage. This is a real issue if you are ill with inflammatory bowel disease, such as Crohn's disease or ulcerative colitis, or severe malnutrition, but it has been exaggerated as a major cause of problems in healthy people. While gut hyperpermeability is a possible factor in poor health associated with eating unhealthy foods and chronic stress, it is massively over diagnosed and linked with false 'miracle cures' for leaky gut.

The power of these polyphenol pigments is a recurring theme in our foods and in this book. Polyphenols explain many real and potential health benefits of plant-based foods. Plants give out clues to their polyphenol content from their shape, size, colour and taste. There is a growing interest in eating older heritage varieties of plants, like purple carrots or potatoes, which are naturally higher in polyphenols, and we are hopefully dumping some blander varieties, where the polyphenols have been lost in intensive breeding. Our tongue and mouth also give us clues to the polyphenol content. Polyphenols are defensive chemicals for a plant, and they are generally bitter and astringent on your tongue, such as strong red wine, good-quality black tea or olives. Through trial and error our ancestors knew that these plants, if they didn't kill you, were probably good for you. We need to regain that skill.

Having a diverse and balanced community of gut microbes is crucial for our health and evidence is accumulating that microbes are also in part responsible for regulating our appetite. When a particular microbe species runs out of its food supply, it will send out signals to the brain asking for more. When a particular species or group is sated and its population has doubled, they fill the available space in the gut community and send a signal to the brain, saying 'No more apples please.' This takes about twenty to thirty minutes – the same time it takes for us to get sensations of fullness after eating.[16] Our microbes have their own evolutionary needs and method of self-regulation. If our microbe community is not well balanced, or we overeat ultra-processed foods, our finely tuned energy signalling system breaks down and we may become overweight or obese. The key to a balanced gut microbiome is a diverse range of whole plant foods and small amounts of fermented foods.

Fermented foods are much more important than we ever realised, both in their health benefits and in the extra flavours and complexity they add. By fermented I mean foods that use live microbes in their production, what used to be called 'cold-cooking', but are also present in the final product. While many foods are made with a fermenting process – sourdough bread, pickles, chocolate, coffee, wine and beer, etc. – only a few actually contain live microbes in the end product. As well as well-known foods like cheese, yogurt and fermented tofu, kefir, kombucha, kraut and kimchi (see page 154) – the K-rations as I call them – are becoming more popular as natural probiotics you can create at home. As they contain live microbes they contribute to your gut microbiome diversity.

Strong health evidence supporting specific types of fermented foods above others is unfortunately still poor, and we often extrapolate from consumption of yogurt, which is a less potent but more accepted and better studied fermented cousin. We now know the microbes from these products definitely make it past our stomach to our colons. Although they only stay for a short while – which is a good reason to eat them regularly – they do have time to stimulate production of helpful chemicals that aid our metabolism. For the microbes to be able to work optimally in our microbial gut garden, we need a combination of the stimulation of regular probiotics plus a variety of good prebiotic foods which act as fertilisers.

Top five tips for healthy eating

1. Foods that are good for your health are also good for your gut microbes.
2. Eat plenty of plants and a variety of them. I recommend aiming for thirty different plants per week.
3. Select plant foods high in the defence chemicals called polyphenols, and fibre.
4. Eat fermented foods regularly.
5. Eat foods in their whole, natural form to maintain the optimal matrix, and avoid UPFs.

4. What foods are unhealthy?

Defining what is unhealthy is surprisingly difficult, but this includes foods that do not benefit our biology in any way. As a general rule, foods made in a factory that are completely lacking in a variety of plant fibre, plant polyphenols or probiotic microbe species will not be good for us if we choose to eat them regularly or in excess. Good examples might be doughnuts, rice cakes, or most protein bars. Another general rule is that foods that get absorbed fast in the upper part of the gut (the small intestine) and rapidly enter the bloodstream as fats and sugars, leaving nothing for the colon (or large intestine), are usually unhealthy. These foods produce sugar peaks and dips and increases in blood fats that the body finds hard to deal with on a regular basis and this, as we have seen, causes overeating and inflammation.[1] Although this is true of some natural foods, such as honey or sweet fruits like dates or figs, most of the foods in this category are 'ultra-processed foods' or UPFs.

But how do we define 'ultra-processed'? Many foods are processed in some way, including some of my favourites, like dark chocolate, raw milk cheese, yogurt and bread, the latter involving fermentation which we have seen is actually helpful for our microbiome, and I'm certainly not suggesting we cut those out of our diets. From my perspective I'm worried about factory-made products with large numbers of ingredients and chemicals – on or off the label – which may be interacting in indeterminate ways to damage our health.

The concept of UPFs was introduced in 2018 by the Brazilian scientist Carlos Monteiro who noticed that although the amount of sugar and salt purchased by consumers was decreasing, the amount of sugar and salt consumed was increasing, which was due to the increased consumption of industrialised foods.[2] The most accepted definition comes from Monteiro's team of scientists (see also NOVA table, page 446):

> The term 'ultra-processed' was coined to refer to industrial formula-tions manufactured from substances derived from foods or synthesized from other organic sources. They typically contain little or no whole foods, are ready-to-consume or heat up, and are fatty, salty or sugary and depleted in dietary fibre, protein, various micronutrients and other bioactive compounds.

This definition is likely to evolve into more of a continuous scale of food processing, taking into account the amount of nutrients and energy and the level of processing of foods. The food industry will have to adapt to this new way of assessing food quality, to avoid their products being classified as UPF.

The simplest way of classifying UPFs is that they are made up of complex mixtures of chemicals and food extracts which don't resem-ble the original parts of whole foods – such as potato starch extract used instead of potatoes. Pringles, the addictive, bestselling 'potato discs', for example, are not officially crisps and are actually made by mixing dehydrated potato, rice and wheat – along with the perfect combination of sugars, fats, salt and enticing flavourings – into a heated molten paste then baking and slicing it. With its aerodynamic shape, and a minimum of twelve ingredients, this is far from a simple sliced potato, and like most other popular synthetic composite prod-ucts (Hula Hoops, Quavers, Doritos), it has virtually none of the vitamins and nutrients of the original vegetable. Meal replacements and slimming liquids also don't have any 'real food' matrix.

A practical way to identify an ultra-processed product is to check its list of ingredients for food substances never or rarely used in kitchens (high-fructose corn syrup, hydrogenated or 'unesterified' oils, and hydrolysed proteins), or classes of additives designed to make the final product palatable or more appealing. There are over 2,000 approved food additives, and even more enzymes, including flavour enhancers, colours, emulsifiers, emulsifying salts, sweeten-ers, thickeners, and anti-foaming, bulking, carbonating, foaming, gelling and glazing agents. UPF labels usually list over ten such ingredients. I have included a table of some common UPFs at the end of the book.

UPFs are designed to be highly profitable (with low-cost ingredients and long shelf-lives), convenient (ready-to-consume), hyper-palatable (addictive) products. Studies have shown that UPFs are so palatable that we regularly eat far more of them than we need. In a randomised clinical study, twenty stable-weight people were invited into a lab and were given either unlimited UPFs or similar but unprocessed foods for two weeks. When left to consume UPFs freely, people on average ate an extra 500 calories per day and had gained 1kg by day six.[3] Those same people were then switched to consuming unprocessed whole foods for two weeks under the same strict lab conditions: they consumed an 'average' level of 2,400 calories per day and lost an average of 1kg. Despite the extra quantities of UPF eaten, both groups rated the two diets as equally pleasant. Part of our pleasure from food comes from how full and content it makes us feel, which is known as satiety. Studies in the 1990s showed big differences in satiety measures with foods that have the same calorie and glycaemic load. It is this difference that food companies exploit to make us eat more of their product. Even between the same kind of food – such as different types of breads – there can be a fivefold difference in how satiating it is. In the ZOE PREDICT study, people who habitually consumed high levels of UPFs, which are less satiating, and low levels of whole foods had a significantly worse blood fat response and inflammation, perhaps explaining why UPFs are strongly linked to heart disease.[4]

UPFs are the source of over half our calories in the UK and US, up from 30 per cent in the early 2000s, and typically contain very low levels of good-quality protein, fibre and polyphenols, as any original plant content has been stripped of nutrients and outer coatings. It requires chemical genius to join together highly refined ingredients which no longer resemble plants and make them taste like the original food with some reasonable texture. Clever food chemists have come up with thousands of chemicals that make food stick together, called emulsifiers (see page 267), or have realistic texture ('carrageenan' or methyl cellulose). Then there are the chemical flavours and enhancers that make you think you are eating something like bacon or pineapple when you are not. These chemicals not only upset our microbes, they also make UPFs addictive as they make these foods hyperpalatable and desirable to eat, driving us to want to eat more of them. The data is still unclear on the exact mechanism by which eating UPFs causes overeating. It could be that the additives and chemicals used in the processing directly affect our microbes or our brains, or it could be the resulting texture of the food: softer, more energy-dense and easier to eat with a more pleasing mouthfeel, combined with the lack of chewing and increased speed of eating which could upset the natural signals of satiety to the brain. Another problem with UPFs is that the sugars are readily available and cause more sugar peaks, and the ZOE PREDICT study showed that volunteers with sugar peaks and resulting dips had more hunger pangs and subsequently overate.[5] Clinical trials are ongoing in the US to explore these mechanisms, but my guess is that *all* will be important factors.

The consumption of UPFs has increased steadily in the twenty-first century and has now reached 67 per cent of food calories in US children.[6] Sales have increased across the globe and more than doubled in South Asia in the last decade.[7] There are distinct links between the countries that consume most of these products and increased rates of obesity, including the US, UK, Canada and Australia, where UPFs are cheap and plentiful. The evidence also shows that removing these UPFs from our diets could be really beneficial. From recent clinical studies comparing different foods with the same calories and components, we now know UPFs make us overeat by around 25 per cent compared to equivalent whole foods.[8] A recent simulation model found that reducing UPFs in children in the US could reduce childhood obesity by 50 per cent in adolescents within a few years.[9]

In Portugal and Italy, where the majority of calories comes from 'real food' and only about 10 per cent from UPFs, there is a lower rate of obesity and more healthy life years on average (a way of measuring added healthy years as opposed to just a longer life). The most bizarre thing about UPFs is that they often strip the core ingredients, such as whole wheat, to make products such as Mother's Pride sliced sandwich loaf, simply to artificially add back those same nutrients and market them as a 'healthy' choice.

Conventional nutritional descriptors are not currently capable of measuring all the detrimental effects/aspects of UPFs, thus manufacturers can misleadingly market them as 'healthy' to an unwitting market. However, specific chemicals in UPFs have been proven to be bad for us. Hydrogenated or trans fats, for example, first created in the 1970s to solidify liquid fats by switching a few chemical bonds, which prolong the cupboard life of margarine, biscuits, savoury snacks and fast food, keeping them soft for months without going mouldy or drying out. The problem is the body couldn't deal with this new form of fat that caused inflammation and millions of deaths from early heart disease. Many countries have banned trans fats completely since the 2000s, but the UK and USA still allow a small percentage of trans fats, probably due to food industry lobbying. Even small amounts of trans fats (1–2 per cent of daily food intake) massively increase inflammation, lipid levels, heart disease and sudden death threefold, not even counting the extra cancers. Some people were consuming 10 per cent of their daily food intakes as trans fats, but the early reports of adverse health effects in the 1980s were largely dismissed as scaremongering. In 2019, the UK suggested a voluntary limit of 2g of trans fats per 100g of fat and better labelling, but still refuses a ban despite expert consensus that there is *no* safe lower limit. New methods of making fats solidify involve interesterification, but despite manufacturer's health claims, the research on their safety for long-term consumption is inadequate.

Nitrates also worry many people. Concerns were first raised when US observational data implicated nitrate (estimated from food surveys) as the factor linking meat consumption with risk of earlier death or heart disease. For a long time, the role of nitrates was difficult to interpret; indeed, hypotheses about their health effects changed from one week to the next, likely because we were trying to pin cause and effect to individual components of food, without considering the whole food in all its complexity.

Nitrates (NO_3) are mostly found in whole plant foods like beetroot, leafy greens and fruits. They are first broken down into nitrite

(NO_2) by bacteria in the mouth, then other microbes in our gut convert them into nitrosamines. Understanding the role of these different metabolites of nitrate is the key to knowing which to worry about. Based on our current knowledge, nitrate-rich whole foods are good for us, whereas nitrites when added to foods or resulting from processing generally are not. Crucially, nitrate-rich foods are high in beneficial chemicals such as polyphenols and fibre, providing an overall protective effect, and they are associated with better heart health thanks to the conversion of nitrate to nitric oxide in the 'wall lining' of our body's blood vessels. Here, nitric oxide maintains healthy blood vessels and prevents clots associated with strokes and heart attacks. Eating more nitrate-rich foods *protects* against many chronic diseases and is associated with a 26 per cent reduced risk of gastric cancer.[10] In animal tests, dietary nitrate improves glucose and insulin balance as much as the diabetes drug metformin and has even greater protective effects on the heart and liver. In short, nitrates are a natural part of whole plants which have fibres, polyphenols and probiotic species of their own. When we eat nitrates in plants, we are eating a lot more than just the nitrates and so the overall effect is a beneficial one.

Nitrites, on the other hand, are mostly found in processed meat and bean products as a result of changing or heating their original nitrate compounds. In these highly processed products nitrates are associated with an increased risk of cancer and other diseases, probably because these foods are lacking in protective polyphenols. Lastly, during ultra-processing, high-temperature cooking and storage nitrites in meat combine with amines in the protein to form nitrosamines. When these nitrates are converted to nitrites (and nitrosamines) outside of our bodies due to food processing they are no longer beneficial for us.

Nitrosamines in processed meats have partly taken over the role of the bad boys in cancer, leading to calls to reduce our intakes. One large observational population study from France suggested that while nitrites explained a third of the increase in breast cancer associated with processed meats, the greater risk may actually be due to increasing levels of nitrosamine in the gut. Another study of half a million Americans (the NIH-AARP study) estimated that about half of the increase in mortality they found with processed meat could be attributed to nitrites.[11] So once again, whole plant foods are protective with their nitrate content, while highly processed meat and dairy products are likely to increase risk with their nitrites and nitrosamine content. The problem is not the nitrate compounds, it is the level of processing of the foods we eat.

The high iron levels in meat have also been suggested (particularly by vegetarians) as a reason for the increase in heart disease or other conditions. Indeed, a substance called heme, which contains iron and transports oxygen around the body, can alter the way we handle nitrogen and has been linked to cancer in some rat studies. However, results of epidemiological population studies are conflicting about the role of iron, and with small effects they can easily be biased. A way round this is to use genes that influence blood iron levels as a proxy for high iron levels (a technique called Mendelian Randomisation). One such unbiased study of 50,000 people found that iron, far from being toxic, was actually slightly protective for the heart. So, iron overload seems to be a diet myth.

Finally, one of the unhealthiest things we can do is consume sugar in sweetened fizzy drinks like Coke, Pepsi or Fanta. This is now strongly linked to risk of obesity, type 2 diabetes and heart disease.[12] Increasingly, as well as added salt and sugar, in response to the demand to reduce sugar content manufacturers are adding artificial sweeteners. These were hailed as miracle products when they were first introduced, but sadly this was wishful thinking. Most of them – saccharine, sucralose, aspartame, acesulfame K (AceK) – were created in labs, often by mistake by scientists working on fossil fuels.

Others are the semi-natural sugar-alcohols, like xylitol used in chewing gums, or are derived from selected genetic strains of plants like stevia. In observational studies, these artificial sweeteners were associated with the same risks of obesity and disease as drinking regular sugar. Better evidence comes from large-scale clinical trials where artificially sweetened drinks have no clear benefit to weight loss, despite the reduction in calories. This suggests they must have negative metabolic effects that offset the lower energy intake. This appears to happen mainly by disrupting the gut microbes, making them lose species diversity and produce abnormal chemicals which upset our normal metabolism and predispose us to type 2 diabetes. Another problem is that these drinks are designed to keep your sweetness threshold high – so you retain a sweet tooth even if you switch from natural to artificial sweeteners.[13] This is a major problem in children who will seek out other sources of sweetness. These artificial chemicals are not inert and although many food companies dress them up as healthy alternatives, they are far from it.

The context of how the food or drink is consumed can also be important in deciding if it is 'unhealthy'. Having a glass of high-sugar orange juice with your meal, or a block of chocolate afterwards with your coffee, will likely do less harm than having it on its own as a mid-morning or late-night snack. This is because although the calorie intake is the same, the sugar spikes and dips will be much greater when the food or drink are taken as a stand-alone snack, resulting in greater hunger levels in the next twelve hours and consequently overeating.[14] It is easy to see why, with food companies pushing a combination of cheap tasty UPFs and snacks, often with misleading healthy labels, we have all tended to put on weight and increase our risk of type 2 diabetes thanks to a rollercoaster of blood glucose and lipid levels and postprandial inflammation throughout the day.

Top five unhealthy foods

1. Ultra-processed foods (UPFs) – with extra fat, sugar and salt as well as other preservatives and additives.
2. Artificial sweeteners in foods or drinks.
3. Highly refined carbs – these are usually UPFs and low in fibre.
4. Foods that produce high blood sugar and blood fat peaks after meals with a lack of natural matrix or fibre.
5. Snacks containing a lot of sugar or low-quality fats – even if they have 'healthy' labels saying they contain protein or 'natural' sugars.

5. Can foods 'boost' your immune system?

With the advent of novel viruses like Covid-19 and the increasing rates of food allergy, we have become much more aware of the importance of our immune system – the natural defence mechanisms throughout the body which defend against attacks from invaders. We now know that our immune system is much more clever and sophisticated than previously realised, and it is key to fighting off ageing and cancer and many other common diseases. Until quite recently it was thought we all had very similar but complex immune systems depending on our age, but developments in technology have allowed us to look more closely and, in fact, we vary enormously.

In 2015, while working with a US group at the National Institute of Health, we performed a landmark twin study on the role of genes and environment on levels of 80,000 different types of immune cells in our blood. We found that around two thirds of our cells were under genetic control, leaving little room for an environmental influence.[1] However, simultaneously, another twin study in California explored a smaller range of cells but tested how they responded dynamically to invaders or chemicals.[2] The findings were opposite to ours: the environment was much more important than genes. So, while both studies were correct, it is becoming clear that how our immune cells respond in real-life situations is probably more important than the resting state. The response of our immune system is largely driven by environmental factors like diet and our gut microbes. And the good news is that these are potentially modifiable.

As newborns we are vulnerable, without any real microbiome or immune defences other than the antibodies passed to us through our mother's placenta and microbes we come into contact with during birth. For the first few weeks we then rely on the immune cells from our mother's milk, and we start to prepare our own microbial garden from the pre- and probiotics it contains, otherwise even a common cold virus could kill us. From an early age our body knows which microbes are dangerous and which are beneficial, including the ones we acquire during the messy process of squeezing through the birth canal and from breastfeeding. Our immune systems deal easily with some infections, skin wounds or spots, blocking off the invading bacteria so they can't spread, and then killing them, producing pus, which is just dead cells.

Other infections from viruses may be harder to fight off as these microbes are much smaller and can disguise themselves as they take over our own cells and replicate. We are prone to several cold and flu virus infections each year and rarely become completely immune as these viruses mutate slightly to regularly create new variants, outwitting our defences and ensuring their own survival. As children, many of us have will have had the viral infection chickenpox, and although it can recur as shingles, we almost never catch it again. We become naturally immune to reinfection as our immune system is now boosted and ready to beat off a second attempt. Vaccination is a man-made process designed to boost our natural immune system by tricking it into responding to a small or a modified, safer form of a virus. The newer technologies developed for Covid-19 vaccines trick our cells into reproducing parts of the virus which our immune systems can then detect and create the necessary antibodies. The first clinical trials to boost the immune system date back to seventeenth-century China; smallpox was rife, so the imperial family put dried scabs up their noses. The Ottoman Empire regularly inoculated against smallpox and it was Lady Mary Wortley Montagu who discovered the practice whilst travelling in Turkey. She tried it out on her own children before introducing it in England in 1721 when six death row prisoners 'volunteered' to have skin and pus from a smallpox patient introduced into an opened vein. All had short-lived symptoms and survived thanks to their healthy immune systems and the small dose ingested.

There are two forms of immune defence. The first is the innate immune system which we share with many other animals. It is a crude but effective blunt instrument, whereby any perceived threat is met by circulating common white cells which trigger a rapid inflammatory response to limit the damage. This is what happens in an allergic rash, when pain, swelling and redness are caused by white cells rushing to the scene and producing chemicals that alter our blood vessels and produce fluid. The second immune defence system, adaptive immunity, is more sophisticated but slower, usually taking around seven days to work. Specialised white cells called 'T cells', 'B cells' and 'natural killer cells' either target the danger directly like assassins or form antibodies to neutralise the virus, then form memory cells to guard against future attacks. These cells lie dormant waiting for the next wave of infection, so that – as with Covid-19 – we are usually resistant to attack by the same variant for six months because we mount such a rapid and precise second response that it can't get a grip on our bodies. This clever system protects us from major infections and death but it can also overreact causing food allergies and some forty autoimmune diseases – coeliac disease, type 1 diabetes, rheumatoid arthritis, for example – where the immune system attacks cells in our own body by mistake. We have seen many more problems of allergy and autoimmunity since the 1970s, possibly because we live in more sterile environments, have less contact with dirt, nature and bugs, use more antibiotics and have a poorer, less diverse, highly processed diet. All of these factors adversely influence our gut microbes and consequently our immune system.

Although I was taught that our main immune organs were in our lymph nodes, spleen or bone marrow, it turns out the biggest immune organ is in our gut – lining most of the small and large intestine, covering an immense surface area of over 25 square metres. The immune system, therefore, is in close and regular contact with the gut microbes which, as well as nourishing the cells of the gut lining, also send chemical signals to dial immune response activities up or down. Certain species of bacteria have tiny little packages (OMVs) on their outer coating that contain microscopic fat particles that can enter the gut wall lining and send all the correct signals to the immune system. The OMVs make contact with certain white blood cells – dendritic cells or regulatory T cells – which then communicate with the other immune cells to elicit a protective response.

Until recently, we scientists had not considered how even from an early age our immune system knows *not* to attack friendly microbes or alien proteins in a piece of meat or a peanut. We now know that the gut microbes have a crucial role in this learning process as they interact every day with the enormous number of immune cells lining our intestines.

In the 1980s we saw that the severe immune deficiency disease AIDS, caused by HIV viral infections, often led to cancers. The cancer spread much more rapidly in AIDS patients than in people with healthy immune systems, so clear links were established between the immune system and the disease. We also now realise that every time our cells replicate, they produce some DNA mutations and that these mutations accumulate to produce microscopic tumour cells throughout our body. Luckily, our immune defences identify these mutant cells as 'alien' and destroy them. But when cancer-seeking immune cells are weakened by disease, poor diet or some immuno-suppressant drugs, these micro-tumours go unchecked and can become life-threatening.

This revelation of the power of activating the immune system is producing medical breakthroughs. Immunotherapy (using our own immune cells to selectively attack malignant cells instead of all replicating cells) is now replacing traditional chemotherapy for many types of cancer. A new breed of drugs called 'checkpoint inhibitors' work by destroying the cloaking device of tumour cells that kept them invisible to our body's natural immune defences. This immunotherapy which boosts our immune defences has transformed the survival rates of some previously incurable solid cancers like end-stage melanoma, lung, kidney, prostate and more recently breast cancer. Checkpoint inhibitors can melt away metastatic tumours in the brain, liver and bones in just a few months and produce miracle cures, as with former US president Jimmy Carter. Sadly, only about one in three people respond so well.

A few small studies suggested this may be due to differences in their gut microbes. With the help of the Seerave Foundation, I formed an international consortium to further explore this hypothesis and finally in 2021, after collecting hundreds of gut samples from melanoma patients undergoing immunotherapy, we got the answer.[3] The varying composition of the microbiome was a key factor in determining survival, and we know that this is driven by diet.

Our immune system not only helps to fight infections and cancers, it may also be instrumental in slowing the effects of ageing. Ninety per cent of deaths from Covid-19 or seasonal flu occur in over eighty-five-year-olds because the immune system performance reduces with age. From our own and other studies we also know that the composition of the microbiome changes slightly with age and deteriorates rapidly over the age of seventy-five. So, how might a weakened and elderly immune system accelerate the rate of ageing? All human cells contain mini batteries of bacterial origin called 'mitochondria' that generate energy for us to function and convert oxygen into hydrogen. A by-product of this chemical change leaves a few molecules, 'free oxygen radicals', floating around, like flying sparks in a metalworks. Too many free radicals can cause inflammation, damage and stress to other cells, so they are usually removed rapidly, with the help of the immune system, which loses efficiency as we age.

Our immune system is also constantly working to alert the body to attend to other vital repairs, but DNA in our cells is simultaneously constantly mutating every time it replicates and causing errors. When we are young, a healthy immune system and the DNA repair mechanism work efficiently, but as we age, they start to fail. The immune system becomes overwhelmed with trying to deal with too many damaged cells at once, so the speed and quality of the repairs gradually deteriorates over time. This failure of the immune system to detect defects in our cells and initiate repairs helps to explain why our bodies age and why we develop cancers with increasing years. The speed at which this degradation happens varies from person to person, but we know that it is more rapid in overweight and obese individuals.

Along with thousands of twins, I have been testing my immune age for the past five years with a blood test which measures small sugar molecules called 'glycans' that adhere to immune cells and change with age.

By analysing the amount of pro-inflammatory glycans attached to an antibody in our blood called IgG and comparing it with others of the same chronological age, we can estimate biological age. According to the GlycanAge test, developed by my colleague Professor Gordan Lauc, I am consistently biologically fifteen years younger than my real age, so I love this test! This allows us a pretty good summary test of a healthy immune system and a poor score is found in people who are overweight, with heart disease, hypertension or diabetes, or a range of autoimmune diseases or cancers. We have recently shown that losing weight can improve this immune marker of age.[4] In the Covid-19 pandemic, obese people did not get the same immune protection from the vaccines as people with a healthy weight. The precise reasons are not totally clear, but diet quality and the gut microbes are likely to play a major role.

There is much talk of foods that boost your immune system. The only way to actually 'boost' our immune system is through infection or immunisation against a certain pathogen. Rather than trying to 'boost' our immune system out of its delicate balance our aim should be to support and balance it. This list of supposedly 'immune boosting' foods often contains berries, wheatgerm, mushrooms, green tea, nuts, seeds, spinach, broccoli and probiotic yogurt, and foods high in specific vitamins. 'Immune boosting' recommendations include a varied diet containing lots of fibre, over six portions of fruits and vegetables a day, and plenty of protein – either from protein supplements or ideally from high-protein plant sources such as lentils, quinoa or tofu. Fish, particularly oily fish, is also on the menu, as are a daily spoonful of mixed seeds, olive or avocado oil and all kinds of spices, especially garlic, ginger, chilli and turmeric. We are told that cinnamon is good at battling inflammation and fighting off bad bugs, rosemary prevents cell damage, and cardamom is a great source of the essential nutrient zinc that is vital to our immune response.

This all sounds impressive and intuitively makes sense. The problem is that when you dig deeper you see that most of these bold and often repeated claims are not derived from proper clinical trials or any solid science. More often than not they are based on small artificial lab experiments, where chemical extracts of the plants, nuts or herbs are found to alter the potency of immune cells, stem cells, cancer cells, blood vessel cells, or a virus or microbe on a plastic plate, by a certain degree. This is the easiest and cheapest way of gathering evidence, but also the least clinically useful and reliable.

The term 'antioxidant' was only coined in the 1980s after discoveries about the workings of the human cell. The term is widely used but few people (including most doctors) know what it really means. Scientists found that many vitamins and chemicals in food could reduce the damaging free oxygen radicals released in normal cell activity and speed up their removal. In 1986, a scientist proposed that many natural vitamins, including vitamin C, could act directly on blood vessels to combat this harmful oxidation, by preventing fats in our blood and low-density cholesterol cells becoming attached to oxygen, and thus reduce build-up of plaque and furred arteries.[5]

But there are two problems with this theory. The first is that when tested in isolation in laboratory conditions most food chemicals can to some extent act as antioxidant sponges and mop up free radicals. The other is that free radicals are not there by accident. Most processes in the body have an evolutionary purpose and free radicals help the body to fight infections and to signal to white cells where to go to fight off invaders or to repair sites of damage. So, while an excess of free radicals may be bad, too low a level is also dangerous. The term antioxidant is now outdated and is too blunt a description for the hundreds of different chemicals that can have a range of effects. Scientific reviews have since argued against a direct effect of many antioxidants as the single factor in improved health suggested by population studies.[6] With the exception of a few of the key vitamins with specific roles such as vitamin K and vitamin A, most antioxidants are simply chemicals derived from or related to plant polyphenols which, as I have described, have a beneficial effect when consumed in a plant-rich diet. We now believe that most of the effect of plant polyphenols is not on the immune system *directly*, but via the gut microbe community, which release key messages to the immune cells lining the gut.

Zinc is an interesting example. It is often added to highly processed foods to allow for 'immune boosting' claims on the label. The original research to support this was performed in the 1980s on a small study of men who had a rare severe zinc deficiency and some abnormalities of their immune cells. This was followed by a few lab tests on immune cells in isolation.[7] But what this tells us is simply that a total zinc deprivation can cause immune problems. Yet somehow, food manufacturers convinced regulators that added zinc can 'boost' our immune systems, even when we don't suffer from the rare zinc deficiency. More recent studies have failed to show any major immune problems in men with mild zinc deficiency. And although no study has ever shown that extra zinc helps prevent any disease, it is very hard to reverse a health claim once granted. Similar claims have been made for added selenium, with a similar lack of conclusive evidence.

The Covid-19 pandemic put the purported benefits of vitamins for the immune system in the spotlight. By 2019 the use of regular vitamin supplements was already high with purchases in around 50 per cent of households in English-speaking countries and in much of Northern Europe, but with the media hype about how they could protect against the virus, vitamin sales went through the roof in March 2020. In the largest study of its kind, after the first wave of Covid-19 in 2020 we surveyed around 2 million people in the US and UK about their Covid infection status via our ZOE Covid app and asked if they had taken regular food or vitamin supplements for at least three months. After adjusting for many potential biases, we found no benefit whatsoever of taking zinc, vitamin C, or garlic supplements in preventing Covid infections. We also analysed reported use of vitamin D, omega-3 fish oils, multivitamins and probiotics. None of these had any preventative effect in men, but there was a small reduced risk of infection in women (7–27 per cent), with probiotics having the strongest protective effects and vitamin D the least.[8]

It is hard to interpret the results. Being an observational study (and not a proper clinical trial) they could be caused by some form of bias, yet could still be instructive as men and women have different immune systems, and hence have different rates of immune-related diseases. Thanks to their reproductive system and the need to interact with and protect a foreign foetus, pre-menopausal females typically have a more resilient immune system than males. When matched for age and weight, females have higher numbers of circulating B cells, which most of the time provides an advantage against infections, but it also leads to a much greater risk of autoimmune diseases than for males.[9] Our ZOE app studies also found that women were much more likely to suffer side-effects of vaccination than men, as their immune systems reacted more strongly. These different immune systems between sexes and the more robust response of women means they could potentially respond differently to supplements but more research is needed to establish what these variances are.

My views on the value of vitamin D supplements have attracted much criticism. For twenty-five years I prescribed it regularly to patients and I even used to take it myself. I then spent many years performing clinical trials and found that levels of the vitamin varied between people because of their genes. But despite many claims for vitamin D preventing everything from osteoporosis to cancer to depression, well-controlled clinical trials so far fail to support any of these benefits. Nevertheless, I'm always open to new data and long-term studies looking at chronic disease outcomes. A meta-analysis of thirty-nine randomised controlled trials of variable quality identified that vitamin D supplements on average modestly reduce the risk of respiratory infections by 3–11 per cent.[10] The finding by my own group that use of vitamin D supplements slightly reduces risk of a positive Covid test matches this data. But this was not confirmed in a clinical trial of high-dose vitamin D injections in Covid patients.[11] In short, additional vitamin D has a trivial effect which, if true, is only seen in women. Regular exposure to sunlight and a diet including vitamin D-rich foods could be – and probably is – much more effective than supplements.

The greatest effect of any supplement in our Covid study was seen when taking a probiotic supplement. I wasn't expecting this, as we did not specify which type of probiotic people took and they vary enormously in quality and amount of gut microbes they contain. Despite this we saw a reduction in risk of 27 per cent in the women we surveyed in the UK, US and Sweden. Even men had a slight benefit from probiotics. As it is an observational study, we are likely overestimating effects or missing some selection bias, but it may be correct, given what we now know about the important role the gut microbiome plays in our immune system function. Probiotics modify the host's gut microbiota and may generate anti-viral metabolites, and they interact with the host's gut-associated immune system. This can result in improved immunity, including better immune responses to the seasonal flu vaccine and possibly anti-Covid vaccinations, creating a good amount of protective antibodies and memory cells ready to fight off future infection. Studies also now support a surprising gut–lung axis, whereby immune effects of gut microbiota and their metabolites can be transferred somehow to the lungs, most likely through movement of immune cells. This could explain why in trials some probiotics also reduce risk and severity of respiratory tract infections, and why certain gut infections can cause lung diseases and can be especially dangerous for people who suffer with lung diseases such as cystic fibrosis.[12,13]

We used to think that stem cells in the bone marrow were the key players in producing the right amounts of immune cells in circulation, but the evidence suggests that the gut microbiome may be more important. We have recently learnt a lot about the link between our immune and microbiome systems from studying cancer patients who need bone marrow transplants after all their immune cells have been destroyed during treatment. From studying 10,000 stool samples and comparing the changes in microbes to the changes in white blood cell counts, we learnt that certain microbe species were central to restoring white cells to normal levels. These microbes acted either directly on the immune system or by sending signals to the stem cells in the bone marrow to precisely regulate the amount of white cells needed.[14] The same study found that when chemotherapy patients were given their own healthy gut microbes, which had been stored by a process called an 'auto-transplant', they were able to regain healthy levels of white blood cells much faster.

Long-term, or chronic inflammation, which can be thought of as an overstressed, overreactive immune system, increases the risk of heart disease and metabolic problems such as obesity, thanks to the complex interactions between the gut lining, short chain fatty acids (SCFAs) and pro-inflammatory chemicals called 'cytokines'.

While anti-inflammatory diets are often promoted in vague terms by the nutrition industry, we do know that the composition of the gut microbiome can crucially modify chronic inflammation. Indeed, certain foods may have a protective role and others a stimulating role. For our PREDICT 1 study, the first phase of the ZOE PREDICT research programme, we asked a thousand healthy people to fill in a detailed diet questionnaire. People who regularly ate a lot of vegetables had lower levels of white blood cells, which meant they had lower levels of chronic inflammation and less risk of disease and infections. We also identified a gut microbe called 'collinsella' that increased white cell levels and risk of inflammation, and was also associated with overeating ultra-processed food.[15] Collinsella likes to feed off a diet of fried starchy potatoes and has been linked in mouse studies to overeating potato crisps and French fries.[16]

Surprisingly, in spite of their high dietary fibre and polyphenol content, consuming fruits has not yet shown a significant beneficial effect in preventing inflammation or heart disease in our studies. This doesn't mean that some fruits are not healthy and more research is needed to understand why, but it may be because some fruits contain a lot of sugar or are consumed in large amounts as drinks. A high-sugar diet has been shown to be pro-inflammatory. On the other hand, it may be due to the certain compounds common in vegetables but *not* in fruits. Another possible clue is the comparatively low dietary nitrate content of fruit (see page 37). Approximately 60–80 per cent of our nitrate exposure comes from vegetable consumption, and this has been linked to better heart health, increased nitric oxide production, reduced inflammation and better immune function.[17]

When we eat meat or dairy products, certain gut microbes break down 'choline', the essential nutrient found in high levels in these foods, into harmless trimethylamine and the more insidious side-product trimethylamine-N-oxide (TMAO). This nasty chemical induces over-stimulation of the immune system leading to inflammation and furring of the arteries as well as causing blood clots and other heart problems.[18] Some of us have the microbes that assist in counteracting this chemical reaction and some of us lack them, potentially explaining why it has been difficult to pin down whether good-quality meat is healthy or not. But in short, it would seem that meat and dairy may be bad for some people and not others.

The gut microbiome and our diets are closely linked, and both of these factors interact with our immune system in complex ways. Immune-'boosting' foods, therefore, are usually simply gut-friendly foods. The many gut-friendly properties of foods are also likely to bring benefits for the immune system which, as we have learnt, is wide ranging in its effects, from reducing allergy and fighting infections, to helping the body's defences against ageing and cancer. So, looking after your diet helps your gut microbes to help your immune system do its job. It is actually quite simple.

Top five tips to support your immune system

1. Eat fermented foods, which contain helpful probiotics.
2. Eat foods rich in a variety of prebiotic fibres, such as leeks, onions, artichokes, cabbages.
3. Eat foods rich in polyphenols, such as colourful blueberries, beetroot, blood oranges, and nuts and seeds.
4. Eat foods that dampen any inflammation after meals such as green leafy vegetables.
5. Reduce consumption of meat and non-fermented dairy to occasional meals.

6. How can we choose better foods?

I used to start my morning before a long, busy day in the hospital wards with a glass of bottled orange juice, a bowl of muesli with semi-skimmed milk and a coffee with sweetener. Before stepping out of my front door, I had eaten four different types of highly processed foods from the supermarket shelves – and no whole plant ingredients. The day continued with a delicious industrial tuna sandwich, a packet of crisps and a fruit smoothie. I felt hungry and tired for most of the day, but I put that down to the nature of my job. Would I have considered myself someone who made bad choices every day at every meal? Of course, not – food choices are a puzzle of availability, convenience, taste and education. I was making choices I believed were best for me given the food and time available to me.

People fail to choose healthy foods for many complex reasons, often depending on upbringing or culture as much as a sensitive palate or nose. We are also influenced by our food environment. If you were brought up in South Korea eating pungent kimchi (see page 155) for breakfast, you would probably struggle to see the bland appeal of cornflakes, toast or All Bran. It took me over thirty years to change my mind about beetroot. Some food preferences and dislikes have a modest genetic basis, but most can be overcome, although even with time, and whatever the benefit, many of us may never be persuaded to eat jellyfish or fried insects.

People can often feel better when they believe they are on a gluten- or lactose-free diet, even when they have in fact unknowingly been eating gluten or lactose. I used to trick my son into eating fish goujons by telling him they were 'underwater chicken', which worked for a couple of years. Our bodies and our minds are in constant communication, and we cannot underestimate the power of our minds.

In a clinical trial for a study of gut health, one in three patients given a placebo tablet reported having worsening gut symptoms, and patients given dummy painkillers reported on average a 30 per cent improvement in pain. If you believe a food will make you feel ill or great, the chances are it will, at least short term. There is a danger that as we read more about the 'risks' of certain foods, we expect everything will make us ill.

We have an illogical approach to the concept of risk, which is partly due to the influence of the media and the dearth of hard facts. We routinely *overestimate* the risks of overdue sell-by dates, raw meat, sulphites, gluten and lactose, or of getting food poisoning by reheating leftovers or eating unpasteurised cheeses or salami. We are probably *underestimating* risks of consuming pesticides or herbicides, infected chickens and eggs, antibiotic-fed animals, snacking, or the long-term effects of artificial sweeteners and other chemicals in ultra-processed foods. We tend to massively *overestimate* the benefits of vitamins, and *underestimate* potential risks of anything labelled a 'health supplement'.

In March 2018 on a skiing trip to Georgia, I was a passenger in a small six-seater helicopter that crashed in the mountains on the Russian border. Miraculously we walked away from the burning wreck unharmed. A few months later I watched the harrowing footage of the helicopter accident that killed the owners of Leicester City Football Club. Never again, I thought, would I contemplate a helicopter ride. The risk must be enormous. However, the statistics showed that in five years up to 2012, there were 4.4 helicopter accidents per 100,000 hours of flying, or around 0.004 per cent per trip. In fact, travelling by car for eleven hours is as risky as flying in a helicopter for an hour. But we all downgrade the risks of getting in a car because we do it so often.

Compared to the dangers of car travel, we shouldn't worry perhaps about eating unpasteurised cheese or kombucha, choking on peanuts, drinking a glass of beer or wine each night, adding extra salt to meals, or even indulging in the occasional rasher of bacon or doughnut. Yet, we are now told there is no safe lower limit for alcohol drinking – so we shouldn't drink. There are no safe limits for walking home at night, but no one tells us not to walk. These guides to risk, with no baseline to compare to, instil unnecessary fear, and distort more sensible messages about healthy eating and moderation.

Most people have trouble distinguishing different types of risk. We may be frightened to learn that eating bacon doubles our (population) risk of some cancer, for example, but might be less concerned if this were qualified by the fact that our personal risk was changed from, say, one in a hundred to one in ninety-eight. Personal risk of getting cancer is very different to the risk of it happening to anyone in your given population – and knowing the difference is important.

Many people refused to take the Covid vaccine on learning there was an up to 1 in 100,000 risk of a potentially fatal blood clot, yet would happily take the oral contraceptive pill with several times greater associated risk, and indeed risked a greater chance of dying from Covid itself, as these risks were not properly conveyed to give context. Dangers or benefits of different foods are usually presented as relative rather than absolute risks, which makes it really hard to assess their impact on an individual. We are not good at weighing up these time-dependent future trade-offs and are easily exploited. Provided food is properly labelled, we should be free, within reason, to make informed choices on which personal short- and longer-term risks to take.

How to sell a miracle food

It is now easier than ever before to get poor-quality or fraudulent research studies published in what appear to be reputable journals. There is a large industry that plays on our desire to believe in wonder products that are too good to be true. Imagine a hypothetical company that represents a collective of farmers who produce a small berry, nut or seed which is proving difficult to sell, either because of competition with a cheaper variety, changing fashions, or because it is very sour or bitter. After discussions with PR consultants, the company decides it is worth investing some money to save the business. They contract an academic nutrition lab to do some studies on the product. The lab staff are happy to help: they will make a small profit, which goes to the university, it helps protect their jobs, and the consequent guaranteed paper will boost their CVs and careers. The company supplying the product and paying for the study will usually not be listed as co-authors on the paper, though should in theory appear in the small print as sponsors.

The academic lab produces a purified berry/nut/seed extract and drops it on ten to twenty test tubes containing different cancer cell types, available by mail order. Alongside this, they may test an extract that they expect not to work, or one with a low concentration of active ingredients. They expect that the magic extract will slow down the growth of some of these cancer cells. But, even if it had no real effect whatsoever, just by statistical chance, it should randomly have an effect on just one cell type, and so they would report that one positive outcome. If the experiment fails to show anything, the lab will just ignore the result, maybe ask for more money and repeat the experiment several times, until something definite is found. These experiments can be done in a few weeks, and written up for a scientific journal in a few more; often for less than £50,000 investment.

If the company has the budget, it might sponsor a rodent study. Lab mice are given the extract for a few months and then killed and the effects on the cancer are examined. Often the doses are very large and unnatural, and if no effects are seen, they can repeat the study with different mice or higher doses, until they do. Usually, this is enough evidence to warrant a glowing press release and a targeted social media campaign boasting of the product's amazing qualities. Companies will sometimes also sponsor professional bloggers to launch products. Thus the farmers' collective increases sales and makes money for the company, all at a fraction of the cost of a national advertising campaign. Hardly any negative studies ever get reported or published.

If the company is really serious about their product and feels it needs added credibility, it may sponsor a small human study of, say, ten people for a few weeks and costing several hundred thousand pounds. This cost will easily double, if done properly with a placebo arm and blood markers at beginning and end. The more blood markers they can afford to test, the greater the chances of one or more of them showing a change in the right direction. These studies often cost too much to repeat, so lab researchers, even if genuinely believing they are independent, often put a positive spin on them, both to get a publication and attract further product studies and to keep their sponsors happy. These subtle manipulations in small studies can be difficult to spot and are easy to get away with. Virtually no food or product research goes beyond this limited stage of testing.

The size of the effects is often too large to be credible when you extrapolate findings from a study to the population. A reported study showed that eating twelve hazelnuts per day improved mortality, which one scientist estimated would add twelve years on average to your life, which is obviously ridiculous.[1] This may not be the fault of the authors or the journalists, but a pushy university PR department keen to get their lab's paper in the press.

There are now hundreds of thousands of specialised scientific journals on food or nutrition which accept such sponsored papers, most of them entirely online and established in the last five years as money-making exercises. Some of them are prepared to cut a few corners. A colleague, psychologist Gary Lewis, submitted a paper to Crimson online publishers who have around fifty journals, including several dedicated to obesity and nutrition. The paper was entitled 'Testing inter-hemispheric social priming theory in a sample of professional politicians'. To his surprise, the paper was accepted after supposedly being peer reviewed within three days, with a request for $581 to cover costs. When he refused to pay, saying he had no funds, the publisher came back with a $99 final offer. He held firm stating that this was ground-breaking research and likely to bring considerable publicity for the journal. The journal agreed to waive the fee, and the paper was published within days, with the promised publicity, but not as the journal had anticipated.

The editor should have spotted something awry when the suggested reviewer was Dr I.P. Daly, and the main author was Gerry Jay Lewis from the Institute of Political and Faecal Science. The results of Dr Lewis's study showed that right-wing UK politicians were more likely to wipe their bottoms with their right hand, and named participants were Boris Jonski, Teresa Maybe and Nigel Farage.[2] The journal subsequently deleted the article from their website, but Crimson's journals are presumably still operating on the same strict scientific principles. There are many similar predatory scientific journals pestering academics with hundreds of emails to submit papers (I get about two per day) as well as other hoaxes. If you have $10,000 you do not even have to submit a paper, some journals (mostly in Asia) will actually write them for you, and you don't even need to think of the subject. It is now easier than ever to be a published scientist.

But it is harder than ever to assess 'real' science as an outsider, and even an insider like me finds it hard to distinguish bona fide scientific journals from bogus. Many have impressive logos and names very similar to serious publications. There are apparently now more 'British Journal of XYZ' variants based in Pakistan than in the UK. Five years ago when I was researching coconut oil blogs and health claims for my last book, many of the Journal references I tried to trace were non-existent.

How to judge a miracle finding

It is not just scientists or their sponsors who are to blame. Journalists will report the latest study as if it is unique and definitive and ignore the previous thirty that may have opposite findings. Scare stories are often published in poor journals then given front page status by an uncritical media – editors know their readers love such food features. But while we should be suspicious of both the 'too good to be true' and horror stories, there is hope. New analytic methods of scrutinising data can help. None of these small studies on their own are likely to be convincing, so we have to combine them in a meta-analysis and look for similarities or discrepancies and evidence of missing unpublished studies. To increase our confidence in the results, these meta-studies should be done by independent researchers, following

guidelines that also judge if the original academic papers are of sufficient quality to even include in the summary.

The other method to assess food and health is to look at large
observational epidemiology studies which often involve hundreds of
thousands of people followed over years to study disease and mortality and not specifically designed for a particular hypothesis about an
individual food. Linking a food with a disease can be biased if these
food choices are also associated with some health benefits or risks;
tomato sauce use may be associated with eating burgers or smoking,
or organic food with being health conscious. But these large studies
have learnt from past mistakes and improved over time, and they can
often adjust for many (if not all) of these so-called confounders. If
you then combine large studies from several countries or across continents with the same result, confidence in the findings increases.
When in the unlikely event you have all the studies pointing in the
same direction, and the effect on health is not trivial, the chances are
that the magic berry or nut is having a real effect. Nevertheless, you
should always ask 'compared to what?'

Food labels and fraud

In the modern world of supermarkets, food manufacturers know
they have to appeal to our senses. Food packaging projects images of
golden cornfields or happy cows grazing to dupe us into thinking we
are eating a natural food rather than a highly refined mixture of unrelated chemicals. We may also be tempted by 'health labels' such as
'low-fat', 'low-calorie', 'high in vitamins', 'no added sugar' or 'free
from'. All these positive messages distract us from thinking about the
quality of the food which would be evident if we were shopping in a
traditional market where we could see, smell and touch the food
itself rather than trusting the packet. Some food labels are specifically
designed to make the food look like it's more authentic and better
quality. 'DOP' on Italian products corresponds to strict rules (in
theory) on provenance and production; the 'Tracteur Rouge' label in

France is all about traditional methods and then there are 'taste awards', 'buyers' choice' and other rosettes that are less about the process and more about the marketing.

In supermarkets we rely on food labels to inform us of the healthy or unhealthy contents. Surveys show that less than 50 per cent of people who read food labels understand them; most shoppers don't bother reading them. Many governments have created 'easy-to-interpret' alternatives to help us understand whether a food is essentially good or bad for us. The most common is the traffic light labelling system, a voluntary scheme designed with food industry stakeholders to encourage healthier formulations (think less sugar, less fat, less salt) and to alert shoppers to foods high in all of the things we are told to eat less of. Unfortunately it is fundamentally flawed, not least because it is voluntary but also because diet Coke or Pepsi cans feature a positive green light, whereas unpasteurised goat's cheese comes up with a dangerous red. The system totally fails to account for processing, fibre content, polyphenol or nutrients, so doesn't help anyone to make informed choices. In Chile, warning labels, similar to those on cigarette packets, let shoppers know which food products to avoid, and have proven to be much more effective.

Ingredient and safety labels are often designed to be hard to read, using small fonts and with deliberate complexity. Occasionally they can be helpful; if only to show the country of origin, total number of ingredients and additives. I will point out tips to look for. 'Free from', or 'natural' labels are what manufacturers strive for, as it helps sales greatly to say a food is GM- or gluten-free, even if the product is meat, dairy or even water, and so could not possibly be a risk. The term 'free from additives' is now common, but the product may often contain even more new strange ingredients in place of red-flag ingredients. These new components are chemicals that exist in nature, and so don't count as 'artificial additives', even though they are made in industrial labs. Food manufacturers legally still use outdated health claims, such as declaring products 'low in cholesterol', or 'high in zinc', without any relevant health evidence to support them.

Labels should in theory be important in countering food fraud which is now an international problem across all food groups. This can

involve alteration or substitution of ingredients or falsifying docu-
ments of origin or authenticity, or simply misrepresenting the contents
on labels. Many foods are exempt or able to disguise what has gone
into the product, or even how old it is by the time it reaches you. Bread
and alcohol do not usually require a label at all. The country of origin
is often concealed: a label on a bottle of olive oil can quite legally claim
it to hail from Tuscany, even if it contains just 1 per cent of Italian oil.
The other 99 per cent will be cheaper sunflower and pomace oils from
multiple countries, reducing its quality and health benefits.[3]

Then there are the scandals of Chinese honey dressed up as European, buffalo mozzarella derived from cows, cheap farmed fish in
sushi, fake sourdough bread, watered-down cow's milk, bog standard
fish roe masquerading as caviar, and horse meat posing as beef. Some
of these food swaps are semi-legal via regulation loopholes; others
are simply frauds run by criminal organisations. In 2014 this cost the
UK food industry alone over £11 billion (and some estimates suggest
20 per cent of our food is not what it seems), and Brexit potentially
made matters worse, reducing access to food-fraud intelligence networks. This problem is bound to keep increasing as our international
food web becomes ever more complex.

Food chains and 'horsegate'

In the world of cheap global food production, we are never sure where
our food comes from. Any single processed product can now have
multiple ingredients from over ten countries. In the 'horsegate' scandal of 2013, cheap frozen lasagne and burgers from several supermarkets
were found on DNA testing to contain horse meat rather than beef,
which understandably upset the sensitive British public. No one had
questioned the obvious: how the meat was so cheap at 30 pence per
burger patty, while the trade price for beef burgers was 55 cents.

The lasagne trail was traced across Europe via companies in Lux-
embourg, France and Romania, and finally traced to an Irish meat
factory, a Danish food producer, a Cypriot food packager in London
and meat companies in Poland. Irish investigators found that the

lasagne contained recycled horse meat from pet ponies and racehorses from Ireland and Poland. Four years later, two of the gang were convicted of passing off 30 tonnes of horse meat as beef, likely just the tip of a global food fraud iceberg.[4]

A 2017 Canadian study showed that one in five sausages contained a different and cheaper meat than on the label. A survey of sixty Indian curry houses in London and Birmingham found that in 40 per cent of samples, lamb curry was replaced or mixed with cheaper meat, including pork meat, which Muslims and Jews do not eat.[5] Similar results come from surveys of Britain's 20,000 kebab restaurants, which vary widely in quality. The meat is usually minced lamb, but genetic testing in 2015 discovered it often contained chicken and pork, as well as a few nasty microbes. Then we have the scandals involving Brazilian companies who supply much of the world's meat. Inspectors were regularly bribed to sign false certificates of origin or pass rotten meat as fresh.[6] Consequently, some countries banned Brazilian meat imports.

The problem is not limited to meat. Recent reports revealed that up to 50 per cent of fish globally is mislabelled, posing as desirable species like Dover sole when we are in fact consuming cheaper, sometimes endangered fish.[7] The scale of fish fraud is staggering, with approximately 12 million tonnes of fish caught illegally every year. The owner of a Yorkshire chain of Indian restaurants was recently jailed for six years in a landmark case for substituting expensive ground almonds with peanut powder without telling his chefs. A thirty-eight-year-old customer who told the restaurant staff he was allergic to peanuts died at home an hour after eating there.[8]

Some food fraud experts have estimated that about 10–20 per cent of the processed foods we eat have some added fake cheaper alternatives, and the scale of the industry makes it impossible to police properly. The longer and more complex the supply chain and the more ingredients used, the more likely the fraud. As supply chains lengthen, this is going to get worse, and the more processed the food, the greater the opportunities.

Independent bodies have been created to help regulate food production. For example, Fairtrade certification is supposed to guarantee fair pay for the farmers who grow bananas and coffee beans; 'free-range' labels reflect that animals are allowed to roam freely for a certain amount of time each day; and the 'MSC certified' seafood label should signify that it has been sustainably fished. No doubt these initiatives were originally launched with honest intent to avoid exploitation, but as with all other regulations the food industry is adept at finding loopholes, so many new certification schemes are hard to verify. Typically also, smaller producers of artisan foods lack the funds to apply for registration for these desirable certifications, so growers of truly organic strawberries in our countryside cannot afford to be certified organic, whilst large supermarket-sponsored farms in Morocco might.

Like many countries, the UK is dominated by a few massive supermarkets, controlling 80 per cent of the food industry with enormous power over farmers and consumers. The more we shop locally or in farmers' markets, the more control we have over the origin of the food. Retail is in a time of great change, with mega-delivery companies such as Amazon selling us groceries directly. But while it is handy to order our boring essentials, like rice, salt, sugar and toilet paper online, we need to be able to trust the person who sells us our food, and looks us in the eye. If you have a local street or farmers' market or a good, reasonably-priced independent shop nearby, try shopping there. The more we promote the time and effort spent by small food producers to provide original or high-quality foods, the more we will see of them and the more we can shift our food culture away from freezer aisles with their plethora of UPF ready meals.

Making the right food choices is not straightforward. Fortunately, for the first time we should soon see new food products whose labels include measures of processing, quality or impact on gut health. But while we wait, we have to be wary and gather data from multiple sources to help us choose what to put in our shopping basket.

Five key factors to consider in making better food choices

1. Labels and certificates can be misleading.
2. None of us is good at estimating risks of food choices.

3. Companies can easily produce data and papers to falsely claim their product is 'healthy' and back it up through marketing.
4. Food fraud is rife and increasing: much of our food is not what it seems.
5. Knowledge of seasonality can help us bypass the labels and enjoy a varied and nutritious diet.

7. How does storing, processing and cooking alter food?

From farm to fork, our food goes through a whole chain of events. Very few of us eat food that comes directly from a field without intervention. As our food is transported and prepared for our tables, its nutrient content and its natural structure, also known as the food matrix, can be changed and sometimes drastically altered, which could impact us too.

Why does the structure of our food matter?

Biology classes at school told us that plants have a different cell structure to animals. One of the main ways plant cells can create impressive structures like artichokes, marrows and walnuts is the most underrated carbohydrate of all: fibre. The plant cell wall is the main source of dietary fibre, which is responsible for much of the structure of plant-based foods, including vegetables, cereals, grains and pulses. Most UK and US adults, however, get much of their dietary fibre from highly processed foods like bread that also contain a lot of starch, which can be easily digested into glucose. Eating large quantities of highly digestible forms of starch causes large and rapid spikes in blood sugar (glucose) levels and is associated with increased risk of type 2 diabetes, obesity and other diseases.

Colleagues from King's College and Norwich compared two types of bread, one made from chickpeas, the other from durum wheat, plants that represent two different methods of storing starch reserves in their seeds or grains. In wheat grains, the endosperm provides the starch and nutrition for the germinating plant. In the chickpea seed, starch is stored in an embryonic leaf structure called the cotyledon. Chickpea cell walls are structured differently and are also thicker, and therefore contain more dietary fibre than wheat. The research found that wheat and chickpeas had markedly different digestion profiles, mostly due to this difference in cell wall structure. Wheat cell walls were broken down by amylase, the main enzyme responsible for digesting starch. But in chickpeas, starch inside the cells was not digested. They reformulated normal white bread and partly replaced wheat flour with chickpea flour, and in tests on volunteers this lowered post-meal blood glucose spikes by 40 per cent on average, although the fibre and carbohydrate content (and therefore calorie count) was much the same.[1]

Food processing techniques change the structure and strength of plant cell walls. Some methods create or maintain the 'cell wall barrier', which greatly reduces starch accessibility to digestion. When starch is not digested it is called 'resistant starch' and considered part of the total fibre counts. This change in the cell wall was also seen in studies of the digestibility of porridges made with differently prepared chickpea powders. Freeze-milling, which damaged the cell walls, led to starch being broken down more rapidly and producing higher sugar spikes than in porridge where the oat cells were left intact, thus retaining a cell wall barrier. I experienced this myself in my own experiments using a continuous glucose monitor when trying different porridges and saw a range of steadily reducing blood sugar spikes from instant oats, rolled oats and steel-cut oats, which all have different cell wall structures but similar fibre count.

These studies raise major doubts about how fibre is currently measured as this fails to account for the cell structure and how it is digested. It also questions the effectiveness of artificial fibre supplements increasingly being added to food to allow claims of healthiness on the label. New ingredients and food processing techniques could deliver more of the benefits of fibre-rich foods, while some methods are providing false reassurance of healthiness because much of the fibre's activity may be lost when cell walls become damaged during food processing and in normal digestion. For the same reason, nor should we assume that smoothies are healthy.

As well as formulation, reheating some foods can change their structure so that they convert more available starch to resistant starch and in theory make them healthier. In 2014, there was lots of excitement when it was claimed that reheating pasta and potatoes will reduce glucose peaks by up to 50 per cent and help diabetes and weight loss. The catch was that this pivotal and influential study was performed on just ten staff in an Italian restaurant for a BBC TV programme and was never published.[2] Quick to spot an opportunity, food manufacturers globally added resistant starch to all kinds of products to promote healthiness. Animal models generally supported the benefits, but human studies have been disappointing.

Storing and preserving foods

While some fruit like apples can improve in flavour and lose tartness with storage over months, the majority of fruits and other plants will naturally deteriorate. Importantly, they also lose half their original polyphenol content. To keep fruits, vegetables and herbs fresh for longer, the trick is to remove any plastic packaging, rinse with cold water and pat dry. Soft stone fruits will last longer in the fridge, but fruits like damper conditions than vegetables, so store them in separate cooler drawers. Fruits like bananas, apples and citrus fruits can be stored at room temperature and placing them in a brown paper bag will speed up the ripening process. (Ripe bananas are big ethylene factories and can speed up the ripening of other fruits if kept nearby.) Store fresh herbs in a sealed container with some damp kitchen roll and they can last for days in the fridge. Potatoes like dark dry places like your food cupboard.

Humans have used many methods to preserve food, especially before refrigerators, from salting, vacuuming, juicing, fermenting, pickling, freezing and canning to drying. More recently food manufacturers have used a range of chemicals and packaging to stop food rotting. People have preserved fruit by drying it in the sun for millennia. Many ripe fruits are 90 per cent water and will spoil quickly unless the water content is reduced below 25 per cent, making it harder for microbes to live on them. Evaporating the water with wind works well, and modern factories combine drying and rapid freezing under a vacuum which avoids heat disruption but causes structural changes. The nutrients in fruits, especially the polyphenols, are generally well preserved with drying and the remaining chemicals can be concentrated up to tenfold. But there are gains and losses in the drying process, depending on the fruit type and method, and vitamin C is usually reduced. The main downside to many commercial dried fruits is the extra sugar often added to 'improve' taste, increase antimicrobial shelf-life, and cynically augment the weight to inflate the price. Dried fruits may look healthy but can produce very rapid blood sugar spikes. Many breakfast cereals claim to contain healthy 'natural' dried fruits, but don't be fooled. Manufacturers of cheap processed cereals, granola, cereal bars, muffins and biscuits use combinations of sugar, corn syrup, gelatine, starch, oil and artificial 'berry' flavours and dyes to create their own mock fruit-flavoured product.[3] Most of these products lack any natural fruit polyphenols.

Canning is generally regarded as a last resort for healthy food, although its reputation is undeserved. It was conceived in the early nineteenth century during the Napoleonic wars by a Frenchman, Nicolas Appert, then improved on by an Englishman, Peter Durand, for the Royal Navy and slowly evolved into the stainless steel or aluminium tin can that we know today. Most fruit or vegetables are canned soon after picking. They are steamed or alkaline-cleaned to remove the skin, cut and added to the can along with brine, water, juice or sugar syrup. The can is then sealed, steam cooked to sterilise the contents and cooled. Much of our misconceptions about canned fruit stem from the loss of vitamin C by heating. But while vitamin C is indeed usually reduced by a third, many fruit polyphenols are often increased, even after many months in the can. Fruit and veg preserved in tins are better for us than we might think.

The sugary syrup or fruit juice in tinned fruit is the main cause for concern, but most of it can be rinsed off. The metal in the cans has also been known to leach into the food, which was a problem in the early days of using lead. Now most cans are either aluminium or tin-plated steel and manufacturers use a thin epoxy lining made from bisphenol A (BPA) to protect the food from the metal and microbes. Unfortunately, this chemical has some unwanted biological effects. In lab animals it has been shown to switch genes that regulate sex hormones on and off (epigenetically) and so affect reproduction and behaviour, and are part of a group of chemicals called endocrine disruptors.[4] BPA is widely used in most plastics, but a particular concern is their use in babies' bottles which has been linked to childhood obesity.[5] Canada banned BPA in 2013, but the US and EU are still dithering. Nevertheless, canning companies have listened to public concerns and by 2018, most had converted to using acrylic and polyester linings and only about 10 per cent of cans still contain BPA. As with most food packaging, we don't know the effects of the chemicals on our bodies, but unless you consume all of your meals and drinks from plastic containers that have been microwaved or survive solely on canned foods, you shouldn't be too worried. I personally avoid heating food in any plastic containers, as heating or microwaving plastic is likely to emit some level of chemicals. You're better off microwaving your meal on a plate.

Jam-making is another way of preserving fruit using heat and added sugar. This usually destroys 90 per cent of the anthocyanin polyphenols and most of the other nutrients including vitamin C. Despite the blood sugar spikes and the lack of fibre, there are some curious exceptions like raspberry jam which retains many nutrients, and some chemicals tend to survive heating such as the naturally tough polyphenol ellagic acid, from tannins in the fruit.[6]

Juicing is another way to preserve the nutrients in fruits and vegetables. Commercial orange juice is often over a year old before you drink it. About thirty years ago juicing was a great idea for getting all the nutrients of fruit into a drinkable format to increase consumption, especially in children. While this helped fruit sales slightly, it reinforced the idea that providing extra nutrients like vitamin C was critical and little else mattered. Our obsession with vitamins distracted us from the far more worrying epidemics of tooth decay and obesity that juice can be blamed for. Now we are starting to realise that it is daft to drink the equivalent of seven spoons of sugar as a vehicle to deliver extra vitamin C that we can easily gain from many hundreds of plant foods. Separating the juice of a fruit from its flesh removes not only most of the fibre strands that protect the sugars from rapid uptake across the gut lining, but many of the polyphenols too (see page 132). Liquidising the whole fruit with its fibre will also retain most of its polyphenols and appears slightly better for health than no fruit at all, highlighting the importance of fruit fibre for overall health.[7] This is still inferior to eating the whole fruit, as mechanically chopping the fibre into small pieces alters its structure, breaks up the cell walls and exposes more sugar for faster absorption. I found that eating the same weight of blueberries mixed in a blender gave me a higher blood sugar thirty minutes later than when eating them whole.

We like the idea of eating fresh rather than preserved fruit, as it tastes better, and we think it is healthier. In 1975 in the US, 80 per cent of fruit consumed was local American, now it is less than 50 per cent. The UK now imports £10 billion more fruit and veg than it exports. Modern fruits have been bred to be long-lasting, but many fresh fruits, particularly berries, will be unsellable within forty-eight hours unless some processing takes place to buy them more time. Within a few minutes of picking, most plants (with a few exceptions like the onion and potato family) start to change their metabolism and structure for the worse, by using up their sugar reserves, switching starch for fibre and reducing water content in order to stay alive. Anyone who has tasted a fig or a plum straight from the tree knows the difference that transporting stone fruits thousands of miles makes to the taste.

As the clock ticks, nutrients and polyphenol content generally declines. Large farms have on-site refrigeration plants to keep the freshly picked fruit at +2°C until it is transported to larger processing plants in refrigerated lorries, and wrapped in plastic to slow down the decline, all costing the fruit and the environment a considerable loss. Carbon dioxide and increasingly nitrogen are pumped into the storage units to further reduce respiration. Only when the berries arrive at the shop is the plastic packaging removed and the clock starts again; although many supermarkets now keep the berries wrapped in their nitrogen rich bubble to avoid spoilage, reducing attractive chemical aromas. Some fruit packaging now also includes anti-ripening enzymes as standard chemicals, with unknown effects on those who consume them.

Freezing food

Frozen food is handy and is a good way to reduce waste. The duration of freezing affects the texture and taste more than the nutrients, as food can slowly absorb other chemical aromas. Vacuum bags help to store food longer but are not ideal if single-use. There is a common myth about never refreezing defrosted food for safety reasons, which leads to a lot of waste, but if you don't leave the defrosted food out for more than two hours this is usually fine.

Freezing meat or fish is generally fine in conserving taste and nutritional content – most of the sushi sold in the UK has been frozen for several months. Freezing doesn't kill most microbes – they hibernate but don't die – so frozen meat and fish must be properly heated before eating.

Nutrients are well conserved in frozen berries. If freezing fruit yourself, adding a sprinkle of sugar will reduce the rate of degradation, ideally on flat trays or containers. Counter-intuitively the faster you defrost small fruit, the less damage to the nutrients and vitamins. Use a microwave if you have one: they are not as dangerous as once thought for our health. For many vegetables including brassicas, freezing is less good for preserving nutrients, though frozen spinach is a useful and notable exception. Frozen broccoli and green beans also compare well with their fresh counterparts, though we should ideally consume our carrots fresh – essential minerals and vitamins are well preserved in frozen vegetables, aside from β-carotene (the polyphenol that gives carrots their colour).[8] Vegetables are best bought fresh-frozen, as those that are rapidly heated or blanched before freezing lose nutritional value as this deactivates the helpful SFN (sulforaphane) enzyme. While we still know little of how freezing affects the hundreds of other polyphenols and other plant chemicals, frozen veg is handy and reduces food waste, so keep some in your freezer to add to meals.

Eggs can be frozen for six to twelve months, but only out of their shell, mixed first and stored in a muffin tray. Alternatively, whole egg yolks can be eaten straight from the freezer as a delicacy.

While you can safely freeze most foods for three to twelve months, do not freeze those with a delicate structure – e.g. lettuce, apples, milks, creams and creamy sauces – as they will disintegrate or separate.

Storing milk

The white colour in cow's milk comes from fat globules and casein protein reflecting a wide range of light, and thinner milks look greyer to our eye. The fact that milk is an emulsion is clear when you freeze it (which is best avoided); the components revert to their original form, the fat globules are disrupted, and the proteins separate out when thawed. When you leave unhomogenised whole milk out at room temperature, the fat layer will float to the surface and can be skimmed off to become cream, and when over-whipped or churned mechanically it becomes butter. When our nomadic ancestors and early farmers started using milk from domesticated animals like goats, cows and camels they would have found this extra creamy butter layer lasted longer than the original milk. Milk spoils easily and left longer, the milk would have soured because of the growth of lactic acid producing bacteria, and as the acidity dropped (to a pH of 4.7), the casein proteins would have curdled, producing yogurt, and if left longer, cheese. These diverse milk products were an instant hit, as they allowed longer-term storage of this tasty energy source. They were also transportable, allowing long migrations.

Many new mums express and store breast milk, but while the energy content and macronutrient composition of breast milk is not significantly altered by freezing, it might have an impact on its complex composition.[9] Human breast milk contains hundreds of different types of nutrients, vitamins, pre- and probiotics and immunoglobulins and the effects of freezing and thawing on the more delicate chemical balance is not known. Regardless, it's still a better back-up option than powdered cow's milk formula.

Fermented foods: a way to store and 'cook'

Microbial fermentation has the combined effect of preserving food and adding health benefits. The fermentation process extracts many of the chemicals and nutrients from ingredients in digestible form before they reach the lower intestine, as well as providing energy for other gut microbes. Our ancestors probably discovered food fermentation by chance when a vegetable, fruit or grain became moist and started to rot, and microbes (yeast and bacteria) in the air or soil, attracted by the aromas and sugars, started to work. The pot of fermenting plants gave off gas and appeared to be 'boiling' and after some strange initial odours, produced something sour but pleasant that kept for months without going off. Before the discovery of microbes, we thought this was a magical or God-given miracle of cold cooking.

Before refrigeration, fermentation was crucial as a means to preserve most vegetables. Around the world there may still be up to 5,000 different variations of fermented foods, in particular sauerkraut (fermented cabbage) in Eastern and Southern Europe, and in Asia, kimchi, the spicy national dish of South Korea made of fermented cabbage, garlic, chillies and other vegetables which, as I have said, is eaten even for breakfast. In the UK until recently we had largely forgotten the art. Some of us may have eaten pickled onions or gherkins, but most of these are pickled in vinegar and pasteurised so devoid of living microbes. There is, however, a growing trend for homemade and artisanal fermented foods.

Fermented milk products such as yogurt have been commonplace for millennia. Fermentation breaks down the lactose naturally which was advantageous as most of our early ancestors lacked the lactase enzymes themselves. By chance it was found that a dry residue of milk could produce a grain-like microbe-rich yeast culture that made kefir, a fermented milk with a much greater range of microbes than the three to four found in yogurt. Non-dairy kefir can be made with water making it suitable for vegans and dairy-free versions of yogurt and other fermented foods are now available. In kombucha, for example, tea is fermented using a 'mother' culture, or 'scoby', that contains a mix of over thirty types of bacteria and yeasts. The discovery of 'cold cooking' by fermentation also unlocked other amazing complex foods such as coffee and chocolate where the bean is naturally fermented before drying and roasting. Before chemical yeasts were invented, we also relied on fermentation from microbes for our breads and cakes. Today sourdough baking has seen a major surge in popularity for its better taste and nutrient profile which aids digestion.

Raw or cooked?

We tend to assume that raw vegetables are always better for us, but in fact, it depends: first on whether the chemical, nutrient or vitamin is generally destroyed by heating, and if so, how much heating is involved. Even lightly steamed vegetables lose 30–50 per cent of vitamin C, and the loss of vitamins increases with cooking time. Microwaves can be very useful for rapidly cooking and reheating food. Their overall effect on nutrients, polyphenols and vitamins is no different from conventional cookers, but the speed of microwave cooking usually causes less damage to some delicate heat-sensitive chemicals.

But while eating vegetables raw is best to retain water-soluble vitamins and nutrients like vitamin C and folate, many of their vitamins and nutrients are only released and properly absorbed into fat, so it is better to cook them with olive oil or butter. Studies have shown that spinach and carrots cooked with oil will unlock valuable beta-carotene, but only if the oil is high quality (i.e. extra virgin).[10] Onions can be tasty when eaten raw in a salad, but they are also delicious and taste very different when caramelised with some extra virgin olive oil. Adding some baking soda helps speed up the caramelisation of the natural sugars in the onions. Try them along with iron-rich vegetables such as cavolo nero – the combination increases our body's ability to absorb the plant iron. Spinach (and sometimes kale) is increasingly eaten raw as baby leaves, but also boiled or steamed. Both are nutritionally excellent. Spinach, as Popeye fans know, is a great source of iron (although oysters and dried apricots actually have more), but the raw form of spinach contains the chemical oxalate which reduces its absorption, making lightly steamed spinach a better option, preferably with a drizzle of extra-virgin olive oil (EVOO) and a squeeze of fresh lemon.

Studies have shown lightly cooked carrots have ten times higher concentrations of beta-carotene than raw ones. Likewise, lycopene, the healthy polyphenol in tomatoes. Swedes, turnips and parsnips also have three times more polyphenols when cooked. But the downside is that important food enzymes in vegetables do get switched off by heating. One example is the enzyme myrosinase. Myrosinase normally unlocks a healthy chemical called sulforaphane (SFN) derived from a chain reaction of healthy (glucosinolate) chemicals in the plant, but is deactivated by cooking in some vegetables including beetroot. Luckily, there is plenty of spare SFN in many other raw vegetables – e.g. onion, garlic and the cabbage family – which are released ten minutes after chopping them up. So, you can easily add some chopped onion or garlic, or even a small piece of your original raw vegetable to your cooked dish and keep it healthy. Once again diversity is key.

What about bone broths, soups and stews?

Bone broths have become popular, thanks to influencers who claim it is the secret to healthy hair, flawless skin, strong bones and an increased ability to stay in crow pose. Most chefs, in contrast, say broth is a made-up term for marketing purposes and call it old-fashioned stock. That said, bone broths are thinner and usually have more meat than stock and have been part of remedial food medicine for centuries, with health reports from China as long as 2,500 years ago. Anyone can make broth at home. Put some bones from any animal in a pot, throw in an onion, a carrot, a tomato and celery, maybe some garlic and spices, add water to cover, put a lid on the pot and leave to simmer for hours. An excellent way to use chicken carcasses or fish bones and reduce waste. But whether bone broth (or stock) actually boosts collagen, plumps your skin or cures migraines is still speculative and its role in immunity is not very convincing. Consuming broth at the beginning of a meal, especially with the addition of spices and fresh vegetables to boost fibre and minerals, does seem to reduce overall calorie intake short term by up to 20 per cent (soup generally has been associated with reduced risk of obesity).[11] I love a bowl of spicy pho and there's no denying the warming and soothing effect that a hearty chicken soup can have when you have a cold. Although there are exceptions, most commercial stock cubes are not recommended as they are often full of sugar and salt, plant extracts, stabilisers and sometimes no trace of real vegetables or meat.

Vegetable soups and stews with legumes and grains such as spelt, rye and pearl barley also have their place in healthy diets. Though the plant foods are boiled, the water-soluble nutrients that survive the heat are consumed as part of the soup, not thrown away as they are when we drain boiled vegetables, for example. A mixed vegetable soup can be an excellent source of diverse fibres, polyphenols and complete plant protein combinations that dispel any myths about vegetarian diets lacking amino acids. The key is variety: plenty of greens, whole grains and legumes and go easy on salt, especially in processed stock. Also avoid too many starches from potatoes, white rice or white pasta.

Pre-packaged and canned soups have none of the benefits of real vegetables. Heinz vegetable soup contains nearly 10g of sugar and only 2.7g of fibre, with almost a third of our daily salt intake. Cup-a-Soup is passed as healthy on the label in terms of fats and sugar, but is high in salt and lists over fifteen ingredients including monosodium glutamate and emulsifiers which are not beneficial in any way. Making a batch of soup at home with any mix of vegetables is always preferable to ultra-processed options in tins or packets; though there are some healthier chilled versions to buy.

Cooking meat and fish

Cooking meat or fish adds hundreds of aromas that are not there in the raw state. Some of these come from the browning or 'Maillard' reaction when the protein and a few sugar molecules in the meat are heated together at over 140°C. As the meat browns, so the number of aroma molecules increases dramatically, making it irresistible. This is why boiled meat or fish (which never gets heated above 100°C) never develops the same flavours and why cooks recommend searing meat and vegetables briefly before adding them to the pot. Many early biblical texts refer to the magical aromas of barbecued sacrificial animals, which apparently kept God happy, though he did not or could not eat the meat himself.

As well as these celestial aromas, among the hundreds of chemicals produced when cooking meat, some are potentially dangerous. Acrylamide is one that hits the headlines. It is produced when the amino acid asparagine combines with some natural carbohydrates due to overcooking. The UK Food Standards Agency warned against eating burnt toast, chips and sausages via a major media campaign in 2017 because acrylamide was categorised as 'carcinogenic' by a WHO/IARC committee. This scare story originated in experiments on a few lab animal using massive doses of the chemical (not the toast) and an observation that cattle grazing near a tunnel in Switzerland developed a mysterious illness that was traced to large amounts of the chemical in a local river. Scientists also found high levels in the local population. But a more careful study found similar levels of acrylamide in people living miles away, who had acquired it from food. Despite the alarm, as is often the case, a review of human studies showed no clear effect on cancer.[12]

Other chemicals on the same 'barbecue toxin' list are polycyclic hydrocarbons. Again the evidence comes from lab studies plus recent observational data of high rates of cancer in firefighters. These findings are unreliable and based on small numbers. You should not worry unless you routinely disguise meat by incinerating it. We are all exposed to hundreds of nasty chemicals every day, and they only cause significant health problems when they are combined with others in high doses, like cigarette smoke. The WHO committee on toxins has *never* found *any* chemical tested on animals completely risk free for cancer. For them every food carries some risk. Despite my misgivings about these reports, I am not advocating eating burnt meat (or toast) every day, not least because overcooking mars flavour; but this is not something to lose sleep over.

A similar level of scaremongering revolves around cooking oils because of their smoke point (the point at which it produces blue smoke) and chemical changes that occur at high temperature. Critics of olive oil assert that its lower smoke point (200°C) is a health problem. These concerns are based on lab experiments where oils are heated beyond the smoke point and the chemicals given off are then collected and analysed, although in real life when pan-frying on high heat temperatures rarely exceed 120°C. But if you do manage to get the oil hot enough when stir frying in a wok, deep-frying, or in an oven at over 200°C, the oil produces other chemicals which may include some which the WHO hit list identified as potentially carcinogenic in lab animals. Some types of olive oil have higher smoke points of over 240°C, but these are highly processed, solvent-treated and best avoided. But more important is oil stability measured when heated at continuous high temperatures (110°C) while exposed to air. The less saturated fat and the more polyunsaturated fatty acids (PUFA) an oil contains, the more easily it will break up into other molecules, as seen with many vegetable oils. These multiple compounds are of unknown health risk and also potentially damaging to food texture, aroma and taste. High-quality olive oil is one of the more stable oils as it contains plenty of saturated fats. This is another reason that a good extra virgin olive oil is my cooking oil of choice, with high-quality rapeseed as a backup.

Food has been cooked in every imaginable way over the centuries, by trial and error and for convenience and taste rather than health. There is no 'best way', and there are numerous exceptions, but in most studies lightly steaming or microwaving (if size permits) is optimal, with sautéing and roasting somewhere in the middle. Nutritionally, long boiling gives the worst results. Of course, you may decide, like me, that microwaving rarely improves the flavour or cooking experience and stick to your preferred method, although the optimum mix of nutrition and taste in the future may well be by cooking most food in a 'sous-vide' vacuum.

Because of Covid-19, we have seen an increase in food delivery services. Unfortunately studies have shown that regularly consuming takeaway meals is bad for us, and the more we eat, the higher our overall likelihood of death.[13] It will be a while before we know all the answers, but we have discussed some of the possible mechanisms involved in optimal foods – texture, additives, microbe heath, etc. – and restaurant food often contains sugar, salt and cream to maximise flavour. In the meantime, takeaway meals should be a treat rather than a daily habit.

*

In summary, how our food is prepared at home, or for us by companies, has a big effect on how it looks and tastes, but many of the modern technologies such as freezing, canning and drying are often helpful in conserving food for longer without harming the nutrients. A good general rule is to avoid overcooking and include a diversity of plants, both raw and lightly cooked or fermented, in your daily diet.

Top five food storage and cooking tips

1. Frozen or canned fruits and vegetables can retain nutritional value and are good options to access out-of-season foods and reduce food waste.
2. Storing, heating and consuming foods exclusively from plastics may not be a good idea – glass, ceramics and wood are safer.
3. Many vegetables are better cooked lightly, and avoid boiling vegetables unless it's for hearty soups.
4. Cook at home as often as possible with whole, unprocessed ingredients using good-quality extra virgin olive oil.
5. Fermenting is a great way to preserve foods and enjoy added flavour and probiotic benefits.

8. What to eat to save the planet?

Today it is impossible to talk about food without talking about the environment and global warming. Most predictions concur that if we don't change our habits fast, by 2050 the Earth will have lost most of its trees and habitable areas and amid climate-related chaos we will have run out of food. A 2018 UN report estimated starkly that just to limit global warming to below 2 per cent, we need to reduce meat eating (especially beef in the West and pork globally) by 90 per cent and increase consumption of protein in beans and legumes fourfold.[1] The UK's 2021 National Food Strategy dedicated a whole section of its report to how to better use our land and focused attention on reducing meat consumption as a vital step to improved health and a healthier planet.

Diet and climate change

The role of food choice on the imminent disaster of global warming has reached centre stage and the 2018 Eat Lancet report marked a step change in our thinking by summarising data on both the positive health benefits and global environmental benefits of shifting to a plant-based diet.

The way we currently grow and feed our livestock is taking up far too much land and killing diversity. Half of our planet's habitable land is used for agriculture, and 80 per cent of the world's farmland is used to raise livestock for meat and dairy, with only 48 per cent of cereals grown for human consumption. Currently 55 per cent of all arable land is used for cattle grazing in the UK. Using valuable space and resources to feed animals to make our protein is a ridiculously inefficient system – producing beef takes as much as 100 times more land than growing peas or soy to produce the same amount of protein. Research suggests that if the entire world adopted a vegan diet, agricultural land use would reduce from 4 billion to 1 billion hectares. Although the exact figures are disputed, meat and dairy farming are estimated to contribute around a quarter of harmful greenhouse gases (GHG) that are warming the planet, not to mention the amount of plant crops and water needed to produce one steak.

Many people feel powerless but we can all help. The greatest action we can take personally to reduce global warming is to eat less meat, although any small change to eating habits can have large benefits. Start with one meat-free day, giving up cheap highly processed meats first. Following the success of sugar taxes, the idea of a meat tax is gaining momentum in some countries, which might just work if it serves to drive up quality and animal welfare and reduce volume. The argument also applies to eating dairy, especially in highly processed foods. That said, the transition to a plant-based world diet will need to be well planned to avoid potential economic downsides.[2]

Better still, the simplest way to reduce your personal carbon footprint is to become vegan.

But as always, it's more complex than that. No food can be exempt from scrutiny of its environmental impact. All of our food choices have some repercussions on the planet and the whole world is not going to suddenly become vegan. We can however make conscious choices. Ranked by their carbon footprint, either per kg of protein or calories, and using soy protein as the baseline, beef is roughly seventy-three times worse: lamb or milk, fifteen times; pork nine; and chicken is six times worse.[3]

Even within types of animal we see large differences in carbon footprints between high-quality beef and poor-quality farming practices. A pasture-grazing British cow will produce five times less carbon than its equivalent in Brazil, so your choice and source of the same meat is also important. Intensively farmed chicken may be one of the most environmentally efficient ways to eat meat, but it would be sad if we used this as a criterion to abandon organic free-range chickens. We are all still being urged to replace meat with fish, but we will rapidly run out of wild fish to catch. We should be treating fish the same way as meat and not trying to push people to eat more, unless it is their only source of protein. Farmed fish now accounts for the majority of fish we consume but it comes with a massive environmental burden. Fish farms devastate the submarine ecosystem, and often precious land and trees, and the farmed fish need to be fed with three times more smaller fish from our oceans. All so we can eat cheap prawns.

The rapid growth in alternative non-dairy drinks and products is partly due to animal welfare concerns but also an increasing awareness of the value of food choice in the battle against climate change. After meat production, cattle dairy farming is next on the global warming list. But although overall some non-dairy alternatives are better in terms of GHG emissions, they also come at a high environmental cost. Almond milk production uses excessive amounts of water and harms bees; many soy milks and others can be highly processed with ten or more ingredients. So they may not be the utopian solution either.

Many plant crops have an environmental impact and are very inefficient to grow. Per calorie, cucumber, celery, lettuce and aubergines are ranked worse than bacon for global warming. Other studies have ranked plants grown in the UK per kilogram; the worst (i.e. least efficient) were sweet peppers, cucumbers and asparagus. The most efficient, by tenfold, included apples, pears and potatoes.[4] With so many variable factors it is difficult to assess these rankings, but they do demonstrate the importance of not relying on monocultures and encouraging diversity.

Eating seasonally and locally is another way to reduce the environmental cost of your food. There are the obvious high costs of transporting specific foods around the world, such as bottled water from Fiji or tropical fruits. But it may be better for retaining carbon to eat imported tomatoes grown in polytunnels in Spain than have them grown locally in less energy efficient ways in the UK. Also, many summer vegetables and fruits and berries can be safely frozen so we can enjoy them over winter.

Food choices also involve the packaging and the risk of food waste. The US daily produces twice as much food as its citizens can consume. Most countries waste over a quarter of their food and many a lot more. It is a complex issue full of contradictions, involving diverse issues such as regulating portion sizes, discount pricing, government subsidies and sell-by dates. We dislike the use of preservatives in food, but they also reduce waste and have been used since ancient times. Organic food has fewer pesticides and chemicals but is more expensive and may go mouldy more quickly, so we may have to cook it faster, and turn the veg into soup. Plastic wrapping may reduce food spoilage but is bad for our environment – at least 14 million tons of plastic waste ends up in the ocean every year, and the microparticles it produces are starting to find their way back to us in the food chain. Although many of us try to recycle these products, globally less than 20 per cent actually reappear as recycled bottles and much of the plastics are simply shipped to Asia for 'recycling' as part of a £250 billion industry which depressingly just ends up being dumped or burned in open fires.[5,6] It is hard to avoid plastic completely but very easy to reduce its use and therefore the proportion that gets dumped. Apart from not buying plastic products, and boycotting retailers who persist in using excessive packaging, lobbying the big four multinationals who control the global market could help make them shift to sustainable materials.

Further ethical concerns are regarding conditions for the workers who produce the food. Should we buy tea bags that cost less than 2p each in the knowledge that sexual abuse is rife on many plantations? Should we keep buying cheap chocolate bars from giant Swiss and Belgian companies that indirectly use child slave labour in Africa to collect their precious beans? Do we want to buy cheap prawns from Thailand when we know a proportion of companies use slave ships to harvest them? As we strive for ever-cheaper food, food chains grow ever longer and more complex, and governments lose control, it will be unwise to rely on what manufacturers tell you. The market is dominated by a dozen multinationals, so these issues of exploitation and our ethical dilemma will continue to grow.

A good reason to go organic?

Antibiotics, herbicides and pesticides in our food are a growing problem. Antibiotics in meat, and to a lesser extent fish, have been shown to be linked to allergies and obesity. They are also responsible for antibiotic resistance, whereby harmful bacteria can become resistant to medicinal antibiotics. Antibiotic use was endemic in the meat industry for decades until the EU banned its use for growth purposes in 2006; the more industry-friendly US waited another eleven years before following suit. Despite bans in Europe, antibiotics are still commonly used to 'prevent infections' in many countries, and there have been a number of documented scandals, and antibiotic resistance is still high. Surveys have been more reassuring in the UK, showing less than 5 per cent of meats sampled in 2017 had detectable levels of antibiotics, with a similar drop in their use in France in the last three years, as the public becomes more aware. Much of the meat we eat is imported or of uncertain origin, however, and other parts of the world are still immune to regulations. Data from 2017 showed that US meat has five to sixteen times the amount of antibiotics as in the UK, particularly beef. Ironically the latest data from intensive poultry farms shows that compared to fifty years ago antibiotics nowadays have only a marginal benefit on growth, due to the many other tweaks and improvements by farmers, geneticists and breeders.

Government safety checks ensure that pesticides act only against enzymes and genes of the bugs that feed off them and not against us humans. While this is true, they are never tested against our own gut microbes and evidence is accumulating of an effect, even if minor in most people. A recent observational study followed 28,000 farmers and found those exposed to high levels of pesticides had a 40 per cent increased risk of an autoimmune condition (rheumatoid arthritis).[7]

European regulators (like their US counterparts) regularly test food samples for 212 common pesticides, supposedly keeping us safe, but 3 per cent of foods tested, including strawberries, regularly exceed the safety limits. But even higher levels are found in spinach, beans, mandarins, carrots, rice, pears and cucumbers. You could be unlucky and unbeknownst to you, have a local producer who is an overzealous pesticide sprayer making you ingest levels several-fold those recommended.[8] Many grains are likely to be imported from countries with laxer controls.

Nearly half of food products in Europe (and more in the US) contain residues of pesticides, with plants that attract the most insects or moulds – strawberries and oats – the most likely to exceed legal limits. Over 90 per cent of UK and US residents have up to sixty different detectable pesticide residues in their blood and urine. Even if you are aware of the problem, low levels are hard to escape as washing only removes some of the residue. Studies show some chemicals are resistant even to industrial cleaning, and many (such as thiabendazole) penetrate the skin. The problem is not limited to a few berries. The top contaminated fruit crops in the US in 2017 included strawberries at number one, with pears, peaches, cherries and grapes as runners up.

European and US regulators monitor levels of pesticides to keep them at 'safe' levels, although whether the bar is set too high for vulnerable groups such as children and pregnant women is an open question. In the UK, children aged four to six get free fruit; in 2017 over 80 per cent of the strawberries, bananas, apples, pears, oranges and raisins they ate tested positive for multiple pesticide residues (although within the current safety limits).[9] Animal studies typically raise concerns for many health outcomes, although translating this to humans is tricky. There have been over twenty observational epidemiology studies (of variable quality) looking at exposure in pregnancy to pesticides suggesting association to retarded mental development and later attention deficit problems in young children.[10]

Glyphosate is the world's favourite herbicide spray and we have all encountered it to some degree, as it is used for both weeding and drying crops before harvesting. In a recent civil appeal case, a California groundsman who regularly sprayed glyphosate (also known as Roundup) and developed non-Hodgkin's lymphoma was awarded damages of $87 million by the jury who ruled that it was 'likely' the

herbicide was responsible. Many governments and the WHO modified their position on Roundup as a probable carcinogen in 2015,
adding it to the list of chemicals we should avoid. Yet tests have
shown that ten common US breakfast foods contain detectable
glyphosate levels with oatmeal having by far the highest levels, as
well as detectable levels in other organic brands.[11]

Whether or not it causes some rare blood cancers if ingested in
small quantities through our food is still uncertain, but it definitely
harms our gut microbes. As our exposures can last a lifetime we
should be concerned about it, especially, ironically perhaps, those of
us who eat more plants. In a recent study, mice were fed food containing Diazinon, a common commercial organophosphate plant
spray. The findings showed it caused considerable harm to the microbiome and their metabolites and, for some reason (possibly due to
small numbers and chance), more so in males than females.[12] Diazinon
reduced levels of a microbe *lachnospiraceae,* which is important in the
human immune system. It is also implicated in depression, and this
raises the possibility of the pesticide causing mild brain effects that
would be very difficult to detect.

Pesticides and herbicides contain chemicals that are supposed to
not target large mammals, but they may cause problems by altering
the genes of microbes they have in common with the insects that the
pesticide was targeting. The so-called safe limits proposed by government agencies for glyphosate are highly controversial, as very little
data exists in humans, and the chemical can remain in soil for several
months depending on conditions. Studies by the FDA show that
glyphosate creeps into most foods tested at some level.

However, the most toxic pesticides, and also the most frequently
detected in food, are organophosphate insecticides, nerve agents such
as Chlorpyrifos – essentially a much weaker form of the infamous
Novichok nerve agent used in the botched assassination attempt of a
Russian former spy in Salisbury. These are widely used in India,
China and the US, rapidly killing many bees and insects. They also
harm fish and other larger animals, particularly marine mammals
such as dolphins and seals. Humans are also affected: there are an estimated 10,000 deaths per year in sprayers and their families. In low

levels, organophosphate insecticides may affect children's brain development and be the cause of over twenty mysterious deaths of Western tourists staying in cheap hotels in Thailand from 2011 to 2015.

There is no international agreement on safe levels of these chemicals and countries vary widely in legal use. Sweden never allowed organophosphates; the EU banned their use in homes in 2008 and completely in 2018. They are still legal across the US and South America where pesticide controls are more relaxed, and commonly used on lawns and golf courses. We know even less about the effects of organophosphates on our body or our microbes.

The widespread use of herbicides and pesticides is also contributing to the gradual reduction in the diversity of our soil microbes. Just as for our bodies, healthy soil needs a rich mix of bacteria and diverse fungi which are harmed by intensive farming, and fertiliser, pesticide and herbicide chemicals. In the future battle with large areas of contaminated land, we may need the power of microbes, such as the bacteria *pseudomonas*, to digest and neutralise the chemicals in the soil.

So, ironically, if we follow the advice to eat a more diverse range of plants all through the year to avoid disease, we may also be exposing ourselves to above-average levels of potentially harmful chemicals.

Organic farming generally does not involve use of standard herbicides and pesticides, genetically modified (GM) products or chemical fertilisers. Organically reared animals are also usually free-range and free from routine antibiotics, although definitions of how much of these chemicals can be used and subsequent labelling are often confusing. Although organic fruit and veg contain five times less pesticides and herbicides than supermarket alternatives, clear health benefits have been difficult to prove. The environmental advantages of converting all our food growing to organic methods are also difficult to prove, as it would likely create crop shortages which would be difficult to compensate for without increased overseas land use.[13] On a slightly more optimistic note, new alternative farming methods, such as no-till approaches where the carbon is kept in the soil, and using cover crops every third year to prevent weeds while the soil regenerates, could prove beneficial.

Are organic plants worth it?

Attitudes to organic foods vary widely. There are, for example, five times more organic shoppers in Austria than there are vegetarians, but five times more vegetarians in Britain, who are more concerned about vegetables and much less about food purity. The US is relatively less concerned about the chemicals and additives to foods and soil compared to Europe.

On my own increasingly rare forays into a British supermarket, I look at the organic fruit and vegetable section and always notice the smaller, dirtier and more natural looking produce. I also can't fail to note that the prices are usually around double those of its heavily sprayed and cosmetically enhanced neighbours.

Organic enthusiasts say their plants taste better and have more nutrients, but hard data on this is hard to come by. In observational epidemiology studies it is impossible to fully separate the reasons people choose organic versus non-organic food and these reasons can cause data biases. Nevertheless these statistics do suggest reduction in allergies, obesity, autoimmune diseases and cancer, but this is really not yet conclusive.

The only small human studies on the health benefits of organic food have been inconclusive, but a few rat studies have shown that consuming organic food resulted in improved metabolic markers of health, equivalent to that of eating extra portions of high polyphenol plants, although the differences were relatively small.[14] A 2014 meta-analysis of 324 studies also found significantly greater concentrations of polyphenols in organic plants, ranging from 19 to 69 per cent increases.[15] It also found higher mineral levels, lower levels of cadmium, a toxic metal, and fourfold lower pesticide levels than in non-organic samples. How to explain this variance? Perhaps pesticides somehow weaken the plant by reducing its need to produce as many natural chemical defences, a bit like stopping exercise and watching muscles wither. Another possibility, with some data to back it up, is that nitrogen fertilisers used in conventional farming force plants to focus their energy reserves on growth at the expense of polyphenol defences.

A study of 58,000 Belgians reported that those eating organic foods were slimmer, but this human data is likely biased by the healthy eater effect. There is better evidence from a meta-analysis that showed higher levels of omega-3 fats in organic grass-fed beef.[16] Yet more significantly, the NutriNet-Santé study followed nearly 69,000 French people over four and a half years to look in detail at organic foods and cancer risk.[17] Regular eaters of sixteen types of organic products – fruit, vegetables, bread, flour, eggs, meat and cereals – had roughly 25 per cent greater protection against several cancers. The data also shows a reduction in risk of breast cancer after the menopause, but not before. While observational and subject to bias from a healthy-eater effect, the results are most convincing for a reduction in non-Hodgkin's lymphoma (cancer of the immune system). Two previous epidemiology studies (also longitudinal and observational – the largest being a UK study of 680,000 women) also showed the same preventive effects after nine years for this particular cancer.[18] So, we should accept the possibility that eating organic plants long term may modestly reduce risk of cancers.

In the absence of more conclusive data, we desperately need proper funded trials of organic vs non-organic food. The EU annual research budget is 145 billion euros; it is a disgrace our governments only spend around 1 per cent of that to properly research the safety of our daily foods.

Until then, what can we do? Paying extra for your organic food is one option, but you will likely still be ingesting some residues, often through contamination from adjacent farms. While ingesting some soil full of microbes in moderation may be a good thing to improve your immune system and gut diversity, it all depends on what else is lurking in the soil. There is inevitably a trade-off. Scrubbing your plants and seeds vigorously to rid them of the chemicals or peeling them may make you feel virtuous, despite reducing the nutritional and microbial value, but this may still not be enough.

However much we wash our plants, we still ingest some microbes. How eating these different microbes affects our health is unclear. The microbes that live on organic fruits and vegetables have (unsurprisingly) been shown to be quite different to those living on pesticide-treated plants. One study compared eleven fruits and vegetables and found quite different microbial compositions, with organic versions having less of the 'Enterobacter' family that causes stomach problems.[19]

Although it is hedging its bets, the conventional food industry currently argues that not using herbicides and pesticides can lead to more ploughing and consequent increased soil erosion and loss of nitrogen. Overall yields of organic farms are around 25 per cent lower than conventional farms, which ironically means they use more land. The relative benefit of organic farming is a complex issue and it is uncertain whether it could be sustained from a global perspective without some major advances, such as genetically modified (GM) or engineered (GE) food, which we will discuss later. GM could be a potential solution to reducing pesticide and fertiliser use long term. But in changing our system of nutrient production to protect our planet's resources, the challenge will be to avoid making different environmental mistakes, such as indirectly destroying native bee diversity by mass almond harvesting, or adding too many chemicals to disguise the taste of plant products, which makes them less healthy than the original dairy or meat product we are replicating.

*

While there are no simple solutions, it is important to know some of the facts behind what is on your plate so you can draw your own conclusions. Understanding where your food comes from, what is in it, and what it might have been sprayed with, is increasingly important and your best insurance policy for good health *and* conscience.

Helping our environment and reducing global warming is not an all or nothing issue. Most of us can make a list of ten things we can do regardless of circumstance, finances and habits.

My resolutions for this year:

1. Learn more about the ethical and environmental issues around the foods I eat.

2. Buy (and freeze) more fruits and vegetables in season.

3. Eat a greater variety of beans and legumes (that fix nitrogen).

4. Reduce red meat consumption to once or twice per month and make it high-quality, local and organic.

5. Buy less cow's milk and fewer milk products, focusing on fermented milks and traditional cheeses.

6. Buy more organic fruits and vegetables.

7. Grow some vegetables and herbs in my garden.

8. Make plants the main component of every meal and learn more recipes.

9. Reduce food waste by buying less, more often and locally and making soups and smoothies with leftovers.

10. Compost food waste to enrich the soil in my garden.

9. How are we all unique?

The Covid pandemic showed us that we all respond differently to this virus in terms of symptoms and in our side-effects to different vaccines. Medicine and the pharmaceutical industry have generally ignored this wide variation in our responses to medications, often seeing it as a minor irritation that gets in the way of definitive clinical trials, clear-cut advice and sales. Consequently, we have got used to relying on 'averages', despite the fact that they are often misleading. This is particularly true when it comes to nutrition and how each of us responds to food. This standardisation has led to nutritional guidelines for calorie requirements that divide all adults into two groups – male or female – and a single group for macronutrients and vitamins.

Until recently it was thought that the main reason we might differ in our responses to food and medicine was genetic. Each of us has different sets and variations of the roughly 20,000 human genes that produce different proteins. Over the millennia, our genes have mutated to allow some of us to digest raw milk easily or enjoy alcohol without going red and falling over. Other genes vary, so that some of us may be so sensitive to caffeine that it makes our heart race and stops us sleeping. Other gene mutations are more idiosyncratic, for example, if you have smelly pee after eating asparagus – think slightly sweet rotten cabbage with hints of sulphur. Or you may be among the one in three people that say you can never smell it. Or you may even be in the one in ten that can only smell it when your partner has just been for a pee before you.

Similarly when one in six people drink beetroot juice, their urine turns red, which is harmless but, if you are not expecting it, can look alarmingly like blood. Although differences in our genes and our microbes are the cause, why we have these chemical differences in our response to asparagus and beetroot remains a mystery, and we don't know why smelly urine could provide any evolutionary advantage.[1]

Pasta-digesting genes

An enzyme called amylase works on the starch in, say, pasta or rice by breaking it down into simple sugar in our mouths and upper part of our gut. My colleague Mario Falchi has shown in clinical studies that the amylase enzyme gene (AMY1) in your DNA might make you thinner. This gene varies widely in populations, depending on exposure to starchy carbohydrates, and is potentially more influential on weight than any other gene found to date.[2] The gene is tricky to measure and the story is not complete, but a Swedish study of over 4,000 people found no overall effect of the AMY1 gene directly on weight, unless you also look at how many starchy foods people are eating.[3] The amylase enzyme is responsible for breaking down the starchy foods into simple sugars which then cause blood glucose spikes. Those who make less of the amylase enzyme will break down starch slower. If eating plenty of starchy foods, having fewer enzymes breaking down the starch means you could eat more pizza before your blood glucose starts to spike. On the other hand, eating a big bowl of rice with plenty of amylase to break it down will cause a big spike in less time.

You can carry out a crude test of your starch genes at home. Put a single dry wheat cracker (ideally something like a Jewish matzah) in your mouth without chewing it and time how long it takes until you taste the sugar being released.[4] Under thirty seconds, you are likely to have multiple copies of AMY1; over thirty seconds, then you have few copies. When we tested a thousand twins, less than 10 per cent tasted the sugar rapidly – most (like me) don't. I didn't feel any sweetness for about a minute, so I probably have fewer copies. Not releasing the sugar early higher up in the digestive tract and instead delivering more starch to your microbes lower down in the gut is probably better for your waistline. Although the science is still evolving, and this test is certainly more for fun, it illustrates how differently we respond to food.

Even if genes control the amount of taste receptors or food prefer-ences, environmental factors can modify them to a large extent, as we have evolved to survive as omnivores, not fussy eaters. Many peo-ple have an aversion to coriander (cilantro) as they are sensitive to some of the chemicals that are shared with soaps. But studies have shown that the brain messages can be overridden if from an early age we associate it with delicious Mexican and Asian meals.

Twin studies, including our own, have shown that genetics only accounts for about half the risk of developing obesity in adults, meaning that around half of our likelihood of developing obesity can be explained by genetic differences between us. Some of this gen-etic component is due to behaviour, which is also heritable, as well as biology, as many of the food choices, habits and preferences we have are strongly genetic.[5] In addition, studies in young infant twins have shown a significant interacting effect of genes and environment – if the family environment or diet is unhealthy, the influence of genes is twice as great. Conversely, in families with low risk for obesity, genes play only a small role and diet plays a major role.[6]

By now you might have got the impression that our gene varia-tions are responsible for most of the differences between us in metabolic and food responses. This is certainly what I believed ten years ago. Then I started looking more closely at identical twins. Although there were plenty of twins who were similar, it was rela-tively easy to find twins who differed from each other, not only in common diseases and mental conditions, but in weight, appetite and food preferences. How could this be? It was hard to blame their fam-ily environment as they had usually been raised together until at least the age of eighteen and sometimes longer. In 2014 we published the first large-scale twin study of the gut microbiome, showing that while there was some genetic influence, the differences were far greater than the similarities. In 2021 we updated this study with deeper metagenome sequencing that showed only a small proportion of microbes were shared between twin pairs – only slightly more than unrelated individuals – with everyone having unique subtypes of strains not found in others. To put this in proportion, we humans are more similar genetically than we believe: we share roughly

99.7 per cent of our gene variants with each other and are on average fifth-cousins (hello cousins!). But we only share around 25 per cent of our gut microbe genes.[7] So, our unique microbiome and the chemicals it produces really do make us more distinctive than our human genes.

Although we start life with a complete set of genes donated from our parents, the same is not true for our gut microbes. As discussed, we are born sterile and acquire them through our nose and mouth during childbirth, then from breastfeeding and touching adults and our surroundings. It takes about three years for these gut microbes to stabilise, but they will be changed by each infection, medication and change of diet or environment, so even infant twins are very different. As we get older, each course of antibiotics or other medication, each bout of diarrhoea, each meal we eat and when we eat it, can alter our microbes to some extent. Where you live also plays an important role, in cities or the countryside, on your own or with a big family, with pets or other animals, and how clean your house and personal hygiene are. While a few microbes are influenced by our own genes, most are not, meaning the environment and food are crucial. When I spent a week in the bush in East Africa eating local plants and animals, I saw large temporary shifts in my microbes that reverted within two days of returning home. Despite these short-term changes, much of our microbiome is pretty stable and, like a fingerprint, we carry our own unique microbial signature for life.

The PREDICT-1 study involved more than 1,000 adults (including hundreds of pairs of twins) who were continuously monitored for two weeks to discover how they respond to different foods. Participants had an initial set-up day in hospital for detailed blood measurements and testing of responses after eating carefully designed set meals. They then continued the study at home, following a schedule of set meals and their own free choice of foods. We measured a wide range of markers of nutritional responses and health from blood glucose, fat, insulin and inflammation levels to exercise, sleep and microbiome diversity. This kind of detailed, ongoing analysis was made possible through the use of the latest wearable technologies. Continuous blood glucose monitors and digital activity trackers meant we could keep track of our participants' blood sugar and activity levels 24/7. Simple finger-prick blood tests also allowed us to measure their blood fat levels on a regular basis. All these measurements added up to millions of data points, which needed to be analysed with sophisticated machine learning techniques (a type of artificial intelligence) in order to spot patterns and make predictions.

The most surprising thing we noticed was the wide eight- to tenfold variation in individual insulin, blood sugar and blood fat responses to the same meals. We also saw large differences even for identical twins. For example, one twin might have healthy responses to eating carbohydrates but not fat, while the other twin was the opposite. Immediately, this told us that we are all unique and no perfect diet or correct way to eat will work for everyone.

Because of the twins' results, we instantly knew that genetics only plays a minor role in determining how we respond to food (less than 30 per cent for blood sugar and less than 5 per cent for fat). It also told us that the many commercial genetic tests claiming to determine the 'right diet for your genes' are ineffective and often misleading. We also discovered that the timing of meals affects nutritional responses in a personalised way. The same meal at breakfast caused a very different nutritional response in some people when eaten for lunch. In others there was very little difference, busting the myth that there are ideal meal times that will work for all. Most people have a lower sugar peak in the mornings after eating the same food, but I was the opposite, showing that for me and some others, especially aged over fifty, having a large high-carb breakfast could be relatively detrimental compared to having it later in the day. Around one in four people had a marked sugar dip three hours after eating breakfast muffins, for example, making them tired and hungrier so they ate up to 20 per cent more food that day, equating to around a 10kg gain in weight annually. This knowledge could be crucial.

Another surprise was finding that the composition of meals in terms of calories, fat, carbohydrates, proteins and fibre (macronutrients or 'macros') also had a highly individualised effect on nutritional responses. Some people handle carbs better than fat, for example, while others have the opposite response. Another factor we are seeing from the ZOE PREDICT studies is that our response to food changes as we age, and in women can alter markedly with the onset of the menopause.[8] What worked for us in our thirties needs to be re-evaluated later in life.

Despite the wide variability between participants, each person's responses to identical meals eaten at the same times on different days were remarkably consistent. This makes it possible, despite the complexity, to predict with high accuracy how someone might respond to any food, and direct their choices, based on knowledge of their blood fat and glucose and gut microbiome test scores, plus other data on sleep and meal timings. ZOE developed a commercial test kit (available on a smartphone app in US and UK so far) that provides personalised scores based on these results for all common foods.[9] Surveys of the experience of the first few hundred users who used the advice on the app to alter their diet, without counting calories, found that 80 per cent reported feeling more energy and less hungry and on average lost around 4–5kg in weight.

Humans are complicated, and there are many things that influence our health. There are the things we can't change, like our age or genetic make-up, and the things we can, such as our choice of food and drink. Then there is our microbiome. As I have discussed, the foods we eat are mixtures of many nutrients that affect the body and microbiome in different ways, so unravelling the relationship between diet, metabolism and health is no simple matter. A detailed study of thirty-four volunteers from the University of Minnesota in which stool samples were taken for seventeen days added yet another layer of complexity, showing that foods with comparable nutritional profiles can have very different effects on the microbiome.[10] Several foods were eaten by most of the participants – such as coffee, cheddar cheese, chicken and carrots – but there were plenty of choices that were unique. The researchers found that while each participant's meals affected their microbiome, with certain foods boosting or reducing the abundance of particular bacterial strains, there wasn't a straightforward correlation that carried over between people. For example, baked beans boosted the proportion of certain bacteria in one person but had far less effect in another. Intriguingly, although closely related foods (such as cabbage and kale) tended to have the same impact on the microbiome, unrelated foods with very similar fats, carbs and protein content had strikingly different effects.

In our 2021 ZOE PREDICT 1 study, as discussed earlier, we looked at the correlation between the composition of the gut microbes of an individual, their diet and their health markers for diabetes, heart disease or obesity. Despite the individual differences as noted in the Minnesota study, we were able to also see some consistent correlations between foods and microbes across not only our initial study participants but also in many other groups from other countries. As I said, this allowed us to identify an initial list of good and bad bugs, and offer advice on how to increase or decrease their levels with so-called 'gut boosters' or 'gut suppressors'. This information can then be personalised depending on your starting levels of these microbes. We are still in the early days of personalised nutritional advice for your microbiome, but it is expanding rapidly as we identify more microbes and will soon extend to personalising probiotics and prebiotic supplements.

Just as we perceive colours and smells differently, we need to realise we are all unique when it comes to food. Some people metabolise food better after exercise, others do better if they eat just before exercising. Just like ourselves, our microbes have circadian patterns that have evolved over millions of years that are hard to tamper with. Working with a study team at Berkeley we found that sleep quality and duration was also important in how we metabolise food the next morning. For most people, we found that avoiding a high-sugar breakfast and instead eating either fats or high fibre, was important in waking up easily and staying alert for the rest of the day. With increasing attention to not just what we eat but how we eat, we are learning that some people do better skipping breakfast and only having two meals a day, while for others it makes less difference health-wise. Extended fasting and shorter periods of eating or time-restricted eating are becoming more popular, but inevitably some people feel this is more natural for them than others. In a few years we will have developed tests to help us understand which category we are each in, but for the moment we need to experiment and keep an open mind.

We are also quite different in how we feel hunger and satiety. Some people seem to be born with voracious appetites, and while a few have recognised genetic conditions from birth, most do not. Our body contains a clever system of gut and fat cell hormones that switch our appetite centre in the brain on and off. People with extreme obesity often have extreme appetites and their hormonal signals are simply not working anymore. When they have a life-saving gastric bypass operation, their blood tests and appetite levels often miraculously return to normal within two days. Doctors who study hormones (endocrinologists) claim that the dramatic change is due to these 'appetite' hormones. But the gut microbes of gastric bypass patients also change dramatically and I believe that as the gut gets rearranged, it is the microbes moving from one part to another which alters the chemical signals to the brain. This is why the long-term success of the operation is related to how long the patient's gut microbes stay in the new state and *not* the gut hormones.[11]

Humans come in all shapes and sizes and so do our intestines; the size of the small intestine, for example, can vary from person to person, sometimes over twofold, from 630cm to 1,510cm. This has an effect on nutrient absorption, as does how quickly you eat and how much you chew your food, all of which vary widely between people and can alter hormone signals of fullness as well as how much time the food spends in your gut.

By now you should realise quite how unique your digestive system is, and with its complex interactions with your genes, your microbes, your immune system, your gut hormones and your brain, why eating food is very personal. The generic 'Eat Well Plate' and its equivalents worldwide are completely inadequate for individuals. Whilst there is some reasoning behind producing a general evidence-based guide for healthy adults, its design and implementation are prone to biases and lobbying which make it problematic. With the help of this book, however, and modern technology such as the ZOE score, you too can create your own evidence-based, personalised nutrition plate.

*

Personalised nutrition in five

1. We all have individual responses to different foods – no two people respond in the same way, not even identical twins.
2. Our response to foods depends on several factors, but is more influenced by our unique microbiome than our genes.
3. Amending your diet can alter your gut bacteria and thus change your response to foods, stress, moods as well as helping weight loss and reducing inflammation.
4. We share virtually all of our genes with each other and only around a quarter with our gut microbes for which we all have a unique set.
5. Our responses to food change with age, menopause and hormone status, stress, sleep quality and illness, making us unique across the course of our lives as well as individually.

10. What is the future of food?

In the eighteenth century Robert Malthus asserted that humans will inevitably go hungry, as the rate at which our population increases is always faster than the rate at which we can produce ample food. This bleak world view has had a major impact on our thinking and despite dire predictions in the 1980s, we now produce food with enough calories (2,800 per person) to feed everyone on the planet. Unfortunately, however, it is not spread evenly and while around 800 million humans are starving, countries like the USA produce at least twice the calories they need each day, and Europe is nearly as bad. If we reduced this overproduction to just 30 per cent, balanced better distribution of supplies, and reduced waste slightly in developing countries, we could save a third of the global food supply. Sadly, as you might have guessed, it is not that simple.

Given the disastrous impact of our food choices and farming practices on the environment, we are likely to see an increasing reduction in meat consumption across the developed countries and a growth in alternatives such as plant-based milks and other alternative dairy-free products. It's also worth noting that increasing our consumption of lentils, pulses, beans, whole grains, nuts, seeds and mushrooms would be a great way to reduce our consumption of animal protein and increase our intake of diverse plants with all their beneficial phytochemicals. The popularity of using these plant foods is growing, but for the majority of us they are not part of our everyday diet, which is a shame for the planet and our health. As well as changing our choices of existing products, we will also need to embrace new technologies and seek out innovative ways of making food.

Where would we be if, in 1909, we had rejected Fritz Haber's novel idea to convert nitrogen from the atmosphere into ammonia for use as a soil fertiliser? This single invention alone is estimated to have increased global food production by up to 40 per cent. But nitrogen fertilisers, despite their success, are also now part of the problem, causing a huge loss of biodiversity, pollution in rivers, and contributing to global warming. Excess fertilisers in soil are converted by microbes into nitrous oxide, a major greenhouse gas which hangs around for a decade and is 300 times more damaging than CO_2. We also have the cost of the considerable fossil fuel needed just to create the fertiliser, about 1–2 per cent of our total carbon emissions. Simply producing all food organically without the use of fertilisers would be a solution. But while this might feed a few rich nations, the rest of the world would probably starve. Is there another solution?

Many legumes have genes that attract nitrogen-fixing fungi species to their roots and so don't need as much fertiliser. Other plants and cereals just need a tweak to three of their genes to be able to fix nitrogen themselves or make them attractive to microbes in their roots which do the same. All this is possible using precise gene editing methods. But although making nitrogen fertilisers redundant seems a pretty good aim for the planet, genetic modification (GM) is still deemed unethical by the EU and groups such as Greenpeace, and scientists are abused and threatened if they work in this area.

Many people in Europe are uncomfortable about GM products because of adverse publicity and effective slogans like 'Frankenfoods', added to distrust of the big conglomerates who in the past have often put greed before public interest. But, their increasing use is inevitable, just as traditional plant and animal breeders continue to find new strains. In the past we were quite happy to accept new varieties created by using gamma rays to cause random gene mutations, but we are now frightened by more sophisticated methods. Importantly, after thirty years, there is no evidence that GM food is unsafe, let alone the new more precise methods of genetic engineering (GE) that use tiny bacterial enzymes like scissors. Because of public opinion and a raft of restrictive legislation and guidelines, few companies (and certainly no small ones) can afford to still be in this business, and there are only around a dozen GM food crops grown globally at scale. Yet we know they work. An EU-funded meta-analysis of 147 GM studies showed that pesticide use was reduced on average by 37 per cent while yields improved by a fifth. The benefits were even greater in poorer countries with problems controlling insects. Overall the current economic advantages have been estimated at around $15 billion annually.[1]

In Brazil around 75 per cent of its major crops – maize, soy and cotton – use GM seeds that contain a special Bt protein that deters most insect pests without the need to spray pesticides. This has increased yields and reduced costs, but there is a catch. Insects need to eat, so they are also evolving ways of surviving, and several of the local pests have become resistant to the Bt protein by changing their own genes. Using genetic engineering of plants as a global food strategy will therefore require regular surveillance of the environment; it will be a continuous arms race against nature. While we have had GM products such as a long-shelf-life tomato and golden rice containing vitamin A since 1994, they have not gained widespread use. We also have bananas resistant to Panama disease, or cassava roots modified to have high iron and zinc levels, which to me all sound relatively beneficial and harmless. But if general public discomfort about GM crops is anything to go by, the reaction to genetically modifying animals for food is likely to be one of horror.

Fast-growing GE salmon is now sold in Canada for fish farms by a company called AquaBounty. Apparently, it tastes the same as ordinary farmed salmon, but it has taken about ten years to convince the US to purchase it and pass FDA approvals as they still treat GE in animals like a veterinary drug. The GE salmon for the US market are housed in a high-security facility in Indiana, with electric fences and CCTV thankfully making escape very hard. All the GE salmon are supposedly infertile females, but miracles do happen, and unlike plants, salmon can swim thousands of miles. So, to be safe, it is perhaps best to keep them away from our oceans and rivers and their natural relatives. Academic groups have also produced GE animals that are genetically resistant to specific infections that cause massive waste or death, such as the virus PRRS in pigs, respiratory flu virus in chickens, or mastitis in cows. Other possibilities include removing horns from cattle or modifying milk genes to prevent lactose intolerance. These are currently seen as not worth the enormous time and money needed to get the approvals, when the public may not buy anyway. In ten years, however, if our resources continue to dwindle, I don't think we can afford to be so fussy.

We are less sensitive to GM when it comes to microbes. Millions of people depend on medicines produced by genetically modified microbes to produce everything from insulin to vaccines. Food companies are cultivating vast tanks of different yeast and fungi that can be used as protein, although they use a lot of energy and plant extracts to produce them. Solar Foods in Finland have developed a low-energy method of growing bacteria from water in the air to make an edible protein called Solein, which is similar to soy. These special bacteria are fed carbon dioxide from the air plus nitrogen and nutrients bubbled through the tanks in water. It was initially developed for a Mars space mission, and has a mix of 65 per cent protein, 25 per cent carbohydrates and 10 per cent fats. The carbon dioxide emissions from single cell cultivation are a hundred times lower than from meat production and ten times lower than from crop production, and the company plans to switch to even more economic solar sources in the future. It has so far been trialled as a base of around twenty foods and Solar hopes it will be commercial very soon. There are other start-up companies with similar plans in the UK and USA and as we learn more about these clever microbes we are likely to find many other ways of using them.

Future burgers

Meat is facing competition from other innovative products. Traditional burger meat, for example, is being bulked up with mushrooms that have a better environmental footprint, with estimates suggesting that replacing just 30 per cent of burger beef is the equivalent of taking 2 million cars off the road. There are also many soy- and pea-based burger products. The US company Beyond Meat uses a base of pea protein, rapeseed and coconut oil, and a large list of additives and chemicals, plus a dash of beetroot juice to make their burger look like red meat. Another fast-growing company is Impossible Foods Inc. of

Silicon Valley, California, founded and run by a gifted Stanford bio-chemist and geneticist Pat Brown, who also invented the first methods for studying gene expression. A strict vegan, Pat strongly believes that reducing meat production is the single most important factor in sustaining the planet. In 2009, he took a sabbatical from his day job to explore alternative foods and with a $3 million seed investment came up with an answer; a plant burger that looks and tastes like meat.

The Impossible Foods burger is made from a protein called 'heme', derived from the pink nodules of fungus found on the roots of the soy plant. Heme contains iron, which also carries oxygen around our bodies in blood, and gives meat its taste and 'bloodiness'. The team isolated the gene that makes heme from the fungus and inserted it into the genome of a common yeast, so it could make it for them. They then grew the yeast in giant vats and mixed this mass-produced plant heme with wheat gluten, potato, coconut oil and spices to pro-duce a burger that has a meat texture, an umami savoury kick, cooking aromas and 'blood' that other veggie burgers lack. It tastes pretty good, though they are continually changing the mix to get it progressively closer to the holy grail of 'real' meaty tastiness. They emit 80–90 per cent less greenhouse gases compared to a normal meat burger, and human trials have shown that even with the extra chemi-cals used to make the patty stick together and taste good, they are still potentially healthier for your heart (based on blood markers) than the original.[2] The genetically modified plant meat burger looks like it is here to stay.

The key, of course, to successfully changing the market is price. These plant-based burgers originally were expensive, but massive scaling and investment from the giants of the meat industry itself, like Tyson Foods and Cargill, has brought the price closer to conven-tional beef. US beef is around $5 per pound, Beyond Meat $9 and Impossible Burger $11, with prices of the plant alternatives likely to fall a further 30–40 per cent in the next few years.

A scientific rival to the 'heme-burger' is the 'stem-cell burger', grown in a laboratory using the same techniques that we are using to grow new cells to treat cancer and Alzheimer's disease and replace vital organs. A group of Dutch scientists, led by academic Mark Post, worked hard for a decade to grow enough animal muscle fibres from a single cow stem cell to make a burger. They grew them in little dishes that have to be nourished with animal fluids (like foetal calf serum, which didn't appeal to vegetarians). This isn't exactly a veggie version, but it's a question of scale. In principle, one cow's stem cells extracted harmlessly could supply a million people in theory, so we could reduce the number of cows on the planet to a single herd of 30,000 pampered animals. In 2013 they produced the first prototype, with a big press launch in London, to scientific, but not culinary acclaim. Each burger then cost around £200,000, and few thought it could ever be viable. They were wrong. With commercial funding, and scaling up, that price would drop fast.

Eight years later there were over seventy companies making meat from stem cells and they have now devised a plant-based feed for the cells and found clever ways of circulating the nutrients and removing the toxic waste. The cost has plummeted and Israeli Future Meat Technologies optimistically claims it can produce a chicken breast for $7.50. One Cambridge company is using pork stem cells to produce bacon, growing the fat and protein separately then gluing them together. Whether it will taste precisely like bacon, or be kosher, is unclear. Other companies are looking to create shellfish and 'ethical' foie gras grown in labs for the gourmet market. If you go to one restaurant in Singapore you can now buy a stem-cell chicken nugget in a bao bun for $23 (albeit sold at a loss) from a company called Eat Just, Inc. Other countries are likely to approve these experimental novelty foods soon. While it will be tough to get test tube muscle to taste or feel like the real exercised outdoor muscle of a beef steak, passable chicken patties, sausages and mincemeat are already achievable. This cell-based method can also be used to make milk as well as dairy derivatives such as cheese, using additional microbe cultures. This will probably taste better than current vegan cheeses and may be indistinguishable from the mass-produced ultra-processed cheese made from excess subsidised milk, which has no great taste anyway.

A new development in the meat-free industry is 3D-printed plant protein steaks. To overcome the lack of texture, this printed 'meat', championed by celebrity chef Marco Pierre-White, offers the holy grail: the consistency and mouthfeel to compete with the real thing.[3] The problem with these products is they are not actually meat. Instead, they should be considered a protein replacement and their health benefits need to be carefully considered. When compared to a real beef burger, the meatless burger has more fibre but also more saturated fat and sodium, and the metabolites of the two products are very different. Many meat-free burgers may essentially be ultra-processed foods with added emulsifiers that could be harmful to our long-term health if eaten regularly, in the same way that ultra-processed meat is harmful if consumed often.

This industry is still in its infancy and may be at the same stage as the electric car industry in the 2000s. A report in 2021 showed that lab-grown meat firms attracted a sixfold increase in investment in 2020 and that, surprisingly, 80 per cent of people surveyed 'would try' meat grown in giant cell culture bioreactors.[4] It just needs to reach the tipping point in price and availability at which people will consider it preferable to chewing on cheap meat from dead animals. Some predict that this will be within five years. The big environmental impact is that we would replace the vast animal facilities of pigs and cattle with huge complexes of industrial bioreactors with wind turbines and solar panels. On a plus side we can manipulate the stem-cell meat to be healthier, by adding polyunsaturated fatty acids such as omega-3, for example, altering the culture medium to replicate the effects of grass, or lowering the fat content.

Another exciting food tech coming to the fore is the use of mushrooms and fermented mushroom products as meat alternatives. Some of these mushroom-growing activities can actually be carbon neutral, and mushrooms can grow quickly and almost anywhere, providing an excellent source of proteins, fibre, polyphenols and vitamin D as well as tasting delicious. We also may have to get used to all our meat and alternative meats being owned by even more powerful food companies and tech giants like Google who can afford the massive investments, but what's new?

Future Foods

Mushrooms, fungi, soy and pea protein can be used to create meat substitutes such as vegetarian mince and sausages but they are often ultra-processed and not necessarily better for our health.

There are trillions of insects that could provide us with a rich sustainable source of cheap protein. People in many Asian countries eat them as healthy delicacies, especially crickets and locusts, which are often otherwise seen as crop pests. Several companies have started selling cricket-protein snacks and a flour that can be produced in tiny urban spaces and added to bread or pastries. Cricket flour has more iron than spinach, twice the amount of protein per gram as beef and as much B12 as salmon. There are now many players in this market, several in the US, with memorable names such as Don Bugito, Bitty Foods, Jungle and Ynsect. The Chapul brand is now sold in the global chain of Whole Foods supermarkets, as this area becomes mainstream. With a bit of processing, you can even eat your favourite matcha-flavoured insects, as well as coconut, ginger lime, peanut butter and chocolate. If you fancy some maggots for tea, South Africa has just the thing. A Cape Town-based company has won awards for their skill in farming and breeding batches of eight billion black soldier flies that become maggots (they prefer to call them larvae) using local waste from restaurants.[5]

These are not the offspring of your ordinary house flies that spread disease, these are larger healthier omnivores. And you don't have to eat them live and wriggling; they are dried and ground into an innocuous powder that is high in calcium and protein, and (apparently) quite edible. Currently maggot powder is being used as pet food, but soon, just like plant burgers, it could be part of all of our diets.

Most of our planet is under water and there are 20,000 types of seaweed of which we have exploited only a fraction for human consumption, but new companies are changing that landscape. Certain freshwater algae can also be cultivated in big volumes to provide protein and act as egg substitutes, as well as the main source of omega-3 and other potential health supplements. Sea grasses and grains too can be cultivated underwater and have high nutrient contents and great potential for trapping carbon that we have only begun to explore.

As we struggle to increase food resources as our population grows, we need to put aside prejudices and be more receptive to meat or protein substitutes, whether from stem cells or dead worms. We also need to adopt innovations that we may not like aesthetically. In China, increasingly, they are making more of the available arable land by covering it in low cost plastic greenhouses that can double or treble yields. (Only 1–2 per cent of its land in 2022, but this is expanding fast.) We already have robots that can milk cows on demand and Iron-ox Co. in the US makes futuristic greenhouses with robot arms and seed trays that are now producing mechanised farmed foods that can provide local and urban solutions on different scales. If successful, efficient mechanisation could address the longstanding problems of the additional labour and transport costs of producing whole plants compared to ultra-processed foods.

I have highlighted the problems of ultra-processed foods and the corporations behind them; but they are aware of their own failings. Every large food company now has a research team looking at the role of the microbiome and personalising nutrition to prepare for the day when the health authorities finally ask to safety test new foods and ingredients for their effects on human gut microbes, rather than just rat livers. They are already adding pro- and prebiotics as an integral part of some new UPFs such as snacks and breakfast cereals to see if they catch on. Bizarrely, a new generation of pasteurised (i.e. dead) microbes may also be used in novel foods because of the tiny proteins they carry on their cell walls – this could have health benefits, such as anti-obesity signalling effects with the dead gut bacteria *Akkermansia*.[6] They are also looking at how food ranges can be personalised for those with health issues. We cannot feed the planet without some reliance on UPFs, so it makes sense to encourage the industry to make them healthier, less addictive and better for the planet.

When I watched *Star Trek* as a kid I imagined what it would be like

in the future to have all our food in liquid form in interesting colours. Companies like Huel and Soylent have tried this complete
nutrient meal replacement approach that claims to offer a complete
package of nutrients so you could exist for weeks, solely on their
liquid food. This has met with some success, at least in young men
working or gaming long hours at their computers. Although most
people do lose some weight short term, this is often because they
don't enjoy eating and so eat less. Humans and their guts were not
designed to eat only liquid food and adding chemical nutrients
rather than real plants may not compensate adequately. We value
the social and emotional advantages of enjoying food together, and
reporters who tried it out said the worst part was missing the communal interactions.

In the previous chapter we discussed our individuality and personalised nutrition. In the future everyone will know how their body
responds to certain foods and will have access to a list of foods ranked
in order of health benefit for their metabolism and microbes. Digital
menus in restaurants might sync with your smartphone or watch to
give personal recommendations, or automated supermarket labels
might change for each customer. But how might this affect our habits
and meal times? Will parents have to prepare four different meals? Or
could this spell the end of the family meal? We don't know how this
could play out in practice, but my hope is that as we all learn the
importance of plant diversity, most meals will be identical and we
will be able to choose add-ons, like fish or chicken (whether fake or
real). More likely we will agree to rotate choices of the communal
meal so we get more variation. The more varied the food, the less
likely it is to cause anyone harm.

Although we have a tough road ahead, I'm actually more optimistic about our food future and our ability to use science sensibly to
help us than I was five years ago. To do this and make the right
choices, we all need to know much more about what we eat and not
let a few companies control our knowledge and dictate our choices.
Eating good and tasty food is still a fundamental human pleasure, and
I believe its importance in our lives will not diminish.

Growing your own and thrifty eating

The future of food looks set to be very diverse. While our labs are creating amazing replacement products using cutting-edge food technology, we are still craving home-grown vegetables, home baking and a closer relationship with nature. During the Covid-19 pandemic, more people grew their own food at home, on allotments, or grew microgreens, cress and salads on kitchen windowsills. Touted as 'the world's most nutritious food', microgreens may be part of the answer to increasing plant diversity, even in a small kitchen and at an affordable cost. Chicken ownership also had an extraordinary boost, with waiting lists for chicks as people who had the space decided to raise their own egg-laying hens.[7] Foraging saw an upsurge, with unprecedented mushroom and wild garlic picking in the UK, and courses on how to forage berries, roots and leaves at an all-time high.

Another trend which is likely to continue, excluding the population hit hardest by the cost of living crisis, for economic, ethical, health and environmental reasons is thrifty, whole-food eating to reduce waste and increase diversity. This includes eating the external dark leaves of a cauliflower, rich in polyphenols and iron, as well as eating all the cuts and entrails of the animals we consume. Recipes to create 'leftover vegetable soups' and 'past-its-sell-by-date fruit crumble' are increasingly popular as the severity of food waste enters our conscience. This has also led to a big increase in home composting.

Personalised, intelligent diets

We are on course to be the first generation to be sicker and die earlier than our parents. But it is not inevitable. There are now hundreds of start-up biotech companies all working on nutrition and microbes, already with billions of pounds of entrepreneurial funding behind them. There are over 800 clinical trials ongoing involving microbes and various diseases, many of which will be successful. Understanding better the complexity of food and how it interacts with our microbes is already producing new treatments to fight many diseases including infections, immune problems and most impressively cancer. Some diabetic patients are now able to live without drugs, just by manipulating the food they put on their plates, reducing those that cause blood sugar peaks and favouring others that keep their levels constant, such as fatty avocados. Pro- and prebiotics are now proven to help many debilitating conditions, and even the extreme makeover of having a faecal transplant is becoming mainstream in treating infections, colitis and cancer.

*

In the not-so-distant future, we will all have the tools to create our own individual evidence-based diets. Just as I now know that grapes and raisins temporarily push my blood sugar levels into the diabetic range, everyone will have access to wearable AI devices to monitor themselves and their metabolic responses to foods. Future advances will allow us to write our own diet books and make choices that suit ourselves, our microbes and the planet in a way that is as unique as we all are.

Top five future food trends

1. Locally grown, seasonal fruits and vegetables will return to our kitchens.
2. We will soon be eating meat, fish and fungi protein grown ethically in labs.
3. Meat and dairy replacements will continue to diversify with greater environmental awareness.
4. Individual diet scores from new tech and AI will replace governmental guidelines and shape our food choices to suit our personal biology.
5. It will be essential to modify UPFs so that they don't cause us harm.

11. So, now what should I have for dinner?

The dreadful mistakes we have been making with food are perhaps most obvious in the diets of our children. All of the foods now identified as harmful and lacking any health benefits are the foods that we often feed children in the UK and US: UPFs in the many forms of crisps, snacks and pizzas, juices, breakfast cereals and fruit yogurts with excessive added sugars, ready meals and processed meats and fish. Clever food marketing and dishonest labelling can fool parents into thinking they are buying food appropriate for their kids, but one in five children under twelve in the US and UK is obese with numbers still growing, especially among the poorest children.[1] We also need to ban the abomination of unnecessary 'children's menus' in restaurants – which do not exist in countries where childhood obesity is unusual – and let children get used to eating real food early in life.

The first 1,000 days – from conception to the child's second birthday – is the most important window where the blueprint for adult health is set and the microbiome is most flexible. By feeding our children fake foods from birth – from ultra-processed formula milk to readymade purée pouches, to white processed bread, croissants, UP veggie sticks, sugar-laden fromage frais, chips and chicken nuggets, all washed down with fruit juice, flavoured milk or even soda – we are omitting the key building blocks for their bodies and brains.

As adults, we have a responsibility to the next generation. Growing social inequality is reflected most starkly in diet, where food insecurity leads to food choices that make obesity and type 2 diabetes nearly inevitable, and those effects are felt by the whole of society as our health infrastructure and economy crumble under its weight. Teaching our children to choose, prepare and eat real food in a family setting is one of the most wonderful lessons we can impart for future generations, and something we should all try to make time for. Keeping close contact with food, handling it and cooking it ourselves, gives us an element of control, appreciation and connection that we might otherwise lose.

Politicians have for decades ignored the devastating impact of poor diets on health, and it is naive to believe that governments will make critical policy steps anytime soon. There have been signs that this is moving up the agenda, such as the commissioning of the 2021 Dimbleby food report mentioned earlier, but as we saw in 2022 with the UK government's wimpy response to it, they are scared of taking any real action to reverse the trends, quoting the 'nanny state' and personal choice. Many of the recommendations they did accept are unlikely to become reality without a tougher stance. My hope and belief is that we can change the system via a ground-up approach, empowering individuals to change their habits and educate others. While researching this book over the past five years I have made many discoveries that have improved my life, and I hope you will gain similar insights too. Because of the very personal nature of food and health and our uniqueness in terms of our microbiomes, I am wary of personal anecdotes, but I am often asked about my own habits and diet, so I want to share them as examples, hoping that some of these ideas and my own food journey may also help you to experiment with yours.

When I had my first medical scare that started my food journey, I was 84kg. I had been slowly gaining weight over ten years without noticing (I thought it was muscle) and my waist had crept up to 4 inches more than my ideal size. My first diet change was fairly simple, to stop eating meat, which forced me to seek out more plants. I had to stop and think before eating food offered to me and ask what exactly was in it. I also reduced my salt intake conscientiously for a month, although I found, like many others, that despite the sacrifice, this had little effect on my blood pressure. As I read more about the benefits of plants, I decided to try a vegan diet. I managed this for just over a month. Although I felt virtuous, it was tough going, not because of missing meat, but because I was travelling for work in the

US with very limited and poor food choices, and because I really missed and craved real cheese.

For the next few years, I settled into a meat-free, plant- and dairy-rich diet, with occasional fish. An organic vegetable and fruit box delivery to my home was really useful. After a while, I switched to the now popular vegetarian organic meal boxes, that come with a complete set of ingredients including herbs and spices and instructions on how to prepare your meal, usually in half an hour. This increased my culinary repertoire and the diversity of plants I was eating every week, which I knew was good for my microbes. I became more adventurous with novel ingredients when eating out and was often pleasantly surprised. Researching more deeply about individual foods helped me to increase my own food diversity further. I would investigate into the far corners of my local Turkish-run greengrocers to find some interesting-looking vegetable, fruit, or variety of mushroom.

I now look at plants differently, selecting varieties that have more redness or colour on the leaves that signal their protective polyphenols, or those that just look fresher. I go out of my way to find odd-coloured vegetables like purple carrots, potatoes and Jerusalem artichokes, and have lost interest in bland iceberg lettuce and cucumbers. I replaced them with the many other diverse members of the cabbage family, which I became less afraid of as I learnt to roast, steam and fry them in interesting ways.

Understanding caramelisation and the Maillard browning reaction really made me want to sear everything at the magic 140°C to get the extra chemicals and flavours in the pan or in the oven. Just boiling vegetables now seems plain wrong. My herb and spice drawer expanded and I started experimenting, by adding sumac to avocado on toast or using a wide range of spices on roasted sweet potato, cauliflower or hispi cabbage. Experimenting with the vegetables left in the fridge to make a curry or Middle Eastern dish became fun. I became fussier with my cooking oils, rarely using anything other than high-quality extra virgin olive oil and avoiding old oil that had started to deteriorate. I am less frightened to liven up a dish and change the acidity with lemon or vinegar, liberally adding yogurt, kefir or sour cream, or adding salt or soy sauce.

My views on meat and fish eating have also continued to evolve. In 2011, I thought the evidence was clear that red meat was bad and fish good. Now the distinction is murkier. Although heavily processed meat appears consistently bad, there is no good evidence that good-quality red meat is worse for our health than fish, at least for most people, and I worry about the sustainability of fish eating. So I eat less fish now, and when I do, I shop at my fishmongers and choose higher-quality varieties from a known local source. I also eat a small amount of high-quality, grass-fed organic meat or salami once or twice a month, which keeps my otherwise low B12 levels steady, helped by occasional organic free-range eggs; but I do now know that I could live meat-free without my world ending.

Learning about all the fats, protein, fibre and other nutrients in nuts and seeds made me add them to many more dishes and try to have a handful most days, whether for breakfast on yogurt, lunch with some fruit or sprinkled on my evening meal. Mushrooms have become more of a regular feature in my diet, and I try to add them to many dishes, picking different varieties in season. They are a great source of protein, fibre, polyphenols and vitamin D, and when mixed with carbs add a delicious umami flavour.

I try to eat at least one fermented food per day, often several, and this can be small amounts, such as a single shot of kefir or kombucha, or yogurt or kraut added to my curry or chilli. I have also started to make my own fermented foods, yogurt, kefir, kombucha, kimchi and sauerkraut (see page 154) and sourdough, albeit with different levels of success (at first, my kombucha mother sank worryingly to the bottom (tip: wait and it usually refloats). Our fridge is permanently stuffed with various mothers, blobs and murky alien liquids in jars. With kombucha, you can literally see the scoby changing the dark tea into a light, complex, sour, sparkling drink over a few days. It is easy to imagine the similar process that goes on in our guts every day.

The latest data also points to the benefits of our gut microbes having a holiday every now and then. As well as reducing my snacking, I give mine a long break on as many days as I can by having a fourteen-hour fast. This is easy to start to do on a Saturday night, by finishing eating at nine and waiting till after eleven the next morning to have Sunday brunch. When I am feeling virtuous or putting on weight, I might have an intermittent fasting day with minimal food.

I like a glass or two of wine and try to pick red most of the time, but I know getting the balance right is a delicate matter. We can all justify our choices, and mine is that it gives me pleasure, and I may be helping my microbes, as most of my intake is polyphenol-rich red wine, with a bit of artisan beer or cider. Along with many millions of people in the UK and other countries, I have tried a non-alcoholic 'dry January', which is a good lesson in self-control. Rather than have one dry month in twelve, though, it is looking healthier to spread out those thirty days over the year, so I try (note the word try) to have an alcohol-free day once a week. The kombucha comes in very handy as an alcohol substitute on those days, plus a fast-improving range of alcohol-free beers.

Helped by our collaboration with Matt Walker, the sleep expert at Berkeley and author of the bestselling *Why We Sleep*, I also discovered the importance of sleep quality and timing in reducing our sugar peaks and in the functioning of our gut microbes. Our microbes need a good regular nap to fit in with their own circadian rhythm and the PREDICT study shows the benefits on our metabolism of going to bed earlier and not eating late at night. I also try to emulate the Hadza who (like our ancestors) go to sleep each night at eleven and wake at dawn to get their 7.5 hours, supplemented by the odd power nap in the afternoon. Foods and drinks can affect sleep quality, which is nearly as important as duration and I have tried to limit drinking alcohol to earlier in the evening to reduce the disruption to sleep quality, and have a herbal tea nightcap instead.

Personalising my diet

I was lucky to be one of the first to take part in the ZOE PREDICT study, so I now have some unique insights into how my microbes and my metabolism respond to a wide range of foods.[2] With the power to measure these scores at home, we are able to keep track of how the scores change as the body changes with age and improved health. My results from the study allowed ZOE to compute individual scores for my foods, ranging from 100 (eat as much as I like) to zero (eat rarely).

On setting up my continuous glucose monitor, my first shock was my blood sugar reading first thing in the morning, which on most days showed I was peaking with high levels that classified me as pre-diabetic. My grandmother died of type 2 diabetes heart complications aged seventy, so there were a few genes running in the family which I likely inherited. With high baseline blood levels, it wasn't surprising I reacted strongly to some starchy foods such as rice and potatoes, though luckily not to all. I also found out that, like most people, I had a larger sugar reaction to my test muffins at lunch than at breakfast. But my peak, unlike most people, was not as high in the evening.[3] This reinforced my instinct that regular large lunches were not ideal for me.

I ate a sandwich at lunch for about twenty-five years and I find warm fresh bread impossible to resist in restaurants, so my high sugar reaction to bread was really annoying. My score out of the 'ideal' 100 was near zero (eat rarely) for most bread types except if packed with seeds or made with rye, especially German style, which I can eat in moderation. I try to eat bread as fermented sourdough with at least some rye (home-baked gives me better ZOE scores), and combined with some fats such as cheese or avocado to reduce the sugar peak. I am still occasionally tempted by a great-smelling warm croissant, bagel or baguette, but am more picky on the quality, making sure it tastes good enough to be worthwhile. Luckily, I have no major peaks with most types of rice and pasta (ZOE scores 30–40), and so generally do well with Italian and Asian meals, although I try to have a greater balance of the vegetable sauce to pasta ratio and have to be careful with sticky rice. I have also learned that buying parboiled rice is much better nutritionally and metabolically than I thought. Gnocchi is now an occasional treat, as it is usually made with refined potato (ZOE score zero), so I counterbalance it with walnuts, mushrooms and broccoli. In Middle Eastern dishes, I avoid couscous other than in very small amounts (score 9), and opt for bulgur wheat (45), pearl barley (77) or quinoa (46).

Of all my meals, breakfasts have perhaps changed most over the last fifteen years. I used to eat different types of muesli (0–4) with orange juice (0). In winter, I often used to swap this for porridge made from oats and thought buying more expensive organic rolled jumbo oats (0–10) was healthy. I now eat steel-cut varieties (40) that need longer to soak and cook and are best made in larger batches. Most days now if I'm eating breakfast, I will have a full-fat yogurt mixed with kefir, mixed nuts and seeds and some chopped fruit or berries, frozen or fresh.

As for fruit, I have now gone for more variety, so that I don't just eat my standard banana every day, which gave me a moderate spike (score 38), while apples (68) and pears (62) are better, as are all the berries (blackberries 77, strawberries 75). Grapes turned out to be my nemesis (36), not helped by the fact I usually ate too many. I still have just a few, accompanied by cheese which helpfully reduces the speed of the sugar absorption. The fats in nuts also seem to help reduce the effect of any fruit. Adding fat to your carbs may not suit everyone though.

In the ZOE PREDICT study, I was keen to explore how my body processed and got rid of the fats in my food, especially as official guidelines suggest I should take statins due to my gender, age and family history of cardiovascular disease. I am in my sixties and fairly fit, with a good set of microbes, my pre-meal morning blood fat levels (LDL and triglycerides) were healthy at the low end of the range, and so I was confident of a good score. But the final results showed my fat responses were in the worst 10 per cent of men; six hours after eating, too much fat was still hanging around in my bloodstream.

This was disappointing. I thought I could handle unlimited fat, but apparently not. I would therefore fare badly on a traditional ketogenic diet, which is ideally 70 per cent fat. I was between a rock and a hard place, unable to eat too many carbs or too many fats. I have to be careful about which fats I do eat, and how many at one sitting. As I eat little meat and consume good-quality extra virgin olive oil, avocados or whole nuts, these high-quality fats are not the problem: my main fat vice is cheese. I could just stop eating it. But that would be a disaster, as I would be missing out on one of my favourite foods and a great source of probiotics. So, now I try to reduce the amount of cheese I eat at one sitting and choose the most ethical and probiotic rich versions I can, giving my body time to digest it. Despite my poor ZOE fat score, I have not stopped eating natural fats in tasty, good-quality foods. I eat butter and full-fat cream and yogurt. I don't drink much milk; but when I do buy it now, it is full-fat organic, or increasingly, fortified oat milk which is better for the planet, but in small amounts, as it spikes my blood glucose.

There is nothing like one's own experience to change habits. I had already cut out orange and other fruit juice, just based on the amount of sugar in it, but confirming that my sugar peaks were as high for Coke or Pepsi rammed the message home. I used to have an occasional diet drink with artificial sweeteners, but now I have seen my own metabolic reaction with sucralose (one of the commonest sweeteners), and read about the effect on microbes, I now try to avoid them, but not obsessively, and don't think the occasional can or additive will harm me, as long as it is not regular. Paying attention to daily habits is more important than striving for perfection. I buy better-quality coffee or tea, as this is likely to improve the levels of beneficial polyphenols and fibre I get multiple times a day. Some speciality coffees are now marketed as being high in polyphenols, and if you enjoy teas, make green tea part of your routine.

My resting metabolic rate and estimated resting energy needs were low compared to most people. This confirmed that I need to be careful about my energy balance and what I eat to not gain weight. I, like many others, found that exercising several hours per week felt good and improved my alertness and fitness, and was undoubtedly good for my heart. But it had no effect on my weight, as the body compensates and tries to maintain the stored fat levels. I now cycle about five hours per week, and swim regularly in the summer which probably helps a bit but I would need to double this before I saw a major effect on weight. Most people cannot exercise to lose weight unless they are regularly running marathons, although some studies show long-term exercise can reduce chances of relapse after an initial weight loss.[4]

*

Writing this book during one of the worst food and economic crises ever, I am very aware of how difficult making food choices can be. Many families have to choose between having a hot meal or a warm shower; I know I am privileged to have access to both every day. The luxury of time to prepare and cook food is also not always available, but hopefully this book will show that expensive 'superfoods' and prohibitive meal plans are not the way to harness the power of foods for our wellbeing. Expensive does not mean superfood, cheap does not always mean unhealthy, and some minimally processed food is perfectly healthy. Processed and pre-packed parboiled rice that can be rapidly cooked in a microwave has a surprising amount of nutrients compared to more expensive rice. Whole plants from the market, vegetable aisle or greengrocers are generally cheaper than meats or convenience foods. Seasonal local berries, and cheaper legumes, nuts and seeds are usually as good as more exotic varieties and can be enjoyed frozen, dried, or even canned. Frozen peas and berries, canned tomatoes and pulses, and even baked beans, depending on the sauce, are both economical and good for you. Even a baked potato or boiled potato with the skin on is perfectly healthy as part of a varied and diverse diet. If buying organic produce is not an option, thoroughly cleaning fruits and vegetables with running water will help reduce the levels of pesticides we consume.

Understanding which foods suit us best is important, but we shouldn't forget that the experience of cooking and eating together is probably as important as the food. Sharing a table or plate with another human is one of the most important social interactions we have. The longevity of the population in areas like Liguria, Sardinia, Okinawa or Crete may owe more to the social side of eating and drinking communally, even in old age. Engaging with food invites others to share your experience, and communal eating improves your wellbeing and happiness.[5]

Nor should we ignore other lifestyle choices which impact our health and interact with our microbes. Obviously smoking is bad for us, and no amount of blueberries can balance the damage of cigarettes. The same can be said of crash diets with processed meal replacement bars and chemical powder meals. Reaching an 'ideal weight' should not be our main aim.

Like many people, I don't always obey my own rules and can find myself tempted or may be in social situations where it is easier to comply than create a fuss. The key is to try to follow as many of the healthy eating rules as you can easily, and don't beat yourself up over the odd lapse if you sometimes fail. Diet over time is more important than absolute adherence every day. No one is perfect and our bodies are designed to accommodate the odd takeaway and birthday cake. It's impossible to follow all the advice in this book – but changing just some of your habits most of the time will help both your health and the planet.

Hopefully you have now gained some important insights into how food is made and what effects the components have on your body and the environment. The next part of the book looks at individual foods in detail, providing you with a personal tool kit to help you make healthy and tasty choices.

Five final tips

1. Aim for diversity in your diet including thirty different plant types each week. Keep a tally on the fridge door if it helps.
2. Treat children's gut microbes and diets with care and teach them about real food.
3. Spread the word that UPFs should be avoided and are making us all sick.
4. Experiment with your food to better understand your body and personal nutrition profile.
5. Think of your food choices as transactions for both your and the planet's future health.

PART TWO
Foods

12. Fruits

Fruit has long been associated with bounty, fertility, abundance, wealth and health. Yet although humans evolved to like and eat many fruits, nowadays many of us are so addicted to gimmicky snack offerings that governments have to encourage us to eat fruit as part of the global five-a-day marketing strategy. Historically, fruit has always been perceived as medicinally important, even more so since the discovery of vitamin C, and most countries still rate fruit and vegetables equally, though some like Australia effectively now rate a portion of fruit as half as healthy as vegetables with their 'Go for 2 & 5' campaign, which recommends two large daily portions of fruit to five normal portions of veg. This was mainly over concerns that the sugar content in many fruits negates some of the other benefits. But what does the data tell us?

Results from 680,000 European and US populations in observational studies have shown consistent, but only modest benefits of eating fruit. Regular fruit eaters have only about a 5 per cent reduction in heart disease per extra (80g) portion eaten. This is credible but small when you also consider that fruit eaters are generally richer, more educated and healthier. This is factored in, but can never be totally removed. In the Chinese Kadoorie Biobank study of over 500,000 people, the differences were much greater than in the west with 30–40 per cent reductions in heart disease across all the ten regions.[1] This is possibly because basal levels of fruit eating were lower, so the potential for improvement (or bias) was much greater.

With abundant fibre, anthocyanins and other protective chemicals, high polyphenol fruits should be the best food for our gut microbes, but is there any evidence? Most observational studies with human microbe data have unfortunately lumped fruits together with other plants. Also, most of the research studies to date have grouped all fruits together, with berries only sometimes separated out. We managed to narrow it down using data from 3,000 of our UK twins. We found better gut microbial diversity in those who regularly ate strawberries, cherries and grapes five to six times a week compared to those who ate them only rarely. Feeding fruit to rodents generally improves their microbes, and one study which fed overweight mice apple pectin fibre for six weeks showed improved microbes and helped weight loss. In another study, when rats were fed the polyphenol quercetin, found in dark red or blue berries or plums (as well as onions and capers), anti-obesity microbes and weight loss increased.

As usual, there are only a few short trials in humans. Studies of dried cranberries showed increases of the microbe *Akkermansia*, often associated with weight loss. Another good gut microbe, *Alistipes*, was increased by red grapes, grape polyphenols and cranberries. Freeze-dried blueberry powder equivalent to one cup of raw blueberries also increased the natural probiotic *Bifidobacterium longum*. Unfortunately, these studies are really just teasers, as none involved more than fifteen participants.[2] While the evidence is incomplete, it currently points to moderate fruit eating being beneficial for health and gut microbes, regardless of your level of obesity or blood sugar.

Everyday fruits

Apples are perhaps the UK's equivalent of India's mangoes, and often viewed as our national fruit. They were cultivated first from wild apple trees in Kazakhstan from ancient Greek times and brought to Northern Europe by the Romans. There are over 7,500 recorded apple varieties (over 2,000 in the UK alone), and many are patented or trademarked such as 'Pink Lady' or 'Gala'. The Victorians ate many more varieties than we do, and used to have apple tasting evenings to vaunt their sophistication and palates, just like we might with wine tasting.

An apple may seem rather simple, but it has twice as many genes as we do, allowing it to duplicate itself and making us humans look rather crude in comparison. These genes give them a huge range of chemicals used for energy, protection and attractive makeup. This allows them fine control over different rates of ripening and an extraordinary range of flavours and textures. Each variety contains different amounts of polyphenols and nutrients, but apples from the same tree will also vary. They are an underestimated source of a fibre called pectin, which is thought to be an important factor in healthy weight maintenance and perhaps even weight loss. An apple a day has been estimated to have a similar health impact to taking a statin.[3] But while it may not necessarily always keep the doctor away, it might keep weight gain at bay.

Apricots are known as 'hasty peaches' as they ripen much quicker and have a shorter lifespan. Most in the UK are now imported, but they don't travel well. They often lack flavour and although colour is a good guide, are hard to select without tasting them. They are best air dried to keep the polyphenols intact with the optional addition of sulphur dioxide if you are fussy about the colour, but when dried have relatively high sugar contents.

Pears have also been cultivated for millennia. While there are believed to be over 3,000 species, and Kew Gardens stocked over 600 in the seventeenth century, most shops now stock only one or two varieties; in the UK, 90 per cent are conference pears. Pears have slightly fewer polyphenols than apples but are a good source of fibre including pectin and are low in sugar. As usual the skin (and core) is worth eating providing ten times the polyphenols of the flesh. They have high amounts of unique 'demethylated' polyphenols but we have no clue what they do. Quince is a distant relative that is hard to eat raw because of very high levels of tannin polyphenols, but when cooked these colourless polyphenols transform both colour, taste and aroma to a beautiful red with pigmented carotenoids. Quince paste goes very well with cheese.

Fresh native plums are hard to find which is a pity as they have the highest polyphenol content of any stone fruit, as well as being high in fibre and vitamin C. Delicate local plum varieties are thin-skinned and juicy and don't survive transportation, unlike imported sturdier, less flavourful varieties.

When dried, plums become the famous prune. They are mass

produced by rapidly dehydrating ripe plums in hot air tunnels, which conserves very high levels of polyphenols and the fruit's dark colour, so they don't need additional sulphur preservatives. Prunes, of course, are renowned as a constipation cure. As such, Americans felt too embarrassed to buy them, so ten years ago the California prune board officially renamed them 'dried plums' and sales soared. Prunes have been used successfully for constipation for centuries, based on the theory that fibre worked to soften stools by retaining water and bulking them up. This is only a minor part of the story: the many prune fibres and chemicals play a key role. One such chemical is sorbitol which we can't digest ourselves, but is fermented by our gut microbes. However, only some people have the specific microbes that can ferment the sorbitol which acts as a strong laxative.

Peaches were probably domesticated 6,000 years ago in China; they slowly reached Europe and the Spanish brought them to North America. Edward I of England apparently had peach trees in his thirteenth-century Westminster garden, but without a royal gardener they are tough to grow in the UK climate, though global warming may help. There are over 3,000 varieties, mostly in China, but at least 300 in the USA. Common varieties have white or yellow flesh, and all share chemicals with almonds, so allergy to both is now quite common. When picking peaches, the smell is a good indicator of ripeness, and they shouldn't have any background green in them. In contrast to the usual colour rule, white-fleshed peaches have greater total anti-inflammatory polyphenol levels than the yellow-fleshed ones, although newer red-fleshed peaches beat both of them. More convenient, less messy to eat freestone peaches have less flavour and chemical complexity.

Nectarines, contrary to popular belief, are not peaches crossed with plums, but mutant peaches, differing only in one tiny part of the furry-skin gene, and otherwise very similar in nutrition, aroma and taste. Strangely, some peach trees can produce nectarines as well as peaches. Other breeding crosses include small flat squashed doughnut-shaped peaches first bred about 3,000 years ago in China. I first discovered them in Barcelona about ten years ago. I loved the taste and the perfect doughnut shape and was hooked, although embarrassingly asked for 'pechos planos' (flat breasts!) rather than the Spanish name 'Paraguayos', as they were erroneously thought to have come from Paraguay.

Citrus

The mandarin, the pomelo and the citron were probably the original citrus fruits from India and China. Jews and then Arabs brought these sour fruits to southern Italy around 2,000 years ago where they were cultivated to produce a sweet orange mutant. Limes are a cross of a citron and mandarin and are the most acidic of the citrus fruits, (8 per cent citric acid), lemons are a cross between a sour orange and a citron, with around 5 per cent acidity, the orange is a pomelo-mandarin hybrid, and the grapefruit, with its distinctive astringent naringin chemical, is a pomelo and orange mix. Other mutations and crosses followed, giving us a wide range of zesty fruits, which with their thick aromatic skins can crucially last through our winters. Oranges have gradually become sweeter and thicker-skinned to help transport, though the artificial ripening process can leave the central fruit tougher and less sweet. Their distinctive colours come from the carotenoid polyphenols that are temperature sensitive – in the tropics citrus ripen while still green, but in colder climes, the green changes to orange. Mandarins, satsumas, more seedy tangerines and their smaller cousin clementines get sweeter and less acidic the longer they are stored.

Grapefruits used to be part of the traditional British breakfast, but with our exposure to sugary cereals and jams, many people now find them too bitter. Though not topping the vitamin C or the total polyphenol charts, they are high in anthocyanins and lycopenes, particularly in the recent red-fleshed mutations from Florida and Texas. Grapefruit consumption has been shown to reduce blood pressure in at least three human trials.[4] The hundreds of polyphenol chemicals in grapefruit can also alter the effects of over eighty-five medicines by disrupting the enzymes that normally break them down. While a few medications become less effective, most become far more potent, especially immune, heart and lipid medications as well as painkillers, sedatives, even Viagra. They also make a shot of caffeine go further. There is much more to citrus fruits than vitamin C, and even if you don't have scurvy, they are powerful medicine.

Although we were obsessed with citrus for historical reasons, we now know many fruits and vegetables have higher levels of vitamin C than oranges or limes, including kale, lychees and strawberries. Probably the greatest concentrations are found in a berry called kakadu plums, known to the local Aborigines from a remote part of Northern Australia, where one tiny fruit gives you a week's supply.

Orange Juice (OJ)

Three times more oranges are now sold as juice than for eating whole. The first juice products appeared after the war in the US as frozen concentrate that you thawed and then diluted. They were succeeded by a pre-diluted, pasteurised long-life version that could be stored in cartons or tins, with plenty of extra sugar and other additives to keep it stable. In the 1980s new processing techniques allowed orange juice to be stored whole (not as concentrate) and sold as 'natural juice', 'not from concentrate'. Most people don't realise these are defined as UPFs. The world's biggest brands are now owned by multinationals – e.g. Tropicana (owned by PepsiCo), Minute Maid (Coca-Cola) – who perfected the mass-market processed OJ that had a good shelf-life and reasonable, always consistent taste. They also managed to add back bits of pulp to give it a natural feel. The oranges, which come from Florida, Brazil or Spain, are sorted and squeezed around a year before the carton of juice arrives 'fresh' in shops. On its journey after pasteurisation, it will sit in massive sterile million-gallon vats deprived of oxygen and filled with nitrogen gas. All this processing destroys its flavour chemicals and some of the nutrients and vitamin C. These have to be added back later in so-called 'flavour packs' which are secret and don't have to be disclosed on packaging, but they contain concentrated versions of the chemicals found naturally in oranges like ethylene butyrate, the 'freshness' chemical. To maintain consistency across seasons, they can add other chemicals, natural colourings and sugars to balance the colour, acidity and sweetness and can be adapted to the sweet-tooth preferences of each country. The business is worth over $4 billion dollars in the USA alone and the scale is massive with every hotel, restaurant and household typically able to produce a glass of orange juice from the fridge on any day of the year, despite oranges being a seasonal fruit. About a third of EU fruit juice is sold as fresh (not from concentrate) and about 50 per cent in the UK.

Concentrate-type juice had a bad name, as the regulations about adding sugar and additives are very lax, and taste was poor, but to reverse sales trends, standards have recently improved and they perform well in taste tests. Frozen concentrate can also surprisingly preserve the nutrients and vitamin C pretty well compared to so-called 'supermarket fresh'.

'Freshly squeezed' orange juice is now big business but has the challenge of a shelf-life of ten to twelve days. But these products are still different to squeezing them yourself; you notice how the solid bits don't separate out and sink to the bottom because the oranges are briefly pasteurised, which kills most bugs (and vitamins), but also deactivates enzymes that normally and rapidly separate out the solids and liquid.

Is orange juice healthy?

Fruit juice, despite the high sugar content, has been promoted as being healthy because most juices (if they actually contain the fruit) have good levels of vitamin C, nutrients and polyphenols. In most countries, a glass of juice is promoted as part of the 'five a day' fruit or vegetable quota. However, while better nutritionally than drinking a can of Fanta or Tango, it is no match for a real fruit – skin and all. In the UK, eight out of ten people drink a juice or smoothie at least weekly believing this is healthy. But since its peak in 2012, concerns over the sugar levels have started to hit sales. Guidelines in some countries have belatedly started to change; now emphasising the importance of eating the whole fruit.

A few clinical trials of OJ have explored its health effects. A 'not from concentrate' orange juice (Minute Maid) versus a high-polyphenol version was tested on 100 overweight Spanish subjects blind and randomised for twelve weeks. Their blood showed improvements in antioxidant profiles, which was highlighted in the paper (part sponsored by Coca Cola).[5] What wasn't highlighted was that they also increased their fasting glucose and insulin levels. Drinking a large glass of orange juice is like eating roughly twelve oranges per day, but without much of the fibre and extra polyphenols from the white pithy part of the fruit. Even if you could eat twelve oranges in that time, it would only have a minimal effect on your blood sugar, whereas the processed OJ is guaranteed to give you a spike and dip, increasing your hunger levels. While short-term studies of juice drinking have not shown any evidence of weight gain, there are crucially no good long-term clinical trials. Without clinical trial data, we have to rely on observational studies like a large American prospective study of 120,000 health professionals, which found whole-fruit eaters had a reduced risk of diabetes and general mortality, while fruit juice drinkers had a slightly higher risk of diabetes and no mortality benefit.[6] Orange juice is not a health drink and should be a rare treat, squeezed at home.

Berries

A berry is usually described as any fleshy fruit that has seeds but no large stone, which includes many larger fruits like bananas, cucumbers and peppers, but here I am focussing on classical small berries with seeds, like strawberries, raspberries, blueberries, cranberries, plus the newcomers, chokeberries, sour cherries, goji, noni and acai.

Blueberries were an original North American berry unknown in the UK before the 1930s. They are now very popular, and available year round thanks to local polytunnels and Southern hemisphere growers. Most of the polyphenol content is in the skin, and lowbush varieties (often misleadingly called wild) have 50 per cent more polyphenol content than the more common highbush types usually found in Europe. They start off green then purple and are usually good to eat when the bottoms are blue. Closely related are bilberries, also known as European blueberries or whortleberries. They look similar to blueberries but with a fuller, more acidic taste.

Raspberries come in two main colours: red, originating wild in Europe, and black in America and Asia. The raspberry family has the highest fibre content because of their high number of seeds, and includes a whole range of hybrid berries derived from crossing blackberries or raspberries, such as loganberries, boysenberries, etc., all with very similar beneficial properties.

Both in fresh and processed forms, strawberries are globally popular. The large, juicy bright red modern berries descend from the wild strawberry, one of the few accessible ancestral berries we can still enjoy. These tiny fruits grow prolifically in woods and hedgerows across most of the world and were often the first berries of the season with a special cultural significance. I even have some plants in my tiny London garden. They were popular in medieval gardens from about the fifteenth century and because of their smell were considered love potions. Unless you pick your own wild strawberries, the ones you buy or eat in restaurants will be costly and usually now grown not in forests, but in plastic polytunnels.

The dominant supermarket strawberry in Europe is still the Elsanta variety, bred by the Dutch in the early 1990s for its hardiness and looks, but not flavour – in blind tasting it loses out to its uglier aromatic cousins. Avoid strawberries with a white ring at the base. These are deliberately picked unripe for decoration not taste; but unlike fruits like peaches and bananas, however long you wait, they will never ripen. If you manage to eat them unripe, as well as lacking taste and aroma, they will also disappoint nutritionally. Insects love strawberries as much as we do, so as discussed (see page 85), pesticides are used on them in greater quantities than nearly any other plant we eat. Wash them just before eating or they will rapidly go mushy.

Strawberries are difficult to grow near the Arctic, so strawberry-loving Scandinavians came up with a solution. Arctic flounder fish have a gene that allows them to produce a sort of antifreeze. Scientists inserted the gene into a helpful bacteria, and this is now sprayed on the strawberry plants, providing perfect insulation against freezing

Nordic conditions. The strawberries are then cleaned, removing the genetically modified bacteria, *et voila*!

Sweet cherries grow readily in cool countries, with the dark red ones being good sources of polyphenols. The distinctive cherry flavour comes from the almond-like benzaldehyde plus terpenes, and is often synthesised in laboratories for processed foods and drinks.

Gooseberries grow wild in Britain and Europe and come in at least three colours. They have failed to achieve 'super berry' status, but rate well for both fibre and polyphenols. Alas, there is no gooseberry board promoting their health benefits but they make delicious pies and jams, as well as dried snacks. Many children were told in England and Canada that they were born under a gooseberry bush, but most of us are not aware that this was nineteenth-century slang for pubic hair – a strange origin for the term 'playing gooseberry' (a third wheel).

Berries are the most talked about and studied fruits for their health benefits. Several berry varieties have been pronounced as the 'health food of the decade' or the 'world's most antioxidant rich food', and each novel berry is routinely given the accolade 'superfood'. One of the first superfood claims came during the American Civil War, when blackberry tea was used as a cure for dysentery. Temporary truces were declared to allow both Union and Confederate soldiers to forage for the fruits. It is unclear if it worked as a placebo or an excuse to walk in the woods, as outbreaks of dysentery still continued.

I tasted my first true organic berry in the East African bush during my brief stay with the Hadza hunter-gatherers. These berries looked like nothing I had seen in my local shops. The commonest at that season, the multicoloured kongorobi, or *Grewia bicolor*, are about the size of a small pea and look a bit like Skittles with golden reds, yellows and greens with a large seed in the centre. They are eaten by the handful and the seeds usually spat out, with an astringent citrus taste mixed with a sweetness that increases when left in the sun to dry. This is probably what our ancestors ate before fruit became unrecognisable through domestication and selective breeding. Although tiny, kongorobi have enormous amounts of protective polyphenols – an estimated twenty times more than modern berries. As well as fibre, the seeds are also packed with healthy fats like linoleic acid.

Typical supermarket berries are less nutritious than the original wild varieties, but they are still a rich source of many nutrients. A single cup of mixed berries delivers twice as much fibre as a cup of chopped bananas or apples, or the equivalent of three slices of whole-grain bread. They are also packed with vitamin C, potassium, folate and polyphenols, one of which, anthocyanin, gives them their vibrant range of colours, and also account for many of their antioxidant abilities. As a group, berries average nearly ten times more antioxidants than other fruits and vegetables (fifty times more than animal-based foods). It is not surprising that they have earned a reputation as a superfood. But let's look at the hard evidence.

As part of our Twins UK study, we looked at the dietary habits of nearly 2,000 women and found that at least one portion of any berries daily was associated with significantly lower blood pressure and blood vessel stiffness. Twins who ate the most berries overall had less body fat and a healthier fat pattern. To check for bias, we compared twin pairs who had been brought up together, where one had high berry intakes and the other low. We confirmed the association with lower fat levels, ruling out genetic, and most social and family factors as an explanation. The differences equated to around 8 per cent lower body and central (visceral) fat in the twin consuming around at least 200g berries three times a week.

What of the claim that berries help our memory and may cheer us up? The evidence comes from some observational studies and short-term trials of variable quality. One US study of 16,000 retired nurses showed berry eaters had delayed brain ageing by 2.5 years, and a weak effect on preventing Parkinson's disease and possibly dementia.[7] A study using a dummy placebo juice showed intriguing differences in brain activity using MRI scans.[8] Some, but not all, randomised studies with concentrated grape juice improved brain skills in normal and memory-impaired elderly adults after three months.[9]

In a randomised study of 120 adults, blueberry powder was found to aid cognition over six months.[10] Better data is found in younger people. Randomised placebo controlled studies in seventy-one young people (which is quite big for nutrition studies) have shown blueberry juice improving mood and attention within a few hours.[11]

This was extended to younger children, showing short-term improvements in intellectual tasks for a few hours. A longer-term study gave juice equivalent to over one cup of berries a day to a group of seven- to ten-year-olds and showed improved cognition but not reading skills.[12] This suggests that blueberry juice could be the perfect pre-exam breakfast; though it's probably easier to go for a bowlful of fresh berries.

Berries supposedly also prevent cancer, but the test tube data doesn't get us much further, as in real life a cancer cell does not directly go head to head with a strawberry. A few small human studies have been performed, none perfect. One enrolled fourteen patients with a genetic condition called familial polyposis coli which is often a precursor to colon cancer to assess the 'cancer busting' effects of freeze-dried black raspberries. The study found all patients taking the raspberries as a suppository 'did well' after nine months.[13] Another Chinese study found similarly unconvincing evidence of the influence of freeze-dried strawberries on prevention of oesophageal cancer.

Weight-loss berries

Billed as 'the Most POWERFUL Weight Loss Supplement on the Market Today!', raspberry ketone tablets are a billion-dollar weight-loss industry in the USA. Ketones are just one of over 200 chemicals that provide the fruit with its vibrant red colour and smell, but supposedly the only one that matters. The 'amazing proof' came from two small mouse studies using ketones; the first from Japan in six mice in 2005; the second from Korea, showing a few mice lost weight and altered some fat hormones.[14] The UK Food standards agency was not convinced by the evidence and tried to effectively ban the product by calling for it to be registered as a novel food; in 2014, objecting to the 'miracle' weight loss claims, it imposed a further ban. A subsequent 2017 study in mice failed to show any of these claimed benefits, pointing out that the doses used previously equated to eating over a kilogram of the commercial tablets.[15] Yet, despite these European bans they are still sold online via Amazon across Europe, showing how difficult it is to stop a bogus product once launched.

This might be harmless fun if it were not for gullible victims. In 2014 Cara Reynolds, a twenty-four-year-old healthcare worker, was upset after a row with her boyfriend and swallowed a handful of ketone slimming tablets. She had a fit, lost consciousness and never woke up. The supplements were found (as many do) to also contain caffeine and the mixture was fatal. The irony was that she was a healthy size and did not need them anyway. These 'natural' pills are still being sold at high prices while the natural source – the raspberry – is comparatively cheap, tasty and healthy as well as being relatively safe to consume in large quantities.

Sour grapes and berries

Usually, the more sour and acidic the berry, the more it is promoted for its medicinal qualities.

Kiwi fruit is a tart berry developed in the 1950s from *Actinidia*, a dull Chinese vine fruit. Since the 1970s, it has been renamed and heavily promoted by New Zealand as a cure for everything. Kiwi is best eaten raw; like pineapple, heating releases dangerous protein-digesting enzymes that damage other food ingredients and can cause a nasty rash. Some studies (well, only one) have suggested that kiwis contain the brain chemical serotonin and can boost sleep. A Taiwanese study of twenty-two insomniacs given two kiwi fruit at bedtime increased their time asleep by 13 per cent, but without a control group this is just another placebo. The study was repeated on a British volunteer for a BBC documentary who claimed it helped him, but, as with most experiments on television, we should remain sceptical.[16]

Another sleep aid with better evidence is sour cherries (also called Montmorency cherries). These bright-red acidic fruits lack sugar, so growers needed to find other uses for them. They naturally contain melatonin whose primary function is as an antioxidant, but also initiates sleep in mammals. Melatonin supplements sold in many countries have been shown to have a modest effect in helping jetlag. There are several uncontrolled studies which are best ignored, but one placebo-controlled trial of twenty people given tart cherry juice or a dummy juice found it aided sleep and increased natural melatonin levels.[17] Another smaller placebo study helped the sleep of eight insomniacs and suggested it was due to different brain chemicals like tryptophan. So, drinking a tart cherry cocktail before retiring is likely to be better for most people than a traditional glass of whisky.

Sour cherries are also said to have 'incredible' effects on athletic performance, infections, heart disease and gout. Most of these claims rest on a few poor studies and I was very sceptical until I read a randomised placebo-controlled study in a reputable scientific journal. Fifteen men with mild hypertension were given a liquid sour-cherry supplement and showed a significant drop in blood pressure of 7mmHg three hours later.[18] The cherry growers subsequently funded a less impressive study showing that the supplements could also improve human gut microbes.

Grapes, technically berries, are the most popular global fruit after bananas and were originally sour. The Romans brought them to the UK where there are now over 500 vineyards producing grapes, though mostly for wine. Since 2007, seedless grapes have also been grown in the UK, as well as other cooler countries. The more grapes there are on a cluster, the lower the nutrient value and the quality of the wine, but they are fine for eating. Grapes used to be the fruit you took to relatives in hospital, but now the health benefits are forgotten. They have high sugar content and modest fibre levels, mainly from the seeds and skins. Red or black grapes have about 30 per cent more polyphenols than white grapes, though neither makes the top berry rankings.

Grape seed contains vitamin E, linoleic acid, polyphenols and condensed tannins, which give grapes, particularly the skin and seeds, their astringency. The most famous polyphenol produced by grapes is resveratrol, which was hailed as a superfood extract and the answer to heart disease. Grape Seed Extract (GSE) is a much-hyped polyphenol supplement similar to green tea extracts. It is supposed to help allergy, immunity and, of course, provide a vital 'detox function'. While theoretically it could be beneficial, the dosage needed is unknown and the only evidence so far comes from second-rate studies in rodents and in test tubes. As for most fruits, swallowing the odd seed from your unpeeled grape is a better option.

Cranberries are particularly tart, containing a natural food preservative, benzoic acid, which stops them going mouldy. Cranberries are famous nowadays not for the traditional sauce to accompany turkey in the Anglo-Saxon world, but for Ocean Spray adverts and the fruit's lauded effects to ease bladder infections. Cranberry farmers saw a gap in the market and turned to science to endorse their product. One in two women suffer from cystitis (or UTIs) at some point in their lives, and many are plagued by it regularly, so a natural remedy avoiding antibiotics would be very popular. Test-tube studies showed that one of the compounds in the berries stopped bacteria sticking to surfaces. This sounded perfect to prevent infections. A series of small studies then followed showing that cranberries may protect (but not treat) women against recurrent cystitis, with an average 30 per cent reduction in new infections.[19]

But not everyone agreed. An independent review by the UK Cochrane database team questioned the size and relevance of any benefit, and a recent well-performed placebo-controlled study of 185 US nursing home residents taking high dose cranberry capsules for a year showed no effect whatsoever.[20] It is also hard to eat so many sour berries, and downing litres of commercial cranberry juice, which is heavily diluted, is unlikely to help much. Cranberries could also mask some symptoms of the urinary infections, like burning, leading to possible kidney problems. The other downside is that the high levels of added sugars in popular juices, needed to mask the sour polyphenols, make it as bad as fizzy drinks. In 2017, EU regulators ruled that cranberry products could no longer be branded as 'medical devices'. So sadly, I can't yet advise cranberries for preventing UTIs.

Superstar cele-berries

Now we come to the real superstars – acai, goji, chokeberry/aronia, and noni (and expect more inedible miracle berries to emerge every year). They have all the classic ingredients: rare, expensive, untested, with a mysterious exotic past, and promoted by celebrities.

Chokeberries are a nearly inedible (the clue is in the name) tropical fruit native to America that is now being cultivated in the UK and other countries where they are known as aronia berries. They have great potential, with a very high total polyphenol content, but there is no scientifically credible data on specific health benefits. Similarly, despite tasting revolting, Tahitian noni berries have built up an impressive internet following helped by talk of a magic compound called xeronine and celeb endorsements, but nothing else.

Acai (pronounced 'a-say-ehh') fruit grow high in Amazonian palms and look like blueberries. When eaten fresh they have a chocolate aftertaste, as they share polyphenols with the cocoa bean, but outside Brazil you usually have to make do with the duller freeze-dried variety. Brazilians supposedly use the juice to prevent flu, fever and pain, as well as gut infections and skin ulcers. According to wellness websites, they are an incredible energy food, good for the heart, impotence, inflammation, anti-ageing, immune boosting, skin health and, of course, weight loss. It is widely claimed that they contain several-fold more antioxidants than blueberries. This is based on wishful thinking – not data. Yet acai is increasingly added to many foods, including an acai-based ice cream, mixed with both artificial fibre and *lactobacillus* probiotics. The only proper study performed (over a decade ago) showed that, just like other berries, after eating, levels of antioxidants increased in the blood. Some of the adverts for acai supplements promise weight loss of up to twenty pounds in one week. This claim is based loosely on an uncontrolled pilot study of ten obese subjects followed for a month, but they didn't even lose weight, merely trivial improvements in a few blood tests. Unsurprisingly, this highly publicised study was funded by a large Californian juice and supplement company.[21]

Another internet superstar is the goji berry, used cheaply in traditional Chinese medicine for over 2,000 years but now generating a $700 million annual turnover. A member of the tomato family, the fresh berry is bright red and large, but in Europe we only encounter them in their shrivelled, dry raisin-like form. Goji has good polyphenol contents with an unusually high carotenoid content, including beta-carotene, beta-cryptoxanthin, lutein, zeaxanthin and lycopene, which we know from other studies may be beneficial for eyesight. They are also alleged to boost the immune system and brain activity, protect against heart disease and cancer, and improve life expectancy – again, all based on thin air and dubious studies. One 1994 study (reported in a Chinese journal) of seventy-nine patients treated with immunotherapy in combination with goji extracts saw their cancers regress.[22] Several other small studies reported subjective improvements in sleep, energy, calmness, exercise and mental concentration, outcomes that are all easily manipulated. One study claimed ridiculously that after only two weeks of taking 120ml of goji juice daily, overweight subjects lost two inches from their waist and burned 10 per cent more calories. At that rate, after a year of therapy, you would disappear. It is probably no coincidence that most of these studies were performed or funded by companies (including GoChi Himalayan goji juice) selling the same products, whose websites are packed with celebrity endorsements of weight loss. A summary of seven of these poor-quality trials on 548 people unsurprisingly saw no consistent effects. [23]

While these are definitely nutritious berries high in polyphenols and fibre (and acai is rich in polyunsaturated fats), they have no clear health benefits over other cheaper and more local berries. Even if the dubious claims were true, health food shops often sell them in a much more diluted form to that used in the trials. For one serving of dried acai berries you could buy ten bowls of fresh blueberries, each with the same or better nutritional value, and with the bonus of some clinical evidence. Carbon footprints, transport costs and pushy pyramid-selling techniques make them even less attractive. The choice of berry is yours.

Tropical fruits

Most fruits from the tropics have been refrigerated, shipped and artificially ripened before they appear in our shops. This global trade has meant we only see a fraction of the original species, and many are going extinct. They are bred for toughness but generally still contain reasonable amounts of vitamins and antioxidants, but are not usually regarded as health foods.

The banana has rapidly become the most popular global fruit, partly because producers have managed to keep prices low but also because few tropical fruits travel as well, even for shorter distances. As a banana ripens once picked, the starch-to-sugar ratio decreases twentyfold; to avoid sugar spikes, eat less ripe greener varieties, but not if you suffer from constipation. As well as high levels of sugar and potassium, which makes it great between sets at Wimbledon, banana has some inulin prebiotic fibre (only usually found in vegetables such as onions, garlic, Jerusalem artichokes (16 per cent), globe artichokes and asparagus that gut microbes love to ferment. But levels are low, and the sugar content of around 12 per cent probably outweighs any benefit purely for its fibre content. Beneficial antioxidants are present, but only a fraction of those found in the smaller local or wild bananas, which are usually sweeter, with more complex aromas, and more nutritious. High ethylene levels mean the fruit ripens quickly, but further ripening can be slowed down by using the refrigerator which doesn't damage the fruit, but does brown the skins. That said, bananas don't like being kept at temperatures lower than about 10°C (which happens routinely in supermarkets), leading to a good-looking but bland, mealy fruit. Ripe or brown bananas also freeze well and are useful for smoothies and to make delicious 'nice cream' (see page 144).

Overripe bananas have a distinctive smell, but nothing like durian fruits, the infamous product of Thailand and Malaysia. They are tricky to transport and banned on many airlines and trains as their odour can be deadly. They grow in a tough thorny green shell and ripen on the tree, and are then dropped into a vacuum-packed bag before being air-freighted. The flesh is like a sweet custard, but the smell is like rotting flesh, topped with mouldy cheese. These strong flavour associations come from hundreds of aroma chemicals, many containing sulphur in common with onions, cheese, rotten eggs, skunk spray and meat.

Mangoes are a much safer option, and used to be considered exotic, although now they are commonplace even in cold countries. Many are picked too early to ever fully ripen before going soft. The fresh aroma and firmness, not the colour, is the best clue to its ripeness. There are over 900 varieties, of which only a handful make it to Northern Europe or the USA. Because of transport costs, tougher, fibrous mangoes are favoured for export, like the crunchy but taste-less Tommy Atkins that dominates the US, and its slightly better relatives, the Kent and Keitt in the UK. (Often, transport logistics and protectionist politics determine which fruit choices we have.) But the tastiest mangoes come from India which has hundreds of local varieties, such as the much-acclaimed Alphonso. The Alphonso is popular in the UK and in season costs less than a pound. (The same fruit would cost over £20 in the US, after gamma irradiation and an air journey, extra customs and health checks, so most Americans never taste a truly delicious seasonal mango.) Fresh mangoes have a moderate GI (glycaemic index) score – GI ranks food from 1–100 on the relative ability of a carbohydrate food to increase the level of glu-cose in the blood: the higher the food is ranked, the quicker it raises your blood glucose levels – though dried mangoes with the same amount of sugar in a higher concentration score higher. They have more vitamin C than oranges and high levels of fibre and more poly-phenols than their local rivals, papayas.

Persimmons (aka sharon fruit) are ancient Chinese fruits that look like a cross between a giant tomato and a nectarine. The flesh is bright orange, due to plenty of carotenoids and lycopene, but is usually sweet and succulent. The ones I bought for the first time recently from a local Turkish shop would have been picked months earlier and kept at zero degrees. These were hard work, with a bitter skin and very astringent taste due to the high levels of tannins and other poly-phenols. Following good advice (on Twitter) I found another batch with a thinner, sweeter skin, but the tip I learnt is to ripen them for a few days next to other fruits full of the natural ripening chemical ethylene. Alternatively, you can deprive them of oxygen in a plastic bag for two days before eating. This tricks the tannins to bind with an alcohol chemical rather than sticking to your tongue.

Passion fruits are a surprisingly good source of iron and fibre due to the high density of seeds.

Melons are over 90 per cent water, along with sugar, vitamins C and A and some polyphenols, with its seeds the main source of nutrients. Melons will keep for two to four weeks after harvest if kept at optimal conditions, but can't be chilled for more than a few days. Lacking starch they don't get any sweeter with time. Cantaloupe melons are probably the most popular worldwide, followed by watermelons, with honeydew also popular in different countries and seasons. The green honeydew tastes great in the Med, but overuse in mass catering means they are only famous for being the most commonly discarded uneaten food waste.

Melon seeds contain L-citrulline, a precursor of nitric oxide, which does have possible interesting side-effects. Citrulline supplements apparently improved erections, more than placebo, in twenty-four Italian men with erectile problems and in thirteen Japanese men already taking Viagra.[24] Rare yellow watermelons contain even more citrulline, but the treatment has so far only been extended to lab rats and its effects on women are unknown, although like Viagra, it is bound to have a powerful placebo effect. Melons can also cause food poisoning outbreaks, as consumers rarely wash the outer skin which can contain pathogenic microbes from contaminated soil. In some countries, they can also be injected with contaminated water to increase their weight.

Imported varieties of pineapple are never picked when fully ripe and have usually been travelling for three weeks before they hit the shelves, so lack the complexity of flavours and aromas of the local ones. Chemists have worked out that the complex but distinctive pineapple flavour is made up, not from one molecule, but from a combination of aroma chemicals (including meaty, cloves, caramel, basil, vanilla and even sherry notes) which are commonly used to make fake pineapple flavours. Pineapple enzymes can attack the lining on the inside of your mouth, providing a bit of pain before the pleasure.

Banana nice cream

Frozen banana 'nice cream' is a great way to store and use ripe bananas: simply chop overripe bananas, freeze them and when you fancy a cold snack, blend them with your favourite nut butter (my choice is Pip & Nut's 100 per cent nut, high-oleic almond butter), or natural full-fat yogurt.

Endangered fruits

There are inherent dangers in relying on just a few highly inbred strains of fruits and their seeds. Most of the world now only eats one variety of banana, the Cavendish, a sterile cross made to maximise fruit and longevity, with tiny useless impotent seeds. Before 1950, most people ate the Gros Michel banana (Fat Mike in French) which allowed industrialised banana production on a massive scale in Central and South America. It was a sweeter, more flavoursome fruit that grew anywhere, but had a fatal flaw. It had no genetic diversity, as all the plants in the world were identical clones of each other, meaning that it could be easily wiped out by a parasite or disease. That is exactly what happened in 1890 when a highly versatile soil fungus, *Fusarium oxysporum* (Panama disease), decimated one banana plantation after another, devastating economies for decades, thus reducing supply and driving up prices. Normally some genetic mutants would be resistant to disease and survive and reproduce, but not with inbred genetic clones. The sneaky fungus lurked in the soil, waiting to kill bananas decades later. Only the Cavendish variety was resistant to this fungus and could be grown anywhere. Now banana forecasters are predicting the same fate for the Cavendish. The flexible *fusarium* fungus has now mutated to infect the Cavendish in Asia and is slowly making its way towards Central America. It's just a matter of time and we have no plan B – so enjoy your bananas while you can.

Storing fruit

In general, fruits from warmer tropical countries like to be stored warm and will do better kept out of the fridge where, if green, they won't ripen and will lose flavour. Apples and pears are better stored in a cool cupboard, cellar, or in the fridge. There is no consensus on storing citrus, which depends on your room temperature and season. Cherries, grapes and delicate berries can be cooled temporarily, but are best eaten immediately.

What's the big deal with fructose? Can you overdo the fruit?

I saw first-hand what happens when I ate a dozen large red grapes as part of my own experiments using a continuous blood glucose monitor (CGM) stuck on my arm. As discussed earlier, a large number of regular blood sugar spikes stresses the pancreas which produces insulin and over time is likely to increase fat deposits and risk of diabetes. My blood sugar rose to within the diabetic range (from under 6 to over 10 mmol) soon after eating my grapes and then rapidly went back to the normal range again. My wife ate the same grapes and had less than half the sugar spike that I had. So, could I blame my body response simply on the sugar content?

I compared my response to different fruits using the Exchange list system, a common clinical tool for diabetic patients that calculates a standardised sugar portion, i.e. the amount of sugars in different foods that all contain eighty calories (15g carbs, 3g protein and minimal fats). According to the list: 17 small grapes is equivalent to one banana/four apricots/¾ cup blueberries or blackberries/1¼ cups strawberries/one small nectarine or peach/1 cup chopped honeydew melon/half a glass of orange juice. Using these equalised portions of fresh fruits, repeating some of them, every morning on an empty stomach I compared my responses.

Grapes still gave me the largest peaks of nearly double my fasting level (although white less than red); melon, peaches, mangoes, bananas, plums and nectarines gave intermediate spikes; berries (strawberries, blackberries, raspberries and blueberries) gave only small peaks of around 20 per cent. Apples or pears, with high sugar and fructose levels, had negligible effects. Dried raisins, as expected, also gave me the same large peak as the grapes, but dried apricots didn't. When I ate red grapes with full-fat yogurt, my glucose spike was much lower; the fat reduces the speed of sugar absorption. Eating grapes with cheese may be another way. Eating fibre- and fat-rich nuts along with the fruit may also reduce the sugar spikes. But the overall lesson was that if I wanted to avoid being diabetic or to control my weight, I should cut down on grapes and choose a diverse mix of other fruits.

Remember, however, these particular fruit and sugar responses may be unique to me, but it highlights the flaws of current 'one size fits all' nutritional advice. The message is that some fruits may suit you more than others.

Studies show that the benefits of fruit increase with extra portions, but the five a day advice leaves many drinking large amounts of sugary juice, or being conned by supermarket labels about how much fruit constitutes a portion (it is 80g). And what if you ate twenty portions a day? Would all that sugar and fructose have an adverse effect?

Fruitarians claim amazing health benefits of only eating fruit, but without any objective evidence; in the same vacuum, health and diet experts generally advise against overeating fruit because of sugar and calories and a decrease in general dietary diversity. People with diabetes are potentially most at risk of extra sugar and routinely told not to overdo the fruit intake. This may not be true. No differences were found in overall blood sugar control in type 2 diabetes patients randomised to eating two to four portions of berries daily over twelve weeks.[25] The Chinese Biobank followed 8,000 type 2 diabetes patients over time and showed that they actually had lower glucose levels and blood pressure, and less diabetic disease complications if they ate more fruit.[26] While we can't definitively answer the question, it appears that fruit itself is not likely to be harmful, but the way you eat fruit and what else you eat certainly could be.

Which fruits should I eat more of?

All fruits contain around 5–15 per cent sugars, fibre and hundreds of polyphenols and other antioxidants which makes eating them good for us. Although we don't know the specifics, somehow our gut microbes sense when easily absorbed sugars are on their way and influence our variable response to different fruits. We know much more about how fibre and polyphenols in fruit interact with our gut microbes, which takes place lower down in the colon. At our crude level of understanding, we assume that more fibre and polyphenols are good for us, with most studies pointing to longer healthier lives for those of us who enjoy plenty of fibre.

Dried fruits have plenty of the nutrients and benefits of fruit if eaten in small amounts. But the drying process leaves relatively higher sugar contents and because they are much smaller you tend to eat a lot more of them than you would when eating the whole fresh fruit, resulting in a much bigger blood sugar spike. So while giving boxes of raisins daily to children may possibly help their iron stores, it is definitely not so good for their teeth or probably their metabolism.

Ranking real foods can suggest we understand more than we do but it does have practical uses, and so I produced a rough table of relative microbe friendliness of fruits (see page 424). I have used simple measures of two of the major factors, total fibre and total polyphenol content, to rank the foods, so you can see the wide range in nature. There are, as with all simplified summary lists, many important caveats. With each fruit having thousands of chemicals, many of which we know little about, total polyphenol scores can be misleading, as key chemicals (like vitamin C or lycopene) can be overlooked.

*

Portion sizes have been made artificially the same (80 grams) which doesn't happen in real life, and most data is shown in the fresh state, not dried. Most data doesn't account for different transport times, storage and seasonality. Finally, drying will always artificially improve the label stats, because as water reduces, the proportions of fibre and polyphenols increase. But have a look at the list, and hopefully it will make you try some new fruits and revisit some you may have forgotten. While there is no such thing as bad fruit, there are a few generic suggestions you may consider. If you are worried about pesticides, buy organic produce, so you can be more relaxed eating the skins. If you like juice, have it in moderation, as even if you consume all the pulp you may not get all the benefits, while absorbing all the sugar. To avoid waste don't be shy about freezing or drying fruit for later use, most will still be healthy. It is useful to remember that a cup of berries has more fibre than a bowl of commercial all-bran cereal, with many more healthy chemicals, most of which are still undiscovered. Fruits have naturally been easy to eat without any training; vegetables may take more effort, but the rewards could be even greater.

My top five fruit tips

1. Eat a diverse range of fruit in its natural form, ideally with the skin on.
2. There are no 'superberries' but all berries are nutritional powerhouses providing the best value for fibre and polyphenols.
3. The global fruit market is reducing the number of different types of fruit: opt for lesser-known species to enjoy different flavours and textures.
4. Frozen and dried fruits are rich in fibre and polyphenols and reduce waste and global warming, but don't overdo them (or fruit smoothies) as they can produce excess blood sugar peaks.
5. Know the origin and season of different fruits and consider their ethical and environmental footprint.

13. Vegetables

A patchy start

Aged about eight, I still remember staring at the plate covered with bright blood-red liquid, obscuring the sad-looking chopped lettuce and cucumber. The blood was coming from three large circular discs of beetroot in my customary school-lunch salad. I wasn't allowed to join my friends outside until I'd finished it. Back then I would do anything to avoid eating beetroot and this experience put me off beetroot and other strange-looking earthy vegetables for over thirty years.

Like many others, my palate is highly sensitive to the geosmin chemical in beet, which lends it the 'muddy' taste. Geosmin is produced both by beet and microbes in the soil, possibly communicating with each other, and can sometimes leach into tap water, causing complaints. Anyway, most children don't want to eat large chunks of earth for lunch, so I would spit out the strangely sweet sickly mixture (beetroot contains as much sugar as an apple). A pity, as I was missing out on a large number of polyphenols with important antioxidants like the family of betaine pigments, and a whole suite of other nutrients like vitamin C, folate, potassium and fibre. Happily, I am now a convert; beetroot can be delicious raw, especially if young and thinly sliced, and has a satisfying crispness with less of the muddy aromas. If not boiled to death, it can also be delicious when cooked, with more complex flavours.

The other thing that really put me off vegetables was the rotten-egg smell of boiled cabbage. This is caused by different sulphur chemical precursors (defensive antioxidants) that combine on heating and are not present in the raw plant. The stronger, rotten-egg smell is only released when overcooking plants genetically derived from the original ancestor, white cabbage – broccoli, cauliflower, Romanesco, Brussels sprouts, bok choy, etc. Steaming these (chopped up small if needed) for under five minutes is less pongy, and retains more nutrients.

Many children dislike vegetables and some people never love them. Sometimes it's because of the way they are cooked, or rather boiled to death. But also as children our genes instinctively tell us to fear green plants; rightly so because less than 1 per cent (around 2,000) of plants are *not* toxic for us. Unlike fruits, which colourfully advertise their sweet edibility, we need to be trained to like veg. Since we discovered fire about a million years ago, we found we could transform inedible toxic plants, yams like cassava, for example, into a great energy source.

Bright and bitter

How do we use our evolutionary skills to pick which vegetable is likely to be the most nutritious? As with fruit, intense dark or bright colours in veg indicate high levels of pigment polyphenols. But the original colours of many vegetables have changed over the centuries, thanks to our breeding and selection skills. Carrots used to be a dull off-white before Dutch gardeners in the seventeenth century developed a bright orange variant to suit their national colours and celebrate the Anglo-Dutch monarch William, Prince of Orange. This added high levels of beta-carotene to the plant, which we use to make vitamin A, important for our brain and eyesight. The Persians (or Indians, it's not clear) had centuries earlier created a dark purple carrot with extra anthocyanin pigments which is estimated to have nine times the level of total polyphenols of our cherished orange variety. Other examples of higher polyphenols in dark-coloured veg include purple potatoes (and sweet potatoes); red cabbage with three times the polyphenols of white cabbage, with green cabbage in between; and red onions, which have slightly more helpful chemicals than yellow, but both are much better than white. You can also now buy purple broccoli, as well as the smaller variant broccolini.

Even with pseudo vegetables that are actually fruits – tomatoes, aubergines, or peppers – pick the darker-coloured varieties, although generally, yellow is usually a better bet than green. So go for colour, although beware, there are always exceptions to the colour rule. The two main asparagus varieties, green and white, are similar but the white ones are grown covered by soil so they never gain the green pigment. Purple asparagus is grown with limited sunlight. In my view, all are delicious if cooked precisely. Studies show that all these plants are healthy, but there are large differences in polyphenol counts, with the greatest levels in the green ones, exposed most to the sun.[1]

Most vegetables we eat have more folate and minerals, protective polyphenols and fibre than ripe fruits, and generally less sugar. Many struggle with the bitterness of some vegetables, often when facing broccoli or the Christmas treat of Brussels sprouts. But many cultures make a virtue of very bitter foods to contrast dishes and extend palates – think French and Belgian baked endives with bechamel, Italian puntarelle (winter chicory) and rocket salads, and Chinese bitter melons, all of which have very high polyphenol counts and are appreciated by our microbes.

Every country has naturally growing dark-green leaves that can be a sustainable and seasonal part of our diets. Whilst spinach and broccoli are great, wild garlic and young nettles are fantastic spring leaves that grow prolifically in woodlands and hedgerows, and are a wonderful way to add sustainable, diverse plants to our diets in a frugal and local way. As well as nutritious weeds, we should adopt a 'whole plant' approach when we eat our veg. The external leaves of a head of cauliflower are delicious and nutritious once the hard stems are removed, the remaining leaf lightly steamed with some extra virgin olive oil and finished with a spritz of lemon. Carrot tops taste a bit like parsley and make an excellent herb to add to soups or fish dishes, adding phytonutrients and fibre. With the right cooking skills, mixed with the right foods, all these bitter tastes become complex and delicious.

Rocket (arugula), watercress and mustard greens may be puny-looking leafy relatives of the cabbage, but their pungent peppery taste provides clues of extra benefit. This is due to abundant polyphenol aldehyde chemicals, although most of the benefits are lost if cooked, so they are best eaten raw in salads. Radicchio, the peppery violet-and-white leafy veg, is so full of these polyphenols that it can be overpowering when raw, so either grill the leaves, add balsamic vinegar, or soak for an hour in ice water as then they become mild and perfect to eat.

As well as the leaf colour, the anatomy of the vegetable provides clues to potential nutrients. In the lettuce family, opt for loose-leaf varieties, with frilly or coloured edges, over the tightly bunched ones. In general, the more tightly-packed leaves near the centre of the plant need less defences, thus contain less antioxidants. In lettuce, for example, this can vary 100-fold from the outer leaves to the centre, so think twice before you discard too many of the tatty darker outer leaves. This is also true for onions, so don't go crazy when peeling away too many layers. Similarly, in root vegetables the centres need the least defences, so in carrots, the watery core is pretty uninspiring. Unfortunately, it is this core section that baby carrots are made from – supermarkets created these artificial miniatures by paring down larger carrots and throwing the good bits away, then selling them at a markup in vacuum bags.

Superveg?

Brassica supplements

Another common health claim is around sulforaphane (SFN) supplements, the substance present in most brassicas, and not the vegetable in its whole form. Along with the usual test-tube studies, there are however some reputable clinical studies of SFN supplements showing some interesting results. The most impressive effect was in autism spectrum disorder: forty young men were followed for eighteen weeks and most improved their symptoms after taking SFN, with average improvements (17–35 per cent) compared to a control group.[2] At follow-up three years later, around two-thirds were still taking SFN believing there was an effect. Other studies in diabetes have shown improvements in glucose as well as cholesterol levels.

Refreshingly, in this area there is actually a published negative study showing no effect on forty high blood pressure subjects.[3] Obviously, these studies are short-term, and need repeating. The optimal doses of both the SFN supplement or the equivalent fresh broccoli or cabbage are unclear. According to one study, you may also need to eat three times more of the artificial supplement to achieve the same benefits as the real vegetable.[4]

Fermentation is our friend: sauerkraut and kimchi

If I had to name one vegetable as the healthiest overall, I would have a hard time as they all have their good points, aside from iceberg lettuce. Because of microbes I would probably say any fermented vegetable, and the world's favourite is cabbage, which is used to make sauerkraut and kimchi.

Sauerkraut

Sauerkraut is a proven cure for scurvy because it has high levels of vitamin C and lasts through winter. Once you ferment cabbage or any other vegetable, the microbes change its chemical composition, and the total number of chemicals increases. After a few days, the levels of healthy glucosinolates (the SFN precursors) drop significantly but are replaced by many other closely related active chemical by-products. On average, sauerkraut contains viable microbes in super-high probiotic quantities ranging from 10 million to a billion bacteria per gram, and you can ingest much more than standard probiotics. A relatively large fraction of these survive passage through the hostile upper GI tract, as they love acid conditions.

Beware most shop-bought sauerkraut; like pickles, commercial sauerkraut is typically pasteurised, which annihilates the hard-working microbes. These are replaced with added preservatives, vinegar and sugar to prolong shelf life. However, making your own sauerkraut is easy.

Make your own sauerkraut

This is a rough recipe which you can adapt to your tastes. You can roughly or finely chop, dice the ingredients, add as much garlic, onion, chilli and other herbs and spices like dill, caraway seeds or juniper berries as you like.

1 cabbage, traditionally white, but red or green also works
20g sea salt (or around 2–3 per cent of cabbage weight)
1 onion
garlic
chilli

Shred and wash the cabbage. In a large bowl, rub the salt into the cabbage. Leave aside for about a hour to draw off some water. Squeeze the cabbage using a sieve to remove as much of the liquid as possible, then stir in the other ingredients and tightly pack this into a big glass pot. Push the cabbage down well and fill the container to the brim with pre-boiled or filtered water. Cover with a tea towel and elastic band. Leave in a warm place for a few days at room temperature. Check the sauerkraut for activity – you should see and hear fermentation starting naturally as the ambient lactic acid bacteria (*lactobacillus*) works its magic. Squash the cabbage down using a wooden spoon and top up the water to make sure the cabbage is always covered, then move the fermenting pot to a cooler spot.

A week later, as the acidity has increased, the microbes producing lactic acid will have broken down the hard structures in the cabbage. The sauerkraut should now be 'al dente', crunchy and tasty.

Fully fermented sauerkraut keeps for several months in an airtight container stored somewhere cool.

Kimchi

Koreans are fanatical about kimchi and can eat it three times a day – even at breakfast. A must-visit for all schoolchildren in Seoul is the Kimchi museum so they acquire the taste early for the national dish. When I first visited Seoul, I'm ashamed to say I wasn't a big fan,

(I found the smell very off-putting, especially first thing in the morning) but am now, though the smell does take some getting used to.

This staple of Korean cuisine is traditionally a mix of green napa cabbage and Korean radishes, with a variety of seasonings including ample garlic and chilli. While there are hundreds of variants made with different vegetables as the main ingredients, most South Koreans eat around 36kg of fermented cabbage yearly in the form of kimchi (that's trillions of microbes) and so it may not be a coincidence that the nation has one of the lowest rates of obesity – less than 5 per cent of the population – of all developed countries.[5] North Koreans are slimmer still, but that is for quite different reasons.

Kimchi, like sauerkraut, is *symbiotic* as it is a combination of a prebiotic and a probiotic, providing us with both the live microbes and the fertiliser to sustain them. In contrast to sauerkraut, however, which contains just five to twelve main bacteria, there are at least twenty-five species of beneficial microbes or yeast in kimchi, feeding off the fibre, sugars and polyphenols. Kimchi is usually a wide mix of vegetable ingredients, and each family has its own recipe. This means that all the vegetable chemicals potentially interact with multiple different microbes to produce multiple new chemicals and metabolites, making it impossible to pinpoint any key ingredient or metabolite. This serves as a good reminder that just as every batch of kimchi is unique, so is the permanent process of fermentation in our gut. The more diverse the microbes we eat and send down for fermentation, the more the range of healthy metabolites we ourselves can produce.

There is a large (mainly Korean) literature asserting that kimchi is good for absolutely everything from weight loss and diabetes to dementia. While most of these studies are pretty rubbish, one credible one showed distinct increases in gut microbes after two weeks of regular consumption.[6] Another in diabetes patients demonstrated health benefits after eight weeks.[7] Kimchi making is the same principle as sauerkraut, but with more ingredients. I went on a kimchi-making course at The Little Duck Picklery in Dalston, east London, where we used the Asian root vegetable daikon (or Chinese white radish), which I prefer (see tip at end).

Make your own kimchi

Slice cabbage (or daikon) lengthways, salt and rinse the cabbage exactly as you would for sauerkraut (see above).

Make a spice paste using carrot, radish, salt, garlic, fish or soy sauce and chilli powder with a teaspoon of rice flour if you like a thicker consistency.

Mix thoroughly and pack the kimchi tightly into a jar to ferment for roughly 5 days.

Enjoy your kimchi with salads, as an accompaniment to meat, cheese or fish and to spice up noodle and rice dishes.

*

As with fruit, I have tabulated the most common vegetables with different polyphenol contents by their colour to help encourage you to eat the rainbow (see table, page 427). As a comparison, I included black beans, a legume that came top of the chart, but avocados, artichokes and red cabbage all did well. There was a fourfold range in fibre, while for total polyphenol we saw a twentyfold difference.

Beetroot, my former foe, also ranks highly. It contains a unique polyphenol, betaine pigment, with strong antioxidant and anti-inflammatory effects, along with high levels of folate and inorganic nitrates: the precursor to a very important signalling molecule – nitric oxide (NO). Among other roles, NO increases the size of blood vessels in muscle to allow more oxygen flow and improve efficiency. Over seventy-five very small-scale studies have shown overall that beetroot juice improves sports performance in healthy adults and athletes by a small but significant amount (even 1 per cent improvement is considered highly significant).[8] Interestingly, beetroot juice seems to add oomph in endurance athletes, but *not* sprinters.

Nitric oxide (NO) works on another notable complaint.[9] One of the subtle signs marking a brothel in Roman times was the beetroot, where apparently preparations of it were used to keep customers perky. Viagra, originally designed to reduce blood pressure, works by increasing levels of NO in blood vessels: giving men erections was a welcome side-effect. So far there is no hard (!) data from clinical trials to support all the similar beet-juice claims on the internet. Like Viagra, the nitrates in beetroot could also reduce blood pressure: twenty-two studies summarised show a useful benefit of around 3.5mmHg (around 3 per cent reduction). But nitrates may only be part of a more complex interaction with other beneficial polyphenols and chemicals in the plant (see page 37), and no one is yet recommending them as a treatment.

Know your onions . . . and garlic

The members of the allium family – onions, spring onions, leeks, chives, garlic – contain large amounts of pungent sulphur compounds which they extract from the soil. They are released from the damaged plant cells on cutting or chopping, with eye-watering effect, and get steadily milder with slow cooking (but not with microwaving). While more nutrients are liberated from the chopped and cooked item, it is a good side bet to also ingest some raw alliums for chemical diversity. Younger onions, chives and spring onions release less sulphur and add piquancy to dishes when raw, some people even munch older onions like apples, but for most of us that is a challenge for the eyes, palate and digestion.

There are many folk remedies for reducing the tears; like pinching your nose, chewing bread or gum, putting a silver teaspoon in your mouth, whistling and sticking your tongue out as you cut (apparently it absorbs the tear-inducing molecules). My favourite google suggestion is to wear goggles to chop your onion which is ridiculous but effective. My tip, goggles or no, is to use a very sharp knife, aligned along the poles between the stalk and the root (rather than around the equator), which helps to minimise damage to the oblong-shaped onion cells. Also, stop chopping before you get too near the hairy root, as this tends to release a higher concentration of sulphur compounds.

Onions are an important source of inulin, also found in bananas, Jerusalem artichokes and garlic, which is associated with a plethora of benefits for our gut microbiome. Eating inulin every day is likely to be beneficial for overall health. The Italians, Spanish and Portuguese, who we have seen have good long-term health on average, use abundant onions in their cooking. The foundation of many dishes is a 'sofrito', a polyphenol- and inulin-rich combination of onion, garlic, carrot and celery with added herbs such as basil and oregano, gently and slowly cooked for at least an hour in extra virgin olive oil. The fragrant and unctuous sofrito forms the base for pasta sauces, fish and meat dishes as well as any soups and stews. Using a sofrito base is an easy way to include inulin to our diets every day.

Garlic, which is really a concentrated onion, is also inulin-rich. As well as successfully warding off vampires, it has long been widely used medicinally in most cultures, for everything from warts and colds to arthritis. There is plenty of testimony that it can cure warts, some weaker evidence that it can help ease the pain of arthritis, and some controlled human studies seem to even support the claims for it as a panacea for colds. Needless to say, only one randomised trial stands up to scrutiny and it still certainly needs replication. This study found that (compared to placebo) after taking garlic extract, 146 people had threefold less cold episodes and days of illness over three months, although it didn't help recovery from an existing virus.[10]

There is also increasing evidence from different sources that garlic may protect against cancers of the intestine, although the evidence of its benefits for the heart is stronger. Over fourteen studies show that garlic improves blood fat levels, and twenty show improvements in blood pressure by around 4 per cent with no significant side-effects.[11] To put this into context, eating garlic has over twice as large an effect on heart health as severe salt restriction (see page 374), and actually improves food, rather than making it unpalatable. Many of these studies were conducted with different forms of garlic (powdered, in tablet form, etc.) or aged garlic extract, not all containing the ingredient allium, which was thought to be the main player, so, again, we don't know which of its thousands of chemicals are most beneficial.[12] It could also be the high levels of inulin fibre, which gut microbes love. As usual, eating the real thing along with other combinations of the onion family is likely to be the best option.

The bland

Lettuce, in one word. My personal award for the least nutritious vegetable goes to iceberg ('crisphead') lettuce, the tightly bunched salad variety that looks more like a pale green cabbage. It was introduced for commercial production in the 1940s in the USA as the only variety bred to survive cross-country transportation (on ice) and came to be synonymous with the classic wedge salad. Since the 1980s it has spread to supermarket aisles worldwide, because of its impressive fridge-life and pleasant noisy crunch and crispiness. It is also easy to wash and trim, with much less waste. In the US, iceberg is the fifth most eaten vegetable (after the potato, tomato, onion and carrot); indeed half its population has only ever eaten this lettuce variety, and other countries are similar. But it has no taste and virtually no nutrients, not to mention a terrible water footprint. In studies, Italian lollo rosso curly loose-leaf varieties (which have red tips and can taste slightly bitter) had 300 times more antioxidant potential than iceberg.[13] If you depended on iceberg for one of your healthy 'five a day' as many people do – you would probably need 500 a day. Other lettuce varieties fare a bit better and provide most of your vitamin K needs and some folate. Romaine or cos lettuce is a mix of a crispy core and loose leaves that are intermediate nutritionally, and round lettuce is only slightly better than iceberg, with a very modest polyphenol count.

Whilst the convenience of having ready-to-go bagged mixed salad leaves is obvious both for time and for increasing diversity, the processing and plastic packaging involved are not environmentally friendly. Instead buy whole lettuces and store them properly to ensure they stay fresh; simply wrap them in damp muslin or paper towels and refrigerate in an airtight container to avoid squashing. If you have the space outdoors, lettuce is cheap and easy to grow.

Cucumber is another contender for the most useless vegetable. Once hailed for its anti-ageing properties, boosting collagen and an ingredient in heavily marketed face creams, it sadly won't halt the ageing process, though placing cool cucumber slices on your eyes after a heavy night may be soothing.

Celery sticks are often touted as the food that you expend more calories eating than you gain by swallowing it. Celery extract is used in some countries as a weight-loss agent but can have side-effects such as severe thyroid problems with rash and palpitations. When juiced, it supposedly provides a 'mega-dose' of antioxidant nitrogens along with the natural laxative, mannitol, with the potential side-effect of repeated loo trips, but this is because it is mainly fibrous strands and water. But when slowly braised, as in sofrito, bland celery has plenty of chemicals that interact with other food chemicals to produce novel tastes and aromas. Per gram it is the biggest natural source of nitrates and shares some volatile chemicals with walnuts, but the rest of its chemical secrets remain hidden. Until we unlock them, a snack of crunchy celery sticks remains a great way of transporting hummus to your mouth.

'Bad' veg?

The most maligned vegetable has to be the potato. Widely perceived as an unhealthy starchy carbohydrate, with a poor GI score of 78/100, it has however more potassium than a banana, is a good source of vitamin C, calcium and iron, and has the same fibre as an apple. After being hugely popular in the Andes, the potato was brought to Britain by Spanish traders (not Sir Walter Raleigh), where being unfortunately related to the deadly nightshade plant, as well as being linked falsely to leprosy, it was thought to be poisonous and ignored for over a hundred years (they're not great for you if you eat them raw or green). When the spud finally took off as the dominant crop, it was responsible for Northern Europe's dramatic population explosion in the late seventeenth and eighteenth centuries. Then in 1845 a nasty mould caused the potato blight and Ireland's disastrous potato famine, decimating the country and populating the Americas.

The potato's popularity soared again when, in the 1960s, fast food and deep-fried chips (French fries) took off stateside, and as a convenient portable meal (no cutlery required), it rapidly became the most consumed vegetable in America and many other countries around the world. Although it retained its rankings, after the 1980s it became synonymous with bad health. Several large observational studies in the US associated eating potatoes daily with increased heart disease, diabetes and obesity. These early studies were likely biased. A Swedish study found no association with heart disease and as more studies were collected, the association disappeared, unless you were eating them fried.[14,15] If boiled, microwaved or baked with their skin left on and eaten as part of a meal, potatoes pose no particular risk for obesity or other cardiometabolic disease. French fries, cheesy chips (poutine) or mashed potatoes, however, should only be an occasional treat. Although overall potatoes score badly on ZOE, some people may be able to eat them more regularly than others, preferably as a cold potato salad with the skin left on. Most governments have excluded the potato from their five a day lists, presumably because we are already eating plenty of them and we should be focusing on increasing variety.

Potato crisps (or in the US, potato chips), thinly sliced potatoes cooked in oil, are the most common savoury snack in the world. The first recipe for hand-made crisps cooked in lard appeared in 1817 and the first commercial crisp was made around 1920 by Mr and Mrs Smith in North London, and for many years were sold with a separate pouch for salt to add yourself. Smiths were bought out by Walkers Crisps, also originally a husband and wife business, and now the largest UK snack company, owned by Frito-Lay, part of the Pepsi-Co empire. The British consume 55g crisps per person each week, that's over two 25g bags, with a fifth of children eating two bags a day, many in their lunchbox. (My brother Andy has been collecting crisp bags since the age of seven, when he used to shrink them to the size of a matchbox in front of the fire. He now has probably the largest collection of crisp packets in the world – over 3,500 different bags valued at £20,000 – and is never happier than when someone sends him a weird pack from an exotic country.[16]) British factories produce six billion packets with over 100 different flavours a year, taking a variety of seasonal potatoes, forcefully washing the starch off, drying and slicing them and frying them for just three minutes at 180°C in 5,000-litre vats of oil.

We are not the world's leaders in crisp eating, however. The Americans, based on revenue figures, consume three times more per head, and the Canadians double, probably because of those massive jumbo-size bags. While the Japanese are also fond of crisps (wasabi flavour) and come quite close to us, in Europe, the French surprisingly beat us in total consumption – paprika and grilled chicken are particularly popular across the channel, as well as 'coq au vin' and 'chips à la truffe' (truffle).[17] Brits will usually eat crisps as an additional snack between meals, while the French generally only eat them as part of an aperitif. Crisps definitely have a low-fibre and high-fat content, but as the French are slimmer and healthier on average than the Brits, despite eating more crisps, it may be hard to blame this food for all of our ills. Maybe it is our rushed food culture coupled with misguided government advice that encourages snacking between meals, which contributes about 25 per cent of our calorie consumption and to the expansion of our waistlines.[18] Many critics have focused on the high salt content of crisps (see page 373) but an individual 25g bag contains a similar amount of salt to many standard bowls of breakfast cereal, and a fraction of what's found in many UPF ready meals, making crisps an unlikely culprit for our high salt intake.

Are more expensive, more 'natural', artisan crisps a better choice? Some of these may be healthier, or more environmentally friendly, such as one brand that salvages ugly potatoes otherwise destined for the dustbin. The oils used in frying can range widely, including sunflower and/or rapeseed (canola) oils in the UK and the US (see page 405), and there are now 'baked not fried' options, which alters the fat content and calories. The quest for the healthy high-fibre crisp has also led to all sorts of processed crunchy products made with peas, lentils, chickpeas and mixed legumes. But despite lower salt and sugar contents, many of these 'healthier' crunchy snacks are still highly processed, often with over fourteen ingredients, emulsifiers and flavourings. So, as with other foods, quality and context are key: let's keep crisps a simple treat – fried potato slices (ideally in extra virgin olive oil) preferably with the skin on with as little tampering as possible.

Avocados

The fattiest vegetable is actually a stone fruit – the avocado, named by Central Americans after the local word for testicle. Avocados come in several shapes and colours and their combination of a creamy flesh and a mild but complex taste is quite unique, while their very high fat content contributes most of the calories, and probably evolved to attract large hungry mammals like us. The rough black-skinned Hass variety has the highest fat content, mainly monounsaturated, as in olive oil. They are also an excellent source of fibre (about 13g in a single large fruit), vitamin C, folate, B6 and plenty of polyphenols. There is little research on the benefits of the avocado, which was ignored for years because of its high fat and calorie content. In France, where it is thought to have medicinal powers, an extract is mixed with soybean to make a 'natural' medicine called Piascledine which has a mild effect in osteoarthritis in controlled trials that I helped design. The exact mix is top secret and the active compounds are unknown, and the effects are modest. Our data suggests that avocados may, in fact, be the perfect vegetable, at least in terms of average ZOE scores.

The main (first world) problem is they are often bought when rock hard, with some never ripening, as they were picked too early or stored cold. Others can take several days to ripen at room temperature; place them in the fruit bowl with bananas to speed this up. Avocado flesh browns rapidly on exposure to air, but this can be delayed by adding a drop of lemon or lime juice or by storing next to chopped onions which emit volatile antioxidants. Guacamole, made with mashed avocados, chilli, garlic, lime juice and a drop of olive oil, contains an amazing combination of polyphenols; just go easy on the nachos.

The dark side to avocados lies in their growing demand. As smashed avocado on toast became the most photographed food in the late 2010s, demand for the exotic food quickly outgrew supply, creating the perfect opportunity for criminals to monopolise supply chains (see also quinoa, page 191). Not only have avocados become a profitable criminal commodity, they also require huge amounts of water, and diverting rivers by bribing local officials and destroying Mexican and South American communities has sadly become commonplace.

Rotten tomatoes

The tomato – like aubergines, courgettes, cucumbers, gourds and squashes – is actually a fruit with seeds and a low sugar content. Like meat, it also has high glutamate levels, making it savoury. Since its arrival in Europe in the sixteenth century, the tomato, with its soft, juicy flesh, has long been the ideal object to harmlessly hurl at prisoners, politicians or failed footballers (the Italian National team in 1966) to show displeasure and disgust. But now, thanks to intensive breeding, most tomatoes we buy are likely to bounce off the victims without staining their suits, and don't go rotten so quickly. In 1879, American growers found a mutant variety that produced a smooth hard surface and all-over even red colour. While unknown at the time, this mutation also reduced levels of the red carotenoid lycopene as well as many chemicals contributing to flavour. This was the fate for most varieties that followed. And as commercially grown tomatoes have become cheaper and more plentiful year round, they have become tougher-skinned and larger, with a marked dilution in taste and nutrients. Most are picked very early from the vine to increase transport life, and then ripened with ethylene in giant warehouses. Tomatoes are originally a warm climate fruit and lose their flavour permanently when kept in the fridge. This is less of a problem for most supermarket varieties that lack any taste in the first place.

Unless you grow your own or shop at organic farmers' markets, we may have to eat double the number of tomatoes we did fifty years ago to compensate for the reduced nutrients. But there is hope. In the 1970s scientists bred the long-life cherry tomato, which has extra sugar but also reasonable polyphenols. The tomato geneticists have now discovered the flavour gene that was switched off by mistake when the first American mutants were produced. They are using recent breakthroughs in gene editing to bring the original flavour and nutrients back, while still keeping the genes that provide hardiness and a reasonable shelf-life.

In Spain, France and Italy, local shops and markets offer ten or more tomato varieties in all shapes, sizes and colours, each used for a different purpose (eaten raw, in sauces, for baking, etc.), and many of them are ugly or deformed, but above all tasty. Are they also good for us?

Tomatoes are our major source of lycopene, a form of carotene (also found in carrots, pink grapefruit, watermelons and apricots). Over twenty-five observational studies showed that on average, high consumers had a 20 per cent reduction in stroke and heart disease and 37 per cent lower mortality.[19] Twenty-one short-term randomised trials found consuming tomatoes or lycopene supplements reduced cholesterol by about 5 per cent and blood pressure by about 4 per cent which is small but credible.[20] Other reviews have queried the quality of these studies, but not how safe and cheap they are.[21] Like other vegetables in the nightshade family, tomatoes are high in plant-protecting lectins, proteins that bind to carbohydrates, and which cause some people problems in digestion. The 'plant-paradox' diet, free of lectin-rich vegetables, was popularised for its supposedly anti-inflammatory effects, reducing gut permeability and improving overall health. For a small proportion of lectin-sensitive individuals, avoiding raw tomatoes is beneficial, but eating cooked tomatoes, which neutralises lectin and releases lycopene and other phytonutrients, even more so.

As for preventing cancer, as well as unsurprisingly inhibiting cancer cells in test tubes and in some animal models, it also halved ovarian cancer in 150 egg-laying hens (who have similar rates to humans).[22] In humans, over thirty observational studies of prostate cancer in over 250,000 men found a consistent reduction in cancer in high tomato-eaters, averaging a 30 per cent reduction per cup of tomato sauce per week. The protection only appeared with cooked tomatoes, not with raw.[23] Lycopene, like many polyphenols, is fat soluble, so dress raw tomatoes, ideally with olive oil, or eat with bread and butter. In contrast there is plenty of lycopene in tinned tomatoes, especially if the skins are left on.

What's the big deal with starch?

Can you eat as many vegetables as you like? The answer is 'it depends'. If you are eating sweet potato, potato and parsnips, then no. These more energy-dense vegetables contain starch which is a complex carbohydrate that is broken down into simple sugars and contributes to a rise in blood glucose and subsequent insulin spikes. Starchy vegetables are not bad per se in moderation and should not be excluded from a healthy, varied diet, but it's best to prioritise green, purple, bitter and non-starchy veg.

Veg galore

Could you, on the other hand, eat as much spinach, onions and broccoli as you like? The answer is 'yes' – though again, for better nutrition and a tastier meal, the best approach is to diversify your plant choice and eat different types of plants together. In fact, rather than gobbling vast quantities of the same one or two vegetables, combining two or more different plant foods is more likely to deliver all of the micronutrients, minerals and amino acids you need – think brown rice and beans, or tomatoes and chickpeas with pasta. For more on food combos, see the next chapters.

*

As you will have gathered, there's no 'bad' vegetable. But we need to be mindful of the choices we make: ensuring we eat different vegetables every day, and eating consciously, seasonally and locally to minimise the environmental impact of our food choices. To avoid unnecessary food waste, eat the *whole* vegetable and buy simple frozen or canned vegetables in water. To make the most of the richness and benefits that vegetables have to offer, we need to rethink the classic 'meat and two veg' approach: instead go for 'four colourful veg and a fistful of protein' – maybe not as catchy, but certainly healthier.

Key tips about vegetables

1. Virtually all vegetables (except iceberg lettuce) are good for you. Bright colours and bitter or strong flavours indicate high polyphenol content.
2. Eat a diverse range of plants each week.
3. Vegetables are a great source of polyphenols and fibre for your microbiome.
4. How we cut and cook vegetables affects nutrients: mixing with fats in oils and fermenting can enhance benefits; light steaming is often optimal – avoid boiling for long periods.
5. Beware of clever marketing of rare and expensive vegetables that may not be any healthier.

14. Legumes (aka pulses)

Legumes include beans, peanuts, lentils and peas, and are also confusingly called pulses. There are over twenty cultivated types, dominated globally by soy as one of the most versatile beans, which, amongst other things, can also be turned into tofu, soy milk, tempeh, soy sauce and biodiesel oil. Most of the beans we eat today came originally from the New World, with a few from Asia, all high in protein, zinc and iron (like meat), and high in fibre, folate and low in fat (like vegetables). They are also often toxic to animals when eaten raw thanks to abundant defensive chemicals, or even cyanide as in some tough-skinned lima beans. Again, the rainbow colour rule also broadly applies to legumes, but they are all generally high in polyphenols, especially lentils, soy and kidney beans.

As hundreds of generations of farmers have discovered, legumes are a very versatile global crop. By mixing with cereal crops in the fields, they provide nitrogen fertilisation, as well as broad nutrition on the plate. Beans and rice are a common breakfast across Central and South America; Indians have their lentil and millet dhals; in the Middle East they relish maftoul, bulgur wheat plus chickpeas; the Japanese their comforting miso soup made from soybeans and barley; and, of course, the British have their exotic baked beans on toast.

Most nutritional guidelines say we should eat more of them, ideally daily. Combined with rice, wheat or corn, they provide most of what our body needs. But, as always there are some downsides to a staple diet of legumes. The thickness of the seed coat can make the nutrients less accessible and take a long time to cook, and so dried legumes often need to be soaked before cooking – a pinch of bicarbonate of soda in the soaking or cooking water creates an alkaline environment which helps to speed things up – though this doesn't necessarily improve absorption of nutrients as suggested on some popular food blogs. The phytic acids in legumes also make absorption of some nutrients more difficult, so you need to mix them with other foods. As with vegetables, the water used to cook raw, fresh legumes should be minimal to avoid damage and leakage of nutrients, and if possible avoid hard water, and although some cooks suggest otherwise, adding salt makes them softer and acidic tomatoes and citrus make them firmer. Another property most share with some veg is their popularity with certain gut microbes, which ferment them and convert the carbs to methane gas, causing wind.

Beans and natural gas

There is some science showing that the longer you cook beans and the more you rinse them, the fewer flatulent side-effects. Eating and chewing them slowly also helps, but some effects may be psychological. One brave group studied over 120 US adults eating half a cup of baked beans, pinto beans or black eyed peas daily for two months versus carrots as a control. As they hoped, beans improved blood lipids, but they were also interested in side-effects. In the first week, nearly 50 per cent reported some change in bowel habit and flatulence with the pinto and baked beans, although less than one in five had problems with black eyed peas.[1] This slowly reduced over time, so that within two to three weeks only one in five reported any problems with the beans and less than one in ten with the lower fibre black eyed peas. While there is big individual variation, it seems that our body gets used to the changes; but secondly, about 10 per cent of the study participants reported new wind problems even with the control carrots, which boast little fibre. A sudden increase in fibre intake will almost always cause changes in the gut in terms of flatulence and transit time whilst our gut microbes readjust, but a turbulent few days is surely worth the long-term benefits of a happy gut and increased polyphenol intake. Better still, studies suggest that we can extract 20–50 per cent more polyphenols if we mix a squeeze of lime and its vitamin C with our beans, which many cultures have been doing for centuries.

Many factors determine how easily we, or our microbes, can extract the nutrients from legumes, but a smaller percentage of people have real problems (not just farting) digesting beans because of overactive fermentation. This can cause IBS-like symptoms that may be due to complex carbohydrates like oligosaccharides (see FODMAP, page 448). Proteins like lectin (see tomatoes), that are also known as anti-nutrients, can make others unwell, though this is very rare and only happens if legumes are undercooked. There is no hard evidence that lectin causes any significant harm in cooked food. For this reason, raw and dried legumes always carry instructions to soak overnight and boil for at least ten minutes, which effectively neutralises all lectins. Tinned beans and lentils are always thoroughly cooked and don't carry any such risk.

In my kitchen, some beans can become dry if overcooked. Others seem to boil for hours yet still annoyingly stay rock hard. Italian friends say that you must never interrupt the cooking of a legume and then resume it, as they will never cook past the point of interruption. The secret to a velvety soft and tasty legume dish therefore lies in a long, slow, uninterrupted cooking process – at least for the Italians and their famous *ribollitas* and *lenticchie di Castelluccio* dishes. But you can cheat by buying pre-cooked canned beans in water (avoid tinned pulses in brine), which are generally excellent value and healthy. As they are usually picked and dried, or canned at source, they retain most of the nutrients, especially if you don't rinse away the slimy starchy sauce, unpalatable to some, however nutritious.

Broad beans, also known as fava beans, however, are best eaten fresh, ideally from your garden and straight from the pod, as they don't always travel well; shop-bought broad beans are often tougher and drier. The fava bean is one of the few legumes indigenous to Northern Europe, and used to be a staple British crop, supplying the protein needs of poor people until the eighteenth century when meat became more available, and it started to carry a stigma of 'poor-man's food'. Although they and other similar pulses are easy to grow and importantly fix nitrogen back into the soil and thus reduce global warming, hardly any home-grown beans are eaten in the UK – most are for animal feed or export. When dried they are frequently used in

Middle Eastern cuisines in dishes such as the traditional *ful medames*, a stew of cooked fava beans served with olive oil, cumin, and other herbs and spices to taste. British beans are now a lucrative export crop to Egypt and Japan, as we miss out on this nourishing and versatile food that others treasure.

Baked beans

In the UK, despite the choice of over twenty varieties of legumes, most are eaten solely as baked beans served on toast or with a jacket potato. This classic British dish was actually invented in America in the late nineteenth century, made famous and exported by J. W. Heinz and since then mocked by the rest of the world. The Heinz baked bean varies slightly around the world in terms of the sauce, although they are usually haricot beans (also called navy beans) from North America. In the massive Heinz factory in Wigan in the North of England, the rehydrated beans are mixed with spices and tomato sauce and packed into three million cans each day. The cans are sealed and then cooked, not by baking, but by steaming at high temperature for twenty minutes to kill all bugs and produce a uniform product that lasts at least eighteen months.

The British buy nearly a billion cans a year and because baked beans are cheap, canned, and contain the twin evils of added sugar and salt, they were long derided as unhealthy. But they are one of the least processed staple foods around, and there is nothing wrong with the beans in terms of nutrients. You actually get around 7g protein and 8g fibre in half a can serving, which is more than four pieces of wholemeal bread, or six bowls of cornflakes. The sugar content was high in many countries for years, but now has been reduced to around 2.5tsp in the UK and Europe – less than half that in the can of spaghetti hoops I not so fondly remember from my youth. For unknown reasons, US baked bean versions are much sweeter, and have around twice the sugar content (5tsp). Cost-wise for less than 50p a can, they are hard to beat for protein and fibre, as the sugar content hopefully continues to fall. Despite our penchant for baked beans, in the UK we eat only a quarter of the European legume average of 800g, with the French eating per head seven times as many as us, and the Italians with their wonderful Tuscan cannellini, borlotti and kidney beans eat ten times more. Americans have surprisingly high intakes of 3kg per person, though I suspect this is largely due to the Hispanic population. But the awards for the world's top bean eaters go to Nicaragua at 18kg and Rwanda at 27kg per person.[2]

Soybeans

Soy is the world's most consumed and versatile legume. Higher in protein and oil than other pulses, they potentially have good amounts of fibre and polyphenols for the microbiome. Alas, cooked up on their own they are disappointing. They taste and smell lousy, as they don't soften up like other beans and there is no starch to modify into sugar. The Chinese and then the Japanese developed clever ways to get round this and use them as one of their staples. The first is to boil very immature seed pods rapidly and eat them like peas in the pod, with salt sprinkled on top; eaten in this way soybeans are called 'edamame'. A small serving as a snack gives you around 11g protein and 8g fibre. Tough soy is also squeezed to extract its 'milk', which when curdled like a cheese becomes protein-packed bean curd or tofu. Tofu is a rare product that probably improves after freezing, making the rather bland product more absorbent, soaking up much-needed flavour from other cooking ingredients. About half of the original nutrients are lost this way, but there are still plenty left. Sales of tofu are increasing in countries such as the UK and although the quality is way behind Japan, certain pre-smoked tofu varieties are very tasty. The final way of improving soy is by fermentation; microbes break down the soy into a range of more pleasant chemicals, by digesting and altering the more bitter ones.

A key microbe in Japanese cuisine is the koji fungus, a white fluffy *Aspergillus* mould that grows on moist rice. The mould is dried into a powder and added to soybeans to make miso paste and the ubiquitous soy sauce used to add umami and depth of flavour to many dishes, although the salt content in some brands can be quite high. Miso powder is thus essentially a soybean probiotic that the Japanese drink daily; it makes a healthy soup or dressing, and as long as you add hot, not boiling water, enough microbes will survive to nourish Japanese guts. Daily consumption of this probiotic food may be a reason for their longevity, rather than fish or sake. Koji can be used to ferment nearly any food that contains some sugars, and it is increasingly used with other vegetables. Some chefs in fashionable restaurants outside Japan are now experimenting with koji on meats to produce novel but risky flavours, while dodging health inspectors.

Fermented bean curd is made by a similar process, usually with two steps. Natto is a slimy, smelly Japanese breakfast dish that looks extraordinary and is made by cooking and fermenting whole soybeans with *Bacillus subtilis* bacteria, that since my trips to Japan has actually grown on me (probably literally). In a small study, a subspecies, *Bacillus natto*, was found to help reduce fat deposits in obese mice, but no human natto studies exist.[3] Tempeh originates from Indonesia and is a fermented soybean cake made with a different mould, *Rhizopus*, along with a host of other bacteria that thrive in the same conditions and sometimes kill off the original microbe. The microbial mix produces a wide range of aromatic chemicals that give a far greater depth of flavour and texture to soy when fermented.

Western soybean products

The least healthy way to eat soy, as most people do in the West, is as highly processed food, usually made from GM crops grown in the Americas. The global soy market for humans was worth $42.1 billion by 2020 and that doesn't count the 40 per cent that is grown to feed animals. There are big increases in traditional soy products such as tofu and miso, as well as soy protein isolates and other forms of ultra-processed soy being used more and more as conscious consumers look for animal protein alternatives. The health benefits of soy are still uncertain, and may be different in Asian and European populations due to differences in microbes and in the various ways it is eaten. Unlike other legumes, soybeans contain chemicals that are converted by gut microbes into mild forms of sex hormones called phytoestrogens or isoflavones. These may be responsible for both the protection against certain cancers like prostate, and a possible increased risk of breast cancer in Europeans, but not Asians.[4,5] Its action as an estrogenic or anti-estrogenic chemical is unproven, so any effect is likely to be trivial in normal quantities if consumed as a whole food in a normal balanced diet. What we do know is that soy is a nutrient-dense source of plant protein that is safe to consume in its natural form several times a week and confers more benefits than consuming animal products in the same quantities. The lesson may be to eat it, not in processed form as protein bars, fillers in low-fat foods, or as cow's milk replacements, but more like the Japanese do in fermented miso soups and straight from the edamame pod as a light snack.

Peanuts

The most commonly eaten nut in the world turns out to be not a tree nut at all. The peanut is in fact an unusual type of pea that grows in the ground, thus its alternative name 'groundnut'. The peanut is sturdy, easily transported and stored, particularly if roasted first, and so spread rapidly around the world from South America to Mexico and the Caribbean to Asia, Europe and then finally the USA. There it has achieved cult status in the form of peanut butter (known as PB), known to every school kid since the Second World War in the guise of the PBJ (jam or jello) sandwich. Surprisingly, the Canadians consume more PB than the Americans, and the Dutch are also big fans because of their colonial connections with Indonesia and its traditional peanut-based sauces.

Overall peanuts are good for us if part of a diverse diet. Like other legumes they are very nutritious: 49 per cent fat, with most in good-quality peanuts being oleic acid, as found in olive oil, as well as 20 per cent saturated fat, 9 per cent fibre, and 26 per cent protein, plus a range of other nutrients, especially iron and manganese. The phytosterols in peanuts are believed to reduce excessive blood fat uptake from the diet, so they could be beneficial for our heart health.

When crushed the nut produces good amounts of cooking oil, arachis oil, and with the mass production of cheap peanuts, particularly in the USA, arachis oil and peanut protein are used globally as additives in multiple foods, most of them highly processed. This may have contributed to an increase in peanut allergy across the world. In commercial production, when the nuts (or I should say peas) are ground into a paste to make PB, the oil from the peanuts is partially hydrogenated to reduce separation and stop it going rancid. Happily, the amount of nasty trans fats contained in most brands is very small nowadays; PB is less processed than you might imagine and is regulated in most countries to contain over 90 per cent peanut, the rest being peanut oil. It is worth checking labels as it can sometimes include palm oil (best avoided) plus variable amounts of sugar and salt. Some excellent, natural PBs are now widely available in the UK. Pip & Nut PB, for example, uses Argentinian hi-oleic peanuts and contains no added sugar or palm oil.

Peanut allergy

Food allergies are a modern affliction. Before 1969, they were unknown in the medical literature and to my classmates when I was at school. Rates have risen rapidly since the late 1980s, however, and over one in fifty kids is now affected. One highly plausible factor in the rise is changing medical advice.

Guidelines in many countries rightly try to encourage breastfeeding for as long as possible, but also advise mothers especially to avoid nuts and peanuts during pregnancy and when breastfeeding. Yet in the UK, only one in three mothers breastfeed for six months, compared to 65 per cent in Norway, and low rates are linked to deprivation. Breastfeeding has the side-effect of delaying weaning infants onto real foods for as long as possible, but this may not be ideal, as mixed feeding from three months is common in healthy populations. It turns out the advice to avoid allergens like peanuts is also wrong for most people. In Israel they often wean their infants onto peanut snacks after just a few months and (probably) as a consequence have hardly any cases of peanut allergy. The same is true in Vietnam and

Thailand where cases are nearly unknown. Ironically, in parts of the world where food allergies are unknown and famine common, peanuts can save lives in infants and act as a very effective nutritional insurance. A peanut bar called Plumpy'nut is a valuable tool for aid workers to help sick or malnourished kids, providing instant calories and protein that most children love.

A key study led by a St Thomas' Hospital colleague, Gideon Lack has shown that introduction of ground-up peanuts in high-risk kids with allergic parents dramatically reduces the risk of them being allergic themselves. A further study has confirmed the results, now in a total of 1,550 children, showing that introducing peanuts at the age of three months reduced later allergy sevenfold.[6] Guidelines in many countries including the US have changed accordingly, with peanuts and egg being encouraged from the age of four to six months. Some forward-thinking companies have created products to make early allergen introduction in children easy, so allergies to peanuts could soon decline.

Chickpeas

These popular legumes are also called garbanzo beans in Hispanic countries (and the US) and were so important to the Romans that Cicero (from the Italian *ceci*) was apparently named after them. The seeds come in different sizes and can be cream or green or black, with a higher level of polyphenols with deepening colour. Their increasing consumption in the West has come about partly from our taste for hummus as well as from publicity around their glucose-lowering effects. Several consistent experiments in animals, and small trials in humans, have shown that when added to the diet the soluble galacto-oligosaccharide (GOS) fibre extracted from chickpeas (or soybeans) can reduce glucose and insulin peaks, suggesting they can in theory reduce diabetes and obesity.[7] The traditional idea was that the fibre works by merely lining the gut wall, reducing the speed of sugar uptake. But soluble fibres don't all have the same effect. GOS extracts from other legumes were not as effective in tests, and this suggests it is a special cocktail of chemicals in the fibre that combine with the gut microbes to produce the short chain fatty acids that send the healthy metabolic signals to the body. The structure is once again important: eating whole chickpeas, rather than pulverising them in a food processor, seems to have the most beneficial effect.[8]

Hummus is the main source of recent increases in chickpea intake in the US and the UK. Despite its culinary reputation, the UK is often the trendsetter for new food trends; the supermarket Waitrose started stocking hummus in the 1980s, well before Middle Eastern food became fashionable in Britain. Now 40 per cent of British fridges feature a pot.

Hummus has a healthy image and it may deserve it. A few human studies have shown that the chickpea purée may reduce glucose spikes better than chickpeas alone. This is understandable as there is more fat in hummus, with added olive oil and tahini (sesame seed paste) which contributes to slower gastric emptying and carbohydrate absorption, as well as other healthy ingredients like garlic and lemon. But with four to five times the amount of fats as chickpeas alone, while hummus improves postprandial glucose levels, it increases calorie intake too. Epidemiological studies in the US have shown that hummus eaters are healthier and thinner and have more fibre than non-eaters, which is likely just due to selection bias.[9] Anyway, I'm going to continue recommending chickpeas and hummus; although for variety, I am also very partial to an Indian chana dhal.

A lesser-known but delicious chickpea product is chickpea or gram flour. Used extensively in Indian cooking to make vegetable samosas among other things, it's also used in parts of the Mediterranean to make high-fibre, high-protein flatbreads such as farinata in Italy. It's becoming of interest as an addition to normal wheat flour to make higher protein breads without impairing flavour and consistency too much (see page 66).

Lentils

Lentils have the thinnest shell of all the legumes, and because of their convex shape gave their name (via Latin) to glass lenses. Having less chemical protection, they are easier to cook and digest. Lentils are proportionally high in protein, fibre and nutrients and gram for gram have more iron than steak or chicken, though you may need a squeeze of lemon or lime to absorb it well. Lentils are an excellent way of adding texture and protein to vegetarian dishes, and are a staple, particularly in India where they are served with most meals in some form.

They come in multiple colours, which can change during cooking, and can be cooked whole or split, the darker ones having the most polyphenols. Like other legumes, they are supposed to fill you up better than other foods, though the data is not that clear. One study compared a fruit smoothie with either a lentil or an ice-cream base and found no differences.[10] Legumes are certainly comparable to meat in head-to-head tests of satiety or fullness.[11] Dried lentils are easy and relatively quick to cook, and slower simmering with spices as in dhal brings out more satisfyingly complex flavours.

The green pea

The humble pea often gets forgotten as a healthy legume, but it's part of the extended legume family with good protein and fibre levels despite its size. My childhood meals were full of shiny bright green peas that came fresh from the freezer courtesy of Captain Birdseye and were sweet and easy to eat. In fact peas, if frozen quickly, have very similar nutrients to those bought fresh, and they actually retain more vitamin C. Most frozen peas are immature types, rapidly frozen at source after blanching, within two to three hours. The bright green colour comes, not from a clever dye or spray, but from the natural chlorophyll, which is retained if frozen quickly.

Marrowfat peas are hard to find but are a very old UK variety of starchy mature. They are best known for making mushy peas and in medieval times 'pease' porridge, a high-protein staple. The French like to fry their peas with butter and onions, often with carrots, and consider our peas 'à l'anglaise', i.e. boiled and served with mint, as rather quaint and eccentric. Whatever type of pea you prefer, including snow, sugar snap or mangetout – which can usually be eaten pod and all – you don't have to worry about the colour, although I haven't convinced my Belgian wife who still avoids the suspiciously bright ones.

Legumes to reverse climate change?

Legumes are believed to be crucial in ensuring food security since they are a critical and inexpensive source of plant-based protein and nutrients. They also play a key role in our health, since their consumption can prevent and help to manage nutrition diseases such as obesity, diabetes, coronary conditions, etc., and crucially, they are a cornerstone of sustainable agriculture. Since they are able to biologically fix nitrogen and free soil-bound phosphorus, they play a key role in climate change adaptation. Legumes have a broad genetic diversity from which climate-resilient varieties can be selected and/ or bred to be grown and enjoyed the world over. Despite these obvious benefits, the per capita consumption of pulses has steadily declined in both developed and developing countries. This trend reflects changes in dietary patterns and consumer preferences for other highly marketed foods, namely UPFs and standard crops such as rice.

*

There are many other beans and legumes that you can try, and if you are not already a fan, it's well worth working them into your diet individually or as a mixture of varieties in salads or stews. If you are still worried about gusts of wind, and despite reassurance of the placebo effect, remember that your gut will usually adapt after the first week, and eating slowly, and possibly adding garlic and turmeric to them may also help. You can also, according to one study, make your wind more fragrant by cutting out or reducing meat protein which produces most smelly hydrogen sulphide.[12] Apparently, vegetarian farts are more pleasant, but I will let you be the judge.

Five tips for world peas

1. Introduce more legumes to your daily diet, such as peanuts at breakfast, and add lentils, peas and beans to lunch and dinner menus.
2. Eat plenty of peanuts during pregnancy and breastfeeding, and include them in early infant feeding to help avoid allergy.
3. Make your own hummus using tinned chickpeas, tahini paste, garlic, olive oil and a squeeze of lemon.
4. Eat legumes dried, canned or frozen: they retain nutritional value and are environmentally beneficial all year round – just make sure they're thoroughly cooked.
5. Chickpea, lentil, soy and pea proteins offer a plant-based, sustainable, environmentally beneficial and versatile alternative to animal proteins.

15. Cereals and grains

We are all urged to eat more whole grains – but how many of us know exactly what this means? Should we be eating more cornflakes, muesli bars, or raw bran flakes and oat cakes, or chewing on corn on the cob? Grains are just a particular type of hard, dry seed that comes from cereal plants like grasses. The seeds of legumes (such as soy, lentils or kidney beans) are often considered as grains, but are in fact a separate food group, as we saw in the previous chapter. It gets even more confusing with another group of plants called 'pseudo-cereals': these are seeds of non-grasses, such as quinoa, amaranth or buckwheat.

Grains are a precursor to the majority of the foods we eat globally – including the big four staples that make up 70 per cent of the world diet: rice (see next chapter), wheat, corn and soy, though increasingly most oats, corn and soy are used for animal feed or in the case of corn for fuel. Some older grains such as barley and rye have been displaced as staples as they are harder to grow and are now mainly used in specialised foods or alcohol. Grain cereals are the basis of a huge range of products including some of the staple foods such as porridge, bread, tacos, rice, pasta, couscous, hummus, dumplings and noodles, and of course beer.

Wheat

There are many species of the wheat family apart from common wheat. Others still cultivated include hard durum, spelt, einkorn and khorasan wheat. Wheat production takes up more land than any other global crop and its flexibility and gluten proteins makes it ideal for processed foods. It has reasonable fibre, and a high protein content depending on the variety (9–14 per cent), although it is low in a few of the nine essential amino acids. In its usual refined state with the husk removed, it is mainly composed of starch carbohydrates with few other natural nutrients. Bulgur wheat is a slight exception to this rule and is a key part of Middle Eastern cuisine, used in dishes such as tabbouleh and kibbeh. Bulgur wheat retains more nutrients than refined wheat and is made from a hard wheat variety that is pre-cooked in water before being dried and crushed (cracked) to form tiny brown grains that are easily cooked by boiling in two to three minutes. It is the equivalent to parboiled rice.

Wheat is usually ground to make flour, but like other grains it can be superheated under pressure to make the soft starch puff up, making puffed wheat, which once sugar or salt are added, is used to make popular breakfast cereals and savoury snacks . But wheat's main attribute, because of the gluten proteins, is its ability to form an elastic doughy paste with water. This simple dough mixture can be heated to make two of the world's great staples: noodles/pasta, and bread. Not all wheat is the same though, as the six main varieties have different qualities and differ greatly between countries and seasons. Durum wheat is the hardest grain with the highest quantity of gluten protein and is preferred for high-quality pasta products. There is also hard red winter, soft red spring and soft white wheat, all grown in different areas and harvested at different times.

Wheat has been vilified by many due to sugar and gluten concerns, but I'm hard pressed to find a qualified nutrition professional who believes wheat is the root of all evil, and that's because it isn't. Certainly the one in a hundred people who have coeliac disease do well to avoid wheat, but in a varied and nutritious diet, wheat is an important source of protein and the key ingredient in sourdough bread which is surely one of life's great delicious pleasures.

Corn

Also known as maize, corn originated as a tough hardy grass growing in Mexico and Peru where it became the cultivated staple of the Incas, Aztecs and Mayans before it was brought back to Europe. It is now the world's biggest grain crop, produced in vast amounts but only about a fifth is eaten by humans, where it appears in our kitchens in many forms, from sweetcorn, popcorn and corn on the cob, to cornflakes, tortillas polenta, corn oil, corn starch and corn syrup. Corn is so successful because it lasts well and is often easier to grow than other cereals. It has a reasonable total protein content, but unlike ancient forms of maize, doesn't have the perfect balance of essential amino acids contained naturally in meat and other plants, so if you solely ate corn you would eventually develop protein problems due to low levels of the amino acid lysine. This is easily remedied by eating a few beans with your corn, as the Central Americans have always done. Corn's nutrients are also harder to extract. Deficiency in niacin (vitamin B3) can cause pellagra (characterised by dermatitis, diarrhoea and mental disturbance), often linked to an overdependence on maize as a staple food. The Aztecs and Mayans understood this and dipped their corn in alkaline ash or lime before cooking to soften up the hard outer shell. This process is called 'nixtamalisation', which as well as making better dough, restored nutrients such as niacin back into the corn starch. The Hurons used to bury the corn in mud for three months for the soil microbes to ferment it, which made it stink but was apparently more tasty and nutritious.

From the thousands of corn types that existed less than a century ago, only a few are now used: dent corn for animals, and popcorn (which is the main wholegrain corn), sweetcorn (also called sugar corn and pole corn), and flour corn for making corn starch and thickeners, all for human consumption. In Northern Italy, polenta is a staple; a cornmeal porridge that is very tasty if cooked well as it absorbs other flavours and sauces beautifully, but as it needs only two minutes to cook it is usually highly refined and unlikely to provide much fibre. But the US has taken corn production to amazing heights of efficiency, ruthlessly using chemistry and genetics to enable it to use its corn reserves as a weapon of diplomacy around the world. The US is the biggest provider of food aid and uniquely deals with famines by shipping millions of bags of stockpiled US corn to disaster areas. Sometimes this saves lives, but other times it causes a collapse in the price of local grains and discourages farming locally. Corn is also an alien grain in the poorest areas of Africa, and many people don't know how to cook with it, and instead it gets used as currency.

The corn industry is heavily controlled and subsidised by US taxpayers at over $5 billion a year. Why the US taxpayer pays for this vast surplus of corn to supply cheap processed foods and cheap sugar is a mystery, but no politician seems ready to stop the subsidies. And as corn yields have increased, protein levels have dropped as starch has gone up. About a third of corn ends up as low-quality alcohol or fuel, a third is used to feed livestock, and around 20 per cent gets used in processed foods. Hardly any ends up as real food. Around 10 per cent is converted to high-fructose corn syrup (HFCS), as a sugar alternative. A chemical reaction converts regular corn syrup containing glucose to the sweeter fructose, which some people believe (fuelled by internet hype), is much more harmful for our metabolism, particularly the liver with increased risk of fatty liver disease.[1] However, the hard evidence for it being much worse than regular sugar in humans is still missing (see page 338).

Sweetcorn

Sweetcorn is a natural genetic mutant unprocessed corn that has been around for several hundred years, originally used as food for pigs, before humans discovered it was a pleasant treat. It is basically the immature grain, eaten as a vegetable and picked before the sugar turns to hard starch. The outer layer of sweetcorn is cellulose, which is tough and indigestible, but still healthy if steamed. Twenty years ago, I never saw baby sweetcorn (just like baby pigeons), but now they are widespread in salads and stir fries, as the centre is soft enough to eat whole. Selective breeding has produced mini immature sweetcorn that unusually for most food advances has about twice the fibre of the oversize adolescents. Clever use of combinations of chemical fertilisers and pesticides are slowly increasing the nutritional content of sweetcorn, increasing its protein and elements like magnesium, which also subtly changes its flavour. Unfortunately, this comes at the price of increasing the sugar content, especially fructose and most baby corn, though they look pretty, lack the flavour of a good-sized corn on the cob with butter.[2]

Popcorn

This comes from the whole kernel of maize, best made from a variety with a particularly tough shell. Evidence suggests the Incas and Aztecs enjoyed popping corn, way before Europeans appeared. The hard shell makes this possible, enabling the centre to heat up rapidly like a mini pressure cooker, producing steam which changes the tough starch and protein to a fluffy texture. Popcorn is now having a renaissance in the UK, even outside the cinema, with sales soaring as a potentially healthier alternative snack to potato crisps, fuelled partly by the gluten-free craze. Some popcorns are slightly healthier if cooked in high-quality rapeseed oil, with only a light dusting of salt and less fat. But depending on the cooking process, oil, salt and sugar added, this can be a very different case. Some traditional pop-corns made with toffee or molasses can be the highest sugar-containing snacks, having over 20tsp sugar per bag, and many new gourmet brands add other ingredients and extra fat and sugar.

Cornflakes

Cornflakes are actually still made of refined corn, not cardboard as has been alleged, although the latter might be healthier as it has less sugar and so avoids the very high GI of cornflakes (81, which is higher than a potato). At the time the eccentric but entrepreneurial Dr John Henry Kellogg produced his cornflakes in 1894, he claimed that eating them would reduce dyspepsia and feelings of lust and mastur-bation. While he never produced evidence for these claims, he did change forever our global breakfast habits.

The profit margins on processed breakfast cereals are large, allow-ing manufacturers to spend about 25 per cent on advertising to keep children hooked. After the nutritious fat-laden parts of the grain are removed, corn grits are superheated in pressure cookers for several hours. The resulting mash is then rolled flat and toasted. The result is mainly toasted starch whose nutritional value is only minimally bet-ter than cardboard, necessitating the addition of multiple fortifying chemicals and high doses of vitamins. In the first half of last century, many people really needed these supplements to fight deficiencies. This is no longer true, with the exception possibly of some people on extreme or very poor diets. But the real value of the extra vitamins in breakfast cereals is not to prevent beriberi, but in marketing, allowing all kinds of dubious health claims to be made.[3] The amount of sugar, salt and added vitamins put back into these cereals can vary widely between countries, depending on taste and politics. Levels of salt and sugar have declined dramatically in some countries, while staying high for the same brand in another country. Iron overload is another potential problem in predisposed people, particularly in countries such as the US that add it extensively and breakfast cereals are an unlikely source, with one large bowl providing nearly the daily requirement.

The one supplement item we all lack, fibre, is essentially missing, probably because no one has been making money from it yet. You would need to eat about twenty bowls of cornflakes a day to get near recommended levels. Frosties (or Frosted Flakes in the US) are made mainly of corn, with a large portion (100g) containing around 37 per cent sugar (around 9tsp) in the UK version with little fibre. Most breakfast cereals are not gluten free because of other additives like malt and barley, which is probably good news for gluten avoiders. Special K is sold as a slimming low-fat breakfast and is one of the bestselling Kellogg's brands in many countries. Apparently, it is Queen Elizabeth's preferred brekkie when not having eggs. It is made of several mixed grains, heated and reshaped under pressure, with rice as the main ingredient, as well as wheat and barley. It still has about 15 per cent sugar, with a not too healthy carbohydrate to fibre (or C:F) ratio of 17:1, meaning you get seventeen doses of sugar for every one of gut healthy fibre.

Oats

Although it grows well in wet northern climes and was a big crop in the Middle Ages, now less than 5 per cent of oats we grow are eaten by humans. Oat lacks flexible gluten to make bread and doesn't store well and goes rancid quickly because the grain contains more fat, and these parts are harder to separate than in other grains. This means they are more usually eaten as the whole grain than other cereals, and mostly as porridge or muesli. Most oats are roasted at a low temperature and then either steel-cut into smaller pieces, or steamed to soften them and then rolled out to thin strips: the thinner they are the more water or milk they can reabsorb and the faster they cook.

In UK prisons up until about twenty years ago, oats were the standard breakfast, such that 'doing porridge' was the slang word for being in prison. Sadly, prison porridge has disappeared and most prisoners in the UK now eat highly processed cereals, bread, margarine and jam for breakfast in their cells instead, apparently because porridge can be used to block up door locks or fermented to produce illicit hooch. Thankfully, elsewhere breakfast porridge oats are enjoying a welcome revival. As well as Scotland, it is very popular in Eastern Europe, parts of Asia, the Caribbean, the US, Scandinavia, along with Ireland and the rest of the UK. It is increasingly seen in a wide variety of flavours and textures as well as mixed with other grains in the latest pop-up cafes and bars, music festivals, and even on trains as 'overnight oats' in dainty pots.

Despite its main use as animal feed, oat has a firm healthy public image, unlike its cousins corn and wheat. Comparatively it has broadly similar nutrients of starch, protein and fibre, but slightly more of the vitamin B biotin and four times the fat content. This healthy reputation is largely thanks to a marvellous PR campaign in the 1980s and 90s that promoted it as a cure for diabetes, blood pressure and high cholesterol. More recently, the first two claims for diabetes and blood pressure have been disproved by large meta-analyses. Some small effect on blood cholesterol still remains, with a few trials showing an improvement in cholesterol profile.[4] This effect on blood fats appears due to a special fibre in oats called beta glucan which lines the gut wall with a slimy layer and so reduces fat absorption.[5] Other studies have shown that the more purified and processed the oat glucan, the less well it works. Oats are not unique and barley, shiitake mushrooms and seaweed also contain this beta-glucan fibre. This fibre may also act directly on the gut microbes, stimulating them to produce bile acids and break down fats more rapidly. This benefit on blood lipids is relatively small but could be useful long term. To get any proven beneficial effects of beta-glucan you need 3–4g per day, which equates to one and a half cups of regular oatmeal and a massive three sachets of instant porridge oats. But good-quality oats are good for your gut microbiota, especially when eaten as the whole grain. Steel-cut oats are the least processed as the oat is roasted and literally sliced up with knives rather than rolled, to retain a greater amount of fibre. They take much longer to cook, so are often best soaked overnight to soften them before using. If like me you have diabetic tendencies, you should be wary of having regular porridge. Diabetes UK and the NHS only recently stopped recommending oat porridge with mashed fruit as the best breakfast, encouraging fat and protein options instead.

Oat milk is now hugely popular as a dairy-free alternative and contains some beta-glucan, although you need to drink about three glasses per day to get near recommended levels.

Granola and traditional muesli are very similar to porridge in terms of health benefits; both contain oats at different levels of refinement and effects, and both have great PR, although the sugar and extra (non-oat) grains and fruit and nut content varies wildly among commercial brands. Generally granola is pre-baked rolled oats, with added sugar, malt, fruits and honey and some oil to bind it together, while muesli has the same rolled oats, is more often uncooked and with less sugary ingredients and can be eaten cold or hot as a porridge. The bestselling muesli brand in the UK is 'Swiss-style' Alpen made by Weetabix. The packet says it also contains some wholegrain wheat flakes as well as rolled oats. It has 2–3tsp sugar per portion and although it has more fibre than most cereals the C:F ratio is around 9:1. A safer option is to make your own granola mix at home.

If every morning we ate wholegrain cereals, the studies suggest this would be good for us. There may be a catch. Not with the sugars, but the chemicals sprayed on the oats. While nearly every grain grown today gets some exposure to pesticides and herbicides, oats, which are often grown in damp conditions, get extra treatment and they also retain and absorb the chemicals more than other plants. The ten most common breakfast foods in the US all contain detectable glyphosate levels, but oatmeal has by far the highest levels.[6] This means that regular porridge or muesli eaters have tenfold higher blood levels of particular chemicals like glyphosate (or Roundup, see page 85). A 2016 UK monitoring program also highlighted breakfast cereals, with glyphosate present in most samples purchased, and the highest levels found in supermarket porridge. Roundup is so ubiquitous that we should take even weak evidence of its harmful effects on our body and microbes and cancer risk seriously, especially if we consume large amounts of oats daily.[7]

Barley

Barley was one of the first cultivated grains and has been a staple for millennia. It grows widely and rapidly, especially in cold wet areas. Although mostly grown for animal feed or as malt for alcohol in the West, it is still cooked as porridge and baked as flatbreads in some countries. Pearl barley is becoming popular in salads and as a wheat alternative. It has the outer husk and bran removed, before it is polished and so ends up nutritionally quite similar to wheat, but is not technically a whole grain. Barley absorbs water and also has some beta-glucan. Animal studies suggest that it may even slow the ageing process.[8] Beneficial effects are likely due to its high fibre, beta-glucan and polyphenol content which our gut microbes love, so add pearl barley to your kitchen staples to replace more starchy rice in risottos, or couscous, and to add to winter soups and stews.

Should we eat more whole grains?

A summary of forty-five epidemiological observational studies in 2016 suggested a modest benefit on heart disease, cancer and mortality associated with eating whole grains in any form. The benefits were around 20 per cent per three extra daily servings, with a weak suggestion in a few studies that rye and oats may be superior.[9] These effects on the population would potentially be massive if everyone switched from refined to wholegrain foods. The Scandinavians have set a goal of eating about five portions per day (75 grams) and in Denmark the population average has doubled in the last ten years to nearly four portions a day. The British, perhaps still confused as to what whole grains are, manage only a meagre 1.5, which is more than double the low level of average Americans.

As we have discussed, seeds are one of the most nutritious food packages we can consume, containing everything needed for the plant embryo to grow. Humans can't eat most grains raw, because of the tough protective shell or husk that our own enzymes can't break down. So to get to the rich supply of protein, fats, vitamins and omega-3 in them as hunter-gatherers, we had only two options; eat those ruminant animals that had evolved the ability to break down the grasses and their seed shells, or find a specialised human solution. This entailed breaking down the seeds by cooking with fire, soaking them or using microbial fermentation. Where there was a plentiful supply of game, fruit and tubers (as with the Hadza even today), there was no need to expend any more thought or energy on this, but some of our ancestors must have run into meat supply problems, and needed more efficient alternatives.

Pseudo grains

Since grains have recently developed a bad name, substitutes collectively called 'pseudo grains' are a frequent new addition to our salads and other dishes. These are seeds from plants that are technically not cereals, though they often behave similarly.

Quinoa

Quinoa, pronounced 'keen-wah' (which is hard to say without sounding posh), is the red, white or black seed of the plant more closely related to spinach and beetroot than wheat or rice which has been cultivated for thousands of years in Peru and Bolivia. It cooks in boiled water in around fourteen minutes or until it turns transparent. It is a great source of proteins (9–14 per cent) including all nine of the essential amino acids in the right balance. It also has more fibre than other grains (5–7 per cent), alongside plenty of nutrients like iron, folate, manganese zinc and the usual B vitamins. It also provides some omega-3 fats. This would certainly keep you going on a desert island far longer than the other cereals.

Quinoa has a bitter protective outer coating that is usually washed off, but as the good bits of the seed are not stripped off like other grains it is also high in polyphenols that have some protective effects against food poisoning. What is there not to like about quinoa, other than the social embarrassment of pronouncing it properly? Well, there is, as often with new foods, an environmental issue. This seed is now extravagantly flown around the world to organic delis as the prices have skyrocketed, making it unaffordable for many; indeed a French company recently launched an alternative 'healthy' Quinoa Crack cereal at around £7 a box.

As for the myriad health claims for any 'superfood', other than their lower sugar and superior nutritional content compared to other grains, most are overrated. There are few human studies to help us, although in one randomised trial thirty-five overweight Brazilian ladies ate either 25g of cornflakes or quinoa flakes daily for four weeks and the quinoa group lowered their LDL-cholesterol levels, but this is hard to interpret.[10] Overweight men from Newcastle ate quinoa bread vs plain white bread for four weeks with no benefit to glucose or lipid profiles.

Amaranth

This is a relative of quinoa that hasn't quite made superfood stardom yet. It comes from Central and South America where it was a staple, as well as a snack, and the leaves, rather than just the seeds, can also be eaten. The seeds are very small, and this may be its drawback. It has plenty of nutrients, protein and fibre, and is finding a cameo role on food labels as an added ingredient to other cheaper, less nutritious cereals.

Buckwheat

Another pseudo cereal that is unrelated to common (gluten containing) wheat or bulgur wheat. It is the seed of a flowering plant originally from China (*Fagopyrum esculentum*), related to sorrel, rhubarb and knotweed, that grows well in colder climes but was largely ignored in the West until recently. The triangular seeds are much larger than quinoa or amaranth, with a nutty earthy flavour and, like its pseudo-cereal cousins, it has no gluten. It takes a bit longer to cook and to make it less fragile it is often blended with wheat to make soba noodles, blinis and flatbreads. Head to head with quinoa, it is nutritionally pretty similar, with less fat and more starch; it has the same good balance of essential amino acids. Although it loses out marginally on protein content and amount of nutrients, it gains by having an even higher concentration and diversity of antioxidant polyphenols, which you notice from some astringency on the tongue. No long-term health studies exist, but at least thirteen small-scale short-term randomised human studies have been published of variable quality. When summarised they show modest (around 10 per cent) improvements over the control diet in blood glucose and blood lipids. It is definitely a healthy gluten-free alternative to many other grains.

Palaeolithic bakers

At some point in early prehistory, someone discovered that grinding up certain wild grass seeds and adding water made a paste (dough), which when heated could be tasty and nutritious. Depending on how the wet mixture was heated, it made a basic porridge or a rudimentary flat bread. We used to think this happened around 8–10,000 years ago, marking the start of agriculture. But it turns out our ancestors were baking flatbread well before the Bronze Age, when we were still hunter-gatherers in the Pleistocene Age and sharing the Earth with other human species like Neanderthals. Cooked scraps of wild wheat and barley from ancient hearths in 23,000 BCE were found buried in the mud of the Sea of Galilee, but it could be even earlier;

14,400-year-old charred breadcrumbs were found on a stone hearth in Jordan.[11] Grains of another ancient wild grain, sorghum, were found on scrapings of heated rocks in a cave in Mozambique, possibly dating to 100,0000 BCE.[12]

These early bread makers used what we now call whole grains. As well as wheat and barley, other grains like corn, rye, sorghum, soy, amaranth, and even acorns with a reasonable protein content can be made digestible by baking. The entire dried seed was crushed to produce a crude greyish flour, so most of the seed's contents, fibre and nutrients were retained. In refined flour, the grain or seed's larger, darker, less digestible husk and germ are removed, which leaves mainly the starchy carbohydrate and protein. The Romans were probably the first to use filtering methods to produce whiter flour. Although imperfect, it was popular and more expensive, and importantly lasted longer because it had less of the fats that make grain go rancid. Globally, the whiter flour was seen as purer and a sign of social status, and only the rich could enjoy it. Two thousand years later at the end of the nineteenth century, steel roller mills were invented, allowing the grain parts to be properly separated. This marked the start of cheap refined flour that could be transported and stored for years to reduce famines and be enjoyed by the masses.

Refined grains

No one guessed that removing the oily and fibrous kernels of the seed would be disastrous, but as large populations started eating exclusively refined grains, cases of severe vitamin deficiency emerged, such as beriberi or pellagra caused by a deficiency of key B vitamins. Today grain companies sell the nutritious kernels to vitamin companies, who then sell the B vitamins, riboflavin, thiamine, iron and folate additives back to food manufacturers. Sometimes big food companies also add extra calcium and vitamin D, which aren't in the original grain in the first place. The only products that are exempt are those that use or claim to use wholemeal flour. We know these additives work to prevent deficiencies, although overdosing may become a modern problem.

Deadly gluten

Many of the commonly used flour types – wheat, rye, barley and oats (but not corn, rice or soy and other legumes) – contain a protein called gluten, which gives dough its characteristic texture and elasticity and ability to hold gas pockets when heated. These properties can be altered by fermentation, salt, or changing acidity or moisture. Gluten is a baker's best friend but has recently become 'one of the greatest and most under-recognized health threats to humanity' according to a bestselling medical author. How did this 'health catastrophe' suddenly arise after thousands of years? Gluten is everywhere – in pasta, bread, pastries, biscuits and hundreds of other foods and sauces – and is one of the most consumed proteins in the world.

In a few rare cases of coeliac disease, switching to gluten-free (GF) foods can be life-saving and can help symptoms of gluten intolerance in a few other people, but it can often cause other nutritional problems. GF products are usually more refined and calorie-dense due to complex substitutions needed to replicate the bouncy structure that gluten provides. Bakers make gluten-free bread by often including rice or millet flour and adding xanthan gum – a complex sugar which works really well as a thickening agent – and emulsifiers to trap the carbon dioxide bubbles escaping from the weak dough. GF diets usually contain more fat and less fibre than those of comparable gluten eaters. Some people lose weight on GF diets because they eat fewer high-energy refined foods (cakes, biscuits, pastas etc.) but only if swapping for healthier alternatives – not 'gluten free' equivalents which are generally less healthy and can adversely affect your gut microbes. Xanthan gum is one of the modern foods which we never ate before, and research published in *Nature* in 2022 suggests that there are specific bacteria that have recently evolved especially to break xanthan gum down in our gut.[13] Whether these necessary adaptations by our gut microbiome are positive for our health or not remains to be seen. GF bread comes at the expense of over twenty added ingredients we know little about, that could irritate your gut more than gluten unless you have coeliac disease.

Gluten-free pasta is not always healthier. A recent Italian study showed that glucose spikes were consistently higher than with the original wheat varieties in healthy students.[14] The results were confirmed in US students, showing glucose spikes 57 per cent higher.[15] Long-term, this could lead to weight gain and greater risk of diabetes. So, again, unless you have coeliac disease, rather than avoid wheat altogether, perhaps choose good-quality al dente durum wheat pastas. GF products are on average also deficient in vitamin B12, folate, zinc, magnesium, selenium and calcium, and a GF diet in individuals who are healthy (non-coeliac) causes the depletion of beneficial gut microbiome species, e.g. *Bifidobacteria*, in favour of bugs you don't want, e.g., *Enterobacteriaceae* and *Escherichia coli*. A Norwegian study challenged fifty-nine self-reported sufferers of gluten intolerance who had changed their diets to eat muesli bars containing either placebo, gluten or fructans (fructose sugar molecules stuck together in long chains). The most common symptoms were induced with fructan bars, followed by placebo, with only a few reacting to gluten.[16] As well as gut symptoms, the bars also induced feelings of weakness and lack of energy. Fructans sometimes have a bad name but are present in small amounts in wheat (around 2–3 per cent), but much more in other foods like rye (6 per cent) and fruit and vegetables high in inulin fibre, all of which are beneficial for gut health. Even if you don't lose microbes on a GF diet, you will be guaranteed to lose some weight – from your wallet. The gluten substitutes can cost up to five times more, fuelling a global market expected to reach $8.3 billion by 2025. Gradually improving your gut health and microbiome diversity is probably the best way to reduce your symptoms of intolerance long-term.

Top tips for cereals and grains

1. Unless you have coeliac disease, choosing gluten-free products is likely to negatively impact your gut microbiome.
2. Oats and barley contain beta-glucan and are good examples of whole grains, especially in the unrefined steel-cut form.

3. Refined cereals are stripped of their beneficial fibres – it's best to eat unrefined whole grains such as natural corn, bulgur wheat and rye.

4. Cereals, pseudo cereals and grains are nutritious but beware of 'superfood' claims.

5. Try traditional varieties such as barley and rye – diversity is key to better health and happy microbiomes.

16. Rice

Around a fifth of the world's calories are eaten as rice, and it is a staple for nearly half the planet. Rice comes originally from a cultivated wild grass, *Oryza sativa*, that is very promiscuous with hundreds of varieties. Outside China, rice was initially a rare treat and evidence suggests it was hardly ever eaten even in the Middle East before the Islamic empire. Then cultivation and science boomed and it was transported to Italy and Spain where it spread to the New World. The original wholegrain rice is brown; when stripped of its outer coat, cleaned or polished it is white rice. As for other grains, when people exclusively ate the more expensive refined version, they developed beriberi due to the lack of nutrients.

Rice can be long grain or short grain and there are thousands of sub-varieties. The stubby shorter-grain rice favoured in East Asia has more amylopectin starch that makes it stickier and softer. Short-grain rice is used for wrapping food like sushi, and a subtype with nearly 100 per cent amylopectin starch is the sticky rice we know from Thai cuisine. This can be very sweet and an especially glutinous japonica variety called *mochigoma* is used in Japan in a variety of desserts and sweet snacks called *mochi*. The harder long-grain rice common in the US and Europe and much of India has more amylose starch and stays separate when cooked. India has many varieties including brown, white, red, black, all with different nutrient levels. Basmati is a long-grain perfumed variety (similar to Thai Jasmine) which has more fibre than polished white rice and is sometimes partially pre-cooked (parboiled). Wild rice is actually not rice. It is a different species of grain entirely coming from marsh grass which was historically harvested by North American tribes and has a hard, dark brown or black outer coating and a softer centre. It can take over an hour to cook properly if not pre-soaked – as I have forgotten on several occasions.

Wholegrain red and black rice are less refined and thus nutritionally more complete and often tastier options than white rice, but they are still seen as 'luxury' alternatives.

Parboiled white rice is pre-cooked by boiling or steaming while still in the husk, and then dried to make cooking easier. It was a slow process until Herr Huzenlaub, a German scientist working in England around 1910, invented a speedy method using vacuum drying. The entrepreneurial Forrest Mars of M&Ms fame bought the parboiling company and moved it to Texas. During the war he launched the bestselling Uncle Ben's range of fast-cooking long grain basmati rice, which can be heated or microwaved for a few minutes, and doesn't go off because the oil is removed. Now nearly half of the rice globally is parboiled. Usually pre-cooked and processed foods lack nutrients or add unhealthy chemicals, but rice is the exception: the Huzenlaub method actually retains nutrients from the bran husk, so that unlike polished white rice, it has around 80 per cent of the nutrients of brown rice.

Pressure cookers on an industrial scale are used to superheat rice, so that the moisture inside produces steam, forcing the internal starch to heat up and soften and puff up with air pockets. This produces a range of puffed rice products including snacks and cereals, such as Rice Krispies which are actually made with refined rice.

Is white or brown rice healthier?

Many people say we should avoid white rice because of the refined nature of the carbohydrates that release glucose too easily, causing blood glucose spikes followed by insulin spikes which over time could lead to obesity and diabetes. White rice has a high GI score of around 73, compared to brown of around 55, so you should always choose brown rice. A few epidemiological studies support this and a 2012 meta-analysis looked at seven observational studies in over 300,000 people over time and found that risk of developing type 2 diabetes increased by 55 per cent in Asian and a more modest 12 per cent in Western populations eating the most white rice.[1] However, the data doesn't quite add up. Countries with the highest white rice consumption like Myanmar and Laos have the lowest rates of diabetes and countries like Japan and Korea certainly have no problem with longevity.

What we also need to consider is the quantity of carbohydrate-rich starchy foods we consume. The PURE epidemiological ten-year study looked at 135,000 individuals across eighteen mainly rice-eating poorer countries. It found that high carbohydrate intake is associated with a higher risk of death.[2] Association does not mean causation and these results don't show us where the carbohydrates come from, although most from the poorer rice eating countries were 'refined', making it impossible to separate the effects of diet from poverty and undernutrition rather than rice itself. Epidemiological studies looking at the difference in diabetes risk in the US show there is a considerably higher risk for the immigrant populations.[3] As this risk difference is less than US-born ethnic populations, we can assume that traditional rice diets are not to blame, but rather socio-economic status and access to fresh foods.

So far, evidence from short-term clinical studies substituting brown rice for white rice in Asians have been inconclusive and the benefits of brown over white rice actually look very minor, although could add up over time.[4] Ironically, rice bran, which is what we remove from rice when processing it for consumption, is thought to contain several fibres that are associated with reduced inflammation, at least in animal models.[5] Once again the discarded 'waste' product of food processing turns out to be the component of the food we should be consuming more of. An extra concern is contamination of rice with arsenic from pollution of water and soil in poor areas of the world such as India and Bangladesh. Levels of arsenic are greater in wholegrain brown rice and its toxicity has been likened to the risk of smoking occasional cigarettes in causing disease and cancer, so regular intakes are best avoided, especially if you are young or pregnant. However, it can be simply reduced by proper washing before cooking.[6] Wholegrain rice has more nutrients, but this is counteracted by many phytates preventing their absorption. Although brown rice has five times more fibre (1g per portion) than white rice, neither is a rich source of fibre compared to other foods. While brown rice comes out on top, as far as choice of starchy foods go, durum wheat pasta might be a more nutritious and better metabolic option for most people.

Risottos are a tasty way to enjoy rice with a wide array of plant ingredients. Italians say that continuously slowly stirring in the stock to the toasted rice is the only way, releasing the starch from the rice to form an unctuously creamy dish. But you can save yourself thirty minutes of muscular stirring and still have creamy aromatic rice. Put the uncooked rice in a sieve over a container and slowly pour the heated stock over it – starch from the surface of the rice will be rinsed into the stock. Put the now starchy stock aside. Gently fry some finely chopped onion and garlic with EVOO, then add the rice to the pan to briefly toast it. Finally pour in all of the starchy stock, briefly stir, then cover the pot and cook on a medium heat for fifteen minutes, before stirring in your prepared vegetable ingredients of choice – mushroom, asparagus, peas, lemon juice and zest, etc. Selecting the starchiest rice is the most important factor in my method and both Italian Arborio and Spanish Bomba paella rice work fine, but Carnaroli and Vialone Nano are even richer and creamier.

Reheat and lose weight

Reheating white rice (like pasta or potatoes, see page 67) was supposed to offer some health benefits by increasing the amount of resistant starch. But don't bank on it. A 2017 blind study in twenty-eight New Zealand volunteers showed no difference between reheated and fresh parboiled rice on glucose response, though both performed better than fresh-cooked white rice.[7] How the rice is processed definitely has an effect, although the significance for our health is not yet known. The participants actually preferred the refrigerated reheated rice to the other two types, perhaps because of the change in starch and texture. If you also prefer your rice reheated from the fridge, most health websites will warn you of the dangers. In the 1980s, several food poisoning outbreaks were traced to restaurant buffets using reheated rice. The culprit was *Bacillus cereus* that loves white rice and forms tough spores which survive cooking and wake up on cooling. These indestructible bugs can start to reproduce if left for more than a day, producing a nasty toxin causing nausea and diarrhoea.

NHS guidelines say to throw away any rice that is not cooled and refrigerated within one hour of cooking and to reheat it within 24 hours.[8] Despite these warnings, I could only find reports of a few hundred infection cases over five years in the UK, and theoretical estimates (guesses) of 27,000 episodes per year in the US, which sound impressive until you realise that 48 million people suffer food poisoning annually.[9] That said, it is always sensible to cool leftovers in the fridge as soon as possible.

Some entrepreneurial companies are looking to replace our rice with 'pseudo' or diet rice, designed to fill us up without making us fat. These products are generally rubbery with no taste and have dubious ingredients. Although they often contain some fibre, they are essentially made from ultra-processed bulking agents which we have not studied, so we don't know how they interact with our gut microbes. For a healthy rice alternative make some cauliflower rice, or simply enjoy a smaller portion of rice along with plenty of nutritious vegetables and spices.

Rice review

1. Parboiled rice is not only easy to cook, it's actually more nutritious than less processed forms.
2. Brown rice has much more fibre than white rice and a better glucose profile.
3. Risotto rice is a great vehicle for vegetables: use a sofrito base and plenty of vegetables and herbs when making yours. To save stirring time, rinse your rice in a sieve and collect the starchy water in a pot below and add it back to the rice.
4. Eating rice every day can cause weight gain and blood glucose peaks, but eaten occasionally it can be part of a

healthy diet, especially when enjoyed with a range of whole plant foods.

5. White rice comes in many forms, with softer starchy and stickier types often causing more blood sugar problems in those that are predisposed to them.

17. Pasta

On 1 April 1957, eight million open-mouthed Britons watched a short BBC documentary on how the spaghetti harvest that year was going to be a bumper crop, and were given instructions on how to grow your own pasta from planting a small piece in a tin of tomato sauce. The fact that millions of people believed this April Fools' Day prank shows how foreign the idea of pasta was to much of the world until recently. Noodles and dumplings are, however, common in many other cuisines. Noodles have been eaten in Asia for at least 4,000 years. Made with softer wheat grains with lower protein levels, they are more difficult to mould into different shapes than the harder Italian durum wheat. The grain varies across China, Thailand, Japan and Korea in terms of the protein content and produces many shapes and sizes of noodle, but they mostly have salt or alkaline salts added that improve structure and are usually cut in strips, cooked fast and often added to soups.

The classic soft wheat noodle is udon, or if made with buckwheat, soba, which is firmer because there is more protein and it is usually mixed with wheat for texture. Ramen noodles are made from harder wheat flour, and mixed with alkaline water to change the colour and texture. Rice noodles and transparent glass noodles are made solely from the starch of ground and boiled mung beans or starchy rice. The rice paper that holds those tasty Vietnamese fresh spring rolls together is also made from this mix.

A few thousand years after the Chinese there are Greek and Roman references to pasta, especially eaten as large sheets, as in lasagne. In modern times pasta was initially eaten by hand as a street food in southern Italy. Pasta used to be a painstaking hand-made process and so was expensive to buy. Some crude machines appeared in the seventeenth century to help shape the dough, but it was still an artisanal street food until the late eighteenth century when someone had the bright idea of adding tomato sauce to it. By 1867, Signor Buitoni of Tuscany had managed to mass-produce a dough and extrude it into shapes, then dry and package it, so it could be simply boiled and served. Over 99 per cent of pasta is now sold dried in this form and if cooked attentively, tastes pretty good considering the time saved and the near infinite storage times.

There are two main types of flour found in Italy: hard high-protein durum wheat grown in the south, and softer semolina in the north, dividing the country into pasta eaters and rice or polenta eaters. There are as many shapes and sizes of Italian pasta as you can imagine. One count put this at 700 known types and more appear every year; but because some have as many as twenty different names, even Italians get confused. The names can be descriptive, such as *lumache* (snails), tagliatelle (torn strips), and penne (quills), but can be old anti-establishment jokes like *strozzapretti* (priest strangler) or visual gags depicting parts of the male and female anatomy. How pasta is dried and shaped has an impact on its flavour, texture and protein compos-ition, as do the durum wheat blends used to make the dough. Usually large thick pasta (cannelloni, shells, macaroni, penne) goes with thick lumpy sauces, and thin pasta eaten with delicate sauces which stick better because of the extra surface area. Egg pasta is often served with buttery sauces in the north, and plain pasta with olive-oil-based sauces. Bolognese sauce is nearly always eaten with tagliatelle in Bologna, not with spaghetti. Several Italian-American pasta dishes don't exist back in Italy, like spaghetti with meatballs or Alfredo sauce, but now have a perfectly respectable culinary life of their own.

Gnocchi ('lumpy' in Italian and slang for 'dishy') dates back to the thirteenth century when it was basically a wheat dumpling, though now it is usually made with potato and sometimes egg. It can be a bit glutinous, depending on the mix, so I have recently started frying them, either dry or with butter and sage first to crisp and brown them, which works for me. Italian nonnas like to cook them quickly in boiling water until they float and transfer them to a warm pan with butter melted with sage strips, and a final dusting of nutmeg, to make a delicious, firm dish instead of gloopy balls of potato dough.

Italians each consume around 23kg pasta per year compared to 9kg in the US. In the UK consumption of pasta is only 3kg per year and decreasing, perhaps because of health concerns. Pasta may not be the UK's main problem, though, as obesity rates are around 50 per cent higher than for Italians who eat seven times more of the tasty dish. This, and Italians' relative longevity and health, is a source of irritation for people blaming carbs, and suggests that other factors are just as important.

Rival pastas

Other countries are equally proud of their lesser-known pasta versions, which are locally famous, and may be as ancient. Catalonian 'fideua' is like chopped vermicelli and served like paella with seafood. Georgians have hand-made 'khinkali', centuries-old ravioli which are similar to Chinese filled dumplings. South Germans, Austrians and the Swiss eat variations of Spätzle, chopped up bits of flattened egg pasta dough, usually fried or put in soups. Couscous, which is often mistaken for a grain from the mystical couscous plant, has an undeserved healthy image, but it is actually a tiny pasta that just requires hot water to soften it for a minute. This early fast food was probably invented by twelfth-century Berbers who worked flour with their fingers to produce these tiny dough balls that are very low in gluten. Wholegrain versions with a bit more taste and slightly longer cooking times now exist. Pearl or Israeli couscous and the slightly larger Lebanese moghrabieh or more fibrous Sardinian fregola are simply pastas with a similar nutritional profile.

Pasta ingredients and health

Pasta produced in Italy is highly regulated to contain at least 97 per cent hard durum wheat content, without additives. Italians are fussy about their pasta and will pay a premium for higher-quality brands. Barilla is one of the bestselling brands in Italy, and is sold in the US and other countries as top of the range, but is seen as basic by Italians who claim to be able to tell the difference between different makes. Some aficionados seek out pasta cut with old bronze dies, which give a slight rough edge to pasta, improving the sauce binding potential and texture on the tongue. The US is the second biggest producer and major importer of pasta and, unlike Italy, has fifteen different possible and confusing categories of quality and additives. Most US pasta is fortified with thiamine, folate and iron and sometimes vitamin D, allowing wonderful health claims without any real science to back them.

Most people would not regard pasta as a health food or aid to dieting, yet a crude Italian observational study in 2016 of around 23,000 people found that eating pasta was associated with lower weight and BMI. The study was partially funded by Barilla – so may not have been completely unbiased.[1] A systematic review and meta-analysis of thirty-two small studies (not funded by Barilla) also found that pasta consumption slightly reduces body weight compared to other carbohydrates, and a study involving 2,562 participants with type 2 diabetes showed that pasta does not impact glucose control or other risk factors (although authored by Italians).[2,3] One US study in children showed that pasta consumption is associated with better overall dietary quality and nutrient consumption, though numbers were small, and it was unclear if the pasta is acting just as a good way of delivering healthy vegetables via the sauce.[4] A national survey of 10,000 Americans found that the type of pasta you choose is an indicator of your health. If you ate macaroni and cheese you were likely to have an unhealthy diet with less fibre, while regular pasta eaters were healthier.[5] Regular pasta has a GI score of around 49, which is not that high, showing that the starch is harder to release than other grains, especially in the more traditional bronze-extruded durum wheat types. It is reassuring, however, that pasta is not especially fattening compared to other carbs. Whole-wheat pasta surprisingly has a similar GI to refined wheat pasta, but may have other benefits from the additional fibre.

Making pasta at home may be fun but is not any healthier than good-quality shop-bought dried varieties. When it was made entirely by hand, fresh pasta would be left to dry in hot weather under the Mediterranean sun so it could then be stored. This drying process makes the starch more resistant and less likely to cause immediate glucose spikes. Adding eggs to fresh pasta increases the protein content and associated vitamins without losing texture, so may be a better option next time you get the pasta rollers out for a special meal.

Alternative healthy pasta

A study of 756 Italian pastas showed wide variation between brands, with organic varieties having lower protein contents and higher fibre, and GF pasta also having more fat and less protein, while there were no consistent differences between dried or fresh pastas.[6] Whole-wheat pasta sales have increased in much of the world – though unsurprisingly not in Italy, where food tradition trumps crude attempts to increase fibre. I partly agree with the Italians, and have yet to have whole-wheat pasta that provides exactly the same pleasure in eating as white durum wheat. That's a pity, as it contains over double the fibre (around 4g) per serving, as well as extra protein and nutrients. Most varieties are still too chewy and gritty with a nutty flavour, and the consistency and taste often can't cope with a tomato-based sauce, but the best one I've tried is Italy's own Rummo brand. If you eat whole-wheat pasta regularly you do get used to the texture, but if you still don't enjoy it, stick with good-quality durum white pasta and simply add more high-fibre vegetables to the sauce instead. That said, many (such as spelt or millet pasta) have greatly improved recently and in the less-regulated US, many multigrain varieties exist and can work with a heavy creamy or meat sauce. You can even get some high-protein and high-fibre microbe-friendly versions made with Jerusalem artichokes, although costs can be prohibitive.

If you, like me, have been tempted by green healthy looking spinach pasta, I have to break the news that it only contains only about 1 per cent spinach juice to give it a healthy colour and not enough to provide significant nutrients or fibre. Most multicoloured pastas sold in Italy are for tourists. *Pasta nera*, made from cuttlefish ink, is a more interesting addition that tastes great, and is usually genuine. Buckwheat pasta, *pizzoccheri* from the Swiss border area, looks like short tagliatelle and is equivalent to soba noodles as it also contains some wheat to keep the consistency. Chickpea pasta has been touted as the nutritional pasta of the future. It is higher in protein and three times higher in fibre and is more environmentally friendly, though has a nutty taste and doesn't hold its texture as well once cooked. Gluten-free pastas used to be revolting but they have improved rapidly and ones I tasted recently from the Seggiano brand (made with a mix of rice and teff, or corn and buckwheat) tasted reasonable. A major problem of all these non-wheat pastas is they quickly shift from hard to mushy, with a very narrow time window when the consistency is perfectly 'al dente'.

Reheating pasta

Pasta is not just about carbs. As well as being a source of fibre, the wheat is also a good source of protein (around 8–13g per portion). The carbs it does contain are mainly in easily digested forms of simple accessible sugars. If reheated after being stored in the fridge overnight, the structure partly transforms into resistant starch and has a small impact on the glucose response.[7] More important may be portion size. Pasta portion sizes are often huge in North America (120–140g), and large in the UK (over 100g) compared to more modest (80g) amounts in Italy, where it is eaten with nutritious sauces and plenty of vegetables.

Some popular international pasta dishes are definitely less healthy. Macaroni cheese has become synonymous with instant comfort food. The dish supposedly originated in eighteenth-century England and became a popular staple in the US after President Thomas Jefferson discovered it on one of his culinary tours. The bright orange mac'n'cheese developed by Kraft in the US is undoubtedly the most famous, and British versions never looked half as bright. The cheese sauce came in a packet, like a chemistry set, and an eight-year-old could make it for their dinner. In 2016 the Kraft company went for an image change and ditched all the synthetic E numbers and chemicals and went for a clean label, using natural annatto, turmeric and paprika to dye the cheese. Nevertheless, as a very occasional indulgent blowout, it's best to make your own macaroni cheese from scratch at home, using best-quality pasta and cheese.

Pasta myths

The first myth is that you need to cook pasta in a vast pot of water that takes forever to bring to the boil. Italian lore affirms that the ideal ratio is 1 litre of water per 100g of pasta, to allow the pasta to cook without sticking, and to ensure the starchy water reaches all parts of the pasta equally, resulting in an al dente consistency. But chefs and pasta aficionados have proven that you can cook pasta in small amounts of water and science has shown that you can cook it below boiling point by simply cooking for a longer time, both of which reduce greenhouse gas emissions.[8,9]

Another myth is that adding salt alters the boiling temperature: it doesn't significantly, but is still key to tasty pasta and should be added to the water at the beginning. Another myth (though not in Italy) is that you should always add oil to the cooking water or the pasta just after draining to stop it sticking together. Oil does work as a lubricant, but also later stops pasta sticking to the sauce and is no better than simply stirring the pasta for the first two minutes. Adding some butter to drained pasta allows the oil in the sauce to stick better to the pasta. The starchy pasta cooking water is often overlooked by many cooks, but adding a couple of spoonfuls to your sauce provides starch as a vital ingredient in holding your sauce together and improving the texture. By a trick of food chemistry, it can create a creamy sauce without cream, for example, with just oil, pepper and pecorino for *cacio e pepe*, or with raw egg, pepper and fried pancetta when making carbonara.

The only rule every Italian agrees on, is NEVER, NEVER overcook the pasta – it must be eaten al dente, so make sure you you test it just before the recommended time. Overcooked pasta has a slightly higher GI score and less nutrients, so is best avoided on a nutritional basis as well as for the sake of our taste buds. All pasta is not created equal. The pasta snobbery to prefer high-protein durum wheat may have some scientific basis as it is more likely to retain its al dente bite. Moreover, bronze-extruded shapes such as penne or rigatoni, compared with flat-rolled shapes, seem to better retain their resistant starches, making the sugars less quickly absorbed. Overcooking your pasta breaks these resistant starches down and makes it more likely to affect your glucose response negatively. Soft 'easy cook' pastas that result in gloopy mac'n'cheese, gluten-free versions, or readymade or pre-cooked lasagnes are more likely to fall in this category.

Instant noodles

The first instant ramen-style noodles appeared in Japan in 1958, and Pot Noodles appeared in the UK in 1977 made by the manufacturers of Golden Wonder crisps. A curiously popular advertising campaign called it the 'slag of all snacks', and for many years it topped the list of the UK's most loathed but most purchased brands. Chicken and mushroom was the most popular flavour and in the 1980s the factory in Wales was pumping out over 150 million meals a year. The chicken variety was perfectly safe for vegetarians, as it contained no chicken, just a fistful of artificial flavourings and colourants, as well as nearly a gram of sodium per pot. I recently tried a new instant noodle brand called Future Noodles that claims to be nutritionally complete and free from the traditional artificial flavours and preservatives we see in Pot Noodles. It wasn't bad and certainly shows that the future of student food is potentially a bit healthier, if a lot more expensive. The irony is that most pot noodle chefs could prepare a healthier instant dish in another few minutes by simply melting butter and black pepper and cheese and adding it to pasta or noodles, although they might need more than a kettle or microwave.

*

While pasta or noodles are not a health food like blueberries or broccoli, there is no evidence they are bad for most people, if eaten as part
of a wider balanced diet. Italians tend to eat it more regularly, often
in smaller quantities with a greater range of sauces than other countries, as part of a Mediterranean diet, with a rich variety of vegetables,
legumes and wine. Which type of pasta you pick is a matter of taste,
price and quality, though it seems dried durum wheat has the most
desirable nutrition profile with higher protein, lower salt and higher
fibre content than others.

Pasta in five:

1. Durum wheat pasta is a high-protein food with around 13
   per cent protein.
2. Couscous is a highly refined fast-cooking pasta more likely to
   spike your sugar levels – opt for the wholegrain version or go
   for a whole grain like bulgur wheat.
3. Noodles can be made from wheat, buckwheat or refined
   plant starches and are softer, usually causing more sugar
   peaks.
4. Pasta can be a healthy part of our diet, especially as whole
   wheat or as a vehicle for plant-rich sauces.
5. Some wheat alternative pastas such as chickpea, spelt,
   buckwheat and lentil are more environmentally friendly and
   can be healthier, but they are harder to cook well.

18. Bread, pastries and biscuits

The smell of freshly baked bread is universally appealing, as is its texture and versatility. Bread is still regarded as a basic human right, and shortages a major cause of riots (as in Venezuela in 2017). In restaurants we illogically often get upset when we are charged for it. Yet, despite being a staple food for millennia and the mantra 'give us this day our daily bread', bread consumption in the UK and many other countries has fallen steadily over the last few decades, particularly among women. The average British male consumes about four slices daily, nearly twice as much as women. Much of our daily fibre comes from bread, so declining levels due to the association with gluten and weight gain are adding to the problem.

Despite the simple ingredients of flour, water and salt, there are a near infinite number of bread qualities and varieties around the world, from flat breads to white fluffy loaves to sourdough. As well as dividing bread into refined white and unrefined wholegrain flour, the other big differences are if the bread stays flat or is fluffed up (leavened) with live yeast or live fermenting cultures that produce carbon dioxide.

Sandwiches and sugar spikes

Until recently I presumed brown bread was healthier than most white bread, and most breads were similar. I am particularly weak-willed when the bread basket is passed round in restaurants, but didn't think I had a problem with bread until I started testing my blood sugar levels regularly as a guinea pig for the ZOE PREDICT study (see page 118). Various commercial brown breads, English-style (i.e.

stodgier) baguettes, dark malted and seeded loaves all caused massive rapid sugar spikes, similar to those seen in diabetes patients.

Sandwiches have been the UK's most popular lunch five days a week since the 1980s when, following the lead of Marks & Spencer with their prawn cocktail filling, they were first mass-produced by supermarkets. The average sandwich takes just three and a half minutes to consume, and is now eaten by 60 per cent of the UK population every day, which accounts for our increasingly short lunch breaks. Of the 4 billion sandwiches eaten each year in the UK, the humble cheese sandwich on brown bread is the favourite, followed by ham and cheese, then sausage, egg and tuna fillings. One in four people will sometimes upgrade for special occasions to smoked salmon or a festive turkey and stuffing, but our habits are worryingly fixed. This addiction costs each Briton on average £48,000 over a lifetime and supports a huge £8 billion industry that is constantly innovating, developing novel fillings, stopping baguettes going soggy, or breeding the perfect thick-skinned tomato that doesn't leak into the bread. The cost is the end of the social aspect of the work lunch.

Eating bread regularly might be fine for many people, but my ZOE result signalled the end of my daily sandwich routine. This was a disaster for me as I really like to eat good bread sometimes. Luckily there was hope. Good-quality wholegrain bread from a small artisan bakery only spiked me to around 9 mmol. But could I do better? A few years ago Vanessa Kimbell invited me to attend her course on sourdough baking and my wife and I learned the rudiments, and we now usually have a large homemade slow-fermented sourdough loaf made with at least 50 per cent whole grains in the breadbin or freezer.[1] I tested my blood sugars with two big slices of the filling bread and a small amount of butter. After a nervous forty-five minutes I did see a peak, but it was a tiny blip to 7 mmol. This was another reason for me to embrace proper wholewheat sourdough, and realise that bread is not just bread. As I have said, real food is never good or bad, but we all have our own personal response to it, and it really pays to understand much more about what you are eating.

Starting with yeast

The use of leavening yeast was first recorded by the ancient Egyptians. Dough left at room temperature will naturally pick up ambient wild yeast spores. These spores love the moist conditions of the dough and after a few days will colonise it, attracting other bacteria to help increase the acidity (producing a sour taste) and deter other less friendly microbes. The yeast produces the carbon dioxide bubbles that get trapped in the gluten structure of the bread. Wild yeast 'starters', though temperamental, can be kept and reused simply by feeding them with more flour and water every week. The starter 'wakes up' with the fresh supply of food and is then mixed with bread dough and allowed to ferment and rise for several hours, before being baked. This was how all non-flat bread (sourdough) was made until about 120 years ago. Before the era of the microscope, the process of a lifeless dough transforming without heat into a bubbling living mass full of flavours and aromas must have looked like magic, which is perhaps why bread was key to many cultural and religious practices, not least as a centrepiece of Christian Mass. In the Middle Ages most bread was brown, with occasional luxury white loaves made for nobility. Hard brown bread was a versatile household object and served not only as food but as a reusable, edible 'trencher' plate, a weapon, or alms for the poor.

Fast bread

The next big change came with the Industrial Revolution when the burgeoning urban population relied on others to make bread for them. These new bakeries cheated on quality, adding fillers such as chalk and animal bones and often bleached the bread. The baking process was very slow and labour-intensive until the next technical breakthrough, which spelled the end of the sourdough process. By 1900 the first commercial yeasts (*Saccharomyces cerevisiae*) were being grown, initially as pastes and then dried powders. In 1920, US companies like Wonder Bread used factory automation to produce the first pre-sliced white bread, with a dozen added nutrients stripped from the original whole grain, and invented the slogan 'better than sliced bread'.

The next bread revolution changed the product forever. Chorleywood process bread is named after a village in Hertfordshire, north of London, where it was invented. Dough was made mechanically by heating and mixing it at high speed with the addition of vitamin C, emulsifiers, enzymes and preservatives. Now they didn't have to wait for the yeast to work: bread could now be made from flour to fluffy soft white loaf, not in days, but in just three-and-a-half hours flat. Speed and cost were prioritised over flavour, texture and nutrition for what we now see on our supermarket shelves as perfectly square, uniform loaves of bread with a long shelf-life.

A major local advantage of the Chorleywood process was that softer low-protein British wheat could be used, rather than importing expensive North American high-protein varieties. More efficient yeasts were also developed to further speed up this process which now accounts for the majority of breads sold in Western countries. At the same time, scientists bred wheat with shorter stems and roots to accommodate the machines, with a stronger gluten structure, giving modern bread its characteristic fluffy and bouncy texture, but less taste and nutrients. With the new roller mills, wheat was ground with steel cylinders, which made dough lighter and easier to work with, especially important for delicate pastries. Many people were happy to be free of the need for home baking.

The darker side of automation was the need to maintain regular flour supplies: farmers sprayed ever more pesticides on wheat and manufacturers added additives and chemicals to the flour to extend shelf-life and improve the physical properties. In the sixties, US companies started using advanced chemistry (adding L-cysteine hydrochloride, emulsifiers, fats and extra yeast) to improve mass-produced bread and reduce the fermentation time to thirty minutes. They also added other enzymes like amylase to speed up the natural process of breaking down resistant starches into simple sugars. Most countries started using a range of enzymes in the process that don't need to be declared on the label. The US rules on bread are still lax, and still allow chemical bleaching with chlorine and peroxides to make bread look even whiter. Now ironically, as more people are preferring brown bread, similar dyes are used to make it appear darker.

This destruction of the bread food matrix – stripping the original wheat grains of fibre and other nutrients and adding a dozen other ingredients with varying effects on our health – might go some way in explaining my poor response to readymade supermarket breads. Some well-conducted studies show that the transit time, glycaemic index and postprandial metabolites differ significantly between artificially leavened industrial bread and true sourdough bread, with even bigger differences seen when the sourdough is left to ferment slowly.[2] In a small study comparing breads, sourdough had the lowest postprandial blood glucose values. After eating sourdough, which has a concentration of total free amino acids much higher than that of baker's yeast bread, the levels in blood plasma remained high for an extended time.

What is healthy bread?

Manufacturers know that discerning shoppers will look for healthier bread, so have devised a number of tricks to fool us. The first is 'freshly baked', whereby supermarkets and bakery chains heat up frozen or partly cooked dough that may be up to a year old to sell as fresh artisan-style on the premises. The UK chain Pret a Manger was found to use one-year-old baguettes made in factories in France.[3] You may feel reassured by the brown wholesome-looking loaf with a few seeds falling off it. But it may be fake. Adding colour to white flour to make it appear darker and wholesome is common, particularly nowadays using 'natural' colourants from dried and purified cheap vegetables and fruits like carrots or raisins.

Like me, you may also be confused by the healthy-sounding terms wholegrain, multigrain, stoneground, bran, wheat bran, malted, harvest, brown, or nutri-grain. They sound impressive but are essentially meaningless and misleading. The term 'wholemeal' is the only one properly covered by UK law (and most EU countries) and states that the flour used in the process must contain the two parts of the kernel of the seed (germ and bran). To be called 'wheatgerm', bread must have some processed wheatgerm added back in, equalling at least 10 per cent of the dry matter of the bread. In the UK there is no regulation of the term 'wholegrain', and it is usually used to disguise the addition of other non-wheat processed seed parts like rice or soy. For US and Canadian bread, the legal term is 'whole-wheat bread' with a few variations, and the word 'whole' has to come before every ingredient to be taken seriously. In many countries, bread is not sold pre-packed, so there is no obligation at all for a clear label and you are reliant on the baker, or more likely the person reheating the frozen dough.

Testing your bread

There are a few ways to assess bread if you don't make it yourself, or have access to a glucose monitor. Start by rolling a piece of bread into a ball and see if it makes a better flicking projectile than a tasty morsel. Or put a small crumb in your mouth and see if it dries up your mouth or makes you salivate, as good breads should. Quality breads should become dry after a week. Check the number of ingredients on the label (if there is one): the closer to three the better. Also check the ratio of total carbs to fibre: a carb-to-fibre ratio (C:F) of less than 5:1 is ideal. You can find brands in supermarkets with healthy ratios of less than 4:1. The malted brown loaf sandwich that surprised me and my sugar level has a ratio of 10:1. This compares well to Mothers Pride (the UK equivalent of Wonder Bread) which is still made at a Glasgow factory with a ratio of 17:1. But this was even beaten by a number of supermarket sourdoughs with even worse ratios.

It is always worth checking ingredients. Many commercial sourdough brands add several chemicals including commercial yeasts to speed up the process, as well as flavourings, or small amounts of lactic acid or sourdough flour to give it that fake sour tang, and emulsifiers and fats. Don't be fooled by the term 'high-fibre' on bread, as the threshold for putting this on the label is pathetically low, being only around 6g/100g, i.e. 6 per cent in both Europe and the US, and often involves a poor C:F ratio. Bakers and manufacturers often add calcium as a dough conditioner as well as sugar to improve flavour or balance. Salt is usually added to bread for flavour, but mainly because it acts as a brake on yeast fermentation. It also improves the physical properties, making the gluten more stable and less extensible. UK bakers have gradually reduced the salt content of bread by about a third since the 1980s, and the anti-salt lobby want it reduced further, although salt-free bread is quite unpleasant, and as I will explain later (see page 375), reducing salt has been oversold as a health benefit.

Another item not on labels are natural phytates, or phytic acid to be precise, which is how plants like nuts, grains and legumes store phosphorus. High levels can negate nutritional benefits by greatly reducing absorption of some minerals like zinc, iron, magnesium and calcium. The effect is much less in long-fermented (sourdough) bread as the lactic acid bacteria break down the phytic acid with special enzymes, and phytate levels may also be lower in wholegrain rather than white flour. How much this causes real life problems is unclear, but some manufacturers are using special lactic acid microbe starter-cultures with these natural enzymes to remove phytates.

Apart from minor fibre content differences, there is less to separate white and brown/wholemeal bread bought in supermarkets than we might think. The average glycaemic load (amount of carbohydrates (in grams) in a single serving, thus likelihood of blood glucose spike) of white bread for most people is within 10 per cent of whole-wheat bread. These are only averages, and some individuals like me can notice bigger differences, as I did with real sourdough.

Many of us have been told that eating our crusts is good for us and makes us taller. This was part folklore and part based on a twenty-year-old German study that found a new 'cancer-busting protein' that was 'eight times more concentrated in the crust than the crumb'.[4] This pronyl-lysine protein turned out to be just one of hundreds

produced by the Maillard browning reaction, some of them potentially good and others bad – and so another myth. Some people also
advise discarding the end slices from the loaf to reduce mould, but
there is no evidence this works.[5] Instead, use the ends to make bread-
sticks and reduce food waste. Simply drizzle with extra virgin olive
oil, sprinkle on your favourite herbs and bake in the oven for a few
minutes until they are crispy.

Burnt toast and sliced bread

Toasting bread is supposed to reduce the GI index by about 30 per
cent and so reduce sugar spikes, based on a 2008 study that also
showed freezing bread beforehand helped even more. This study was
never replicated and turns out to be another myth. The structure of
the starch does not change apart from losing water content, and so
doesn't alter the sugar response or calories. Toasting your bread does
have some possible adverse effects as it increases the potential carcinogen acrylamide (see page 77) that the WHO gets excited about,
but it is not something I would lose sleep over. I worry more about
the increasing amount of additives in many sliced loaves, supposedly
for our benefit, that could have adverse consequences. Sliced bread
comes with extra chemical additives just to prevent the bread sticking together and going mouldy, so if you want fewer chemicals,
don't buy it pre-sliced.

Sourdough and slow fermented bread

Most coeliacs would be horrified at the thought of trying wheat
bread again, but some small Italian studies found that four out of six
sufferers could tolerate long-fermented sourdough bread.[6] Microbes
in sourdough help degrade the gluten into smaller fragments than
in normal bread, which are less allergenic. The study makes the
point that all bread and gluten is not the same, with implications for
all of us.

Sourdough is the antithesis of the modern Chorleywood white loaf. It is not hard to make, but takes careful planning, good ingredients and plenty of natural microbes. Its name comes from the dough and the bread tasting sour because of the acid produced by the yeast and other microbes. A whole matrix of microorganisms is present in any natural sourdough starter, including acid-loving bacteria and fungi that break down fibres, feast on sugars, produce healthy metabolites, and enhance the vitamin content found in the grain itself. The fermenting mixture is left for twelve to thirty-six hours before baking, depending on conditions. It lasts well for several days and the amount and type of wholegrain to white flour can be modified, as can the length of fermentation. I have found it is great fun to keep experimenting with the mixtures of flours and fermentation times to produce original flavours and textures each time. Colleagues at my hospital recently compared the effects of sourdough on gut microbiota from patients with IBS and controls. They 'significantly lower cumulative gas' in the IBS subjects compared to mechanically produced bread. If bread is left to ferment for longer, its carbohydrates will reach the lower gut in a pre-digested state and gut bacteria won't overreact. This is good news for IBS sufferers who, as well as avoiding dairy, often give up all bread and grains in desperation but may be able to tolerate sourdoughs.

Sourdough researchers around the world are getting together to explore the microbe composition of different sourdough starters, showing major differences in both the common yeasts and bacteria, which combine in different ways to produce the chemicals to make great bread.[7] Sixteen expert sourdough makers from around the world were asked to prepare a dough using identical flour that was sent to them in their home country. They then brought them to a gathering at Puratos, a giant bakery firm near Liege in Belgium with a library of over 1,300 sourdough starters. The microbes both on the bakers' hands and in the starters were analysed. Each baker's hands (after washing) were home to many more *lactobacillus* species than on the average hand. Eating sourdough after baking it at 200°C will kill any friendly microbes, so can't directly have any benefits. But as these microbes are considered probiotics, the act of making sourdough rather than actually eating it could possibly make you healthier. Many of the mother starters were found to be very different, reflecting not only the original destination, but also the personal microbes of the bakers. When you bake sourdough yourself, it will be a very personal bread, the flavour reflecting the chemicals of your own microbes. It may turn out to be a healthy hobby, with many sourdough aficionados likening sourdough preparation to a mindfulness meditation practice which requires presence and patience.

With all the advantages of high fibre, long fermentation time and natural ingredients, eating sourdough should logically be great for your health and gut microbes. Israeli colleagues performed a small but detailed study of twenty healthy volunteers who ate either extra-artisanal sourdough bread or standard factory white bread for a week, then had a break, and swapped breads for a further week. To their surprise, they found no significant differences in the gut microbe response or in other blood markers of health. This may have been because there really is no health difference or more likely because the study was too small and short. Regardless of the bread type, the composition of the gut microbes in each subject accurately predicted the glucose response to the bread, some people having a potentially healthier short-term response to the white bread, and others the sourdough.[8]

Luckily, personalised nutrition means we may soon be able to have our loaf personally selected. An unusual fermented loaf is salt-raised bread. A hundred years ago a Virginia scientist took swabs from an infected wound containing *Clostridium perfringens* (aka the flesh-eating bug responsible for gas gangrene) and for some reason decided to make bread from it. He first poured boiling water over the flour and milk mix to kill off the usual lactic acid bacteria and allow the new flesh-eating microbe to take over. The microbe was very happy, as it is adapted to live in soil and some people's intestines, and while in the hot milky flour it produced a flammable gas containing hydrogen and carbon dioxide making the bread rise. This sourdough has a select following today in the US with a distinctive cheesy taste and unwashed feet aroma which appeals to some palates and dangerous food fanatics.

French bread culture

French bread has been much eulogised by French writers, who all sadly agree the average modern baguette is 'not what it once was'. The baguette appeared in the late nineteenth century, and wasn't officially recorded until 1920 as a bread as its slim size was much too tiny to support a hungry family who would have needed about ten per day. Before the baguette took over, the French ate large sourdough rounds, and the word for a baker, *le boulanger*, means someone who makes large balls of dough. Despite grumbling about declining quality, the French consume about 320 baguettes each second and on average eat much more bread (58kg per year) than the Brits or Americans. Around 83 per cent of French people still have bread at least daily, compared to only 45 per cent in the UK.

Bread is still a key part of French culture and most of the population live within a five-minute walk of a *boulangerie* (there are over 30,000). In the US there are around 9,000 bakeries for five times the population and in the UK, three quarters of bread is produced by just three giant industrial bakeries that control the market. Unlike English speaking countries, most French (86 per cent in recent surveys) believe bread is a healthy part of the diet. The French baguette is strictly controlled in France where it has to weigh exactly 250g, is made only from wheat flour, yeast, water and salt with no other additives, and is usually baked in a steam oven. Unless it is baked on the premises, it cannot be called real bread. Even with strict rules, quality in France varies enormously and connoisseurs look for a dark crust, with a soft chewy interior with uneven holes and a fruity smell as evidence of slow fermentation. Braille-like dots on the base are a sign of mass production. UK supermarket baguettes typically have an unhealthy C:F ratio of 15:1 and of unknown contents. Italian baguettes are a slightly different shape and often last a bit longer, and unconstrained by bread laws they can add milk and oil. They have less salt (and taste) and in my opinion are best used to mop up large amounts of healthy olive oil and sauces.

Many French and Spanish buy their bread twice daily to have it fresh, and vending machines have recently appeared in Paris, because real baguettes go stale quickly. Most people wrongly assume it is due to dehydration, but hermetically sealing bread doesn't prevent it going hard. The structure of the starch becomes more crystalline with time. A slightly stale baguette can be rescued if there is still some water in the gluten by reheating it to 60°C. Keeping bread in the fridge speeds up this crystallising process, and putting it in plastic encourages moisture build-up and attracts unwanted microbes. Instead, wrap in a clean, dry dish towel at room temperature.

Infinite bread variations

Rye grain is harder to refine and separate from the nutritious husk. It also likes cold damp conditions and is mainly used for alcohol and making the ancient black rye bread known as *Schwarzbrot* or Pumpernickel (in German, 'devil's fart'). It is still very popular in Germanic and Scandinavian countries where the crop grows easily, and immigrants took rye bread to America where it was paired with pastrami. It is tough to cook pure rye bread as it has weak gluten proteins, making it harder to rise, so it is often mixed with other grains. It can be made as sourdough by long fermenting and slow cooking to improve flavour, but remains dense, lacking the air pockets produced with wheat gluten. It has a different carbohydrate composition and takes up and retains moisture four times more than wheat because of a particular sugar called arabinoxylan, so the bread can last several weeks.

Rye may have some health advantages. A slice or two of black rye bread at night with the evening meal is quite common in many countries and several clinical studies compared this to eating regular white bread. It appears to better prevent hunger pangs and produces better metabolic and microbiome responses than the equivalent wholewheat bread.[9] In our ZOE PREDICT studies, rye bread breakfasts produced one of the lowest glucose spikes in our volunteers. Its benefits could be because of its unique water-absorbing qualities within the gut. Pumpernickel earned its name presumably because of the high fibre content (C:F Ratio 5:1) and its satanic black colour.

Unfortunately, Germans have higher than expected levels of the herbicide glyphosate which, as for oats, may be due to greater use of the chemical in rye compared to wheat, which could be a reason to prefer organic.[10] A certain fungus called ergot also likes damp rye (and barley), and before fungicides often contaminated the crop, producing chemicals that caused a whole range of unusual symptoms, such as madness and gangrene. The strange outbreaks of convulsions and hallucinations may have caused quite a few people to have been burned for witchcraft as in seventeenth-century Salem. The fungus is also the basis for the hallucinogen LSD.

Some more ancient, tougher grains from the wheat family such as einkorn or spelt are increasingly being added to doughs. They are high in both fibre and protein content and contain different amino acids and polyphenols to modern wheat. They also have gluten, but in lower amounts so are harder to work with and make rise. Any additional nutritional advantages only come with using the whole grain that adds a nutty flavour to breads.

Flatbreads were the original bread made simply using fire-heated rocks, flour, water and salt, still eaten today, and usually unleavened as in chapati, tortilla and pitta. They have a similar range of C:F ratios to yeasted bread, depending often on how much sugar is added or the type of grain used, with corn being lowest. The commonest flatbread in the US is of course pizza, which uses a leavened dough similar to that for normal bread with a high-protein content, and sometimes the addition of sugar to increase the browning reaction on the crust. The dough is often chilled and sometimes frozen before use.

Common thinner flatbreads in the Americas include the traditional tortilla, a thin, versatile bread made exclusively of maize before Europeans arrived with their wheat. Today, so-called 'tortilla wraps' can be found in every sandwich shop and petrol station, with a slightly 'healthier' image than their fellow bread equivalents, but some of these wraps contain more calories and carbohydrates than an equivalent two slices of bread, with some popular wraps at an impressive 300 calories! After bread, wheat-flour tortillas are the second most sold bakery item in the United States. The industry has grown at a rate of 10 per cent per year in the last ten years. According to the US Department of Agriculture, tortillas are manufactured from refined and bleached wheat flour, and contain 10.5g and 2.4/100g of protein and dietary fibre content, respectively. It's no surprise that manufacturers try to improve the protein and fibre profile of these wraps, leading to more processing to enrich their product with everything from soybean protein extract to carrot juice.

In India, the bread traditions vary along a north-south/wheat-rice axis, with wheat-based flatbreads a staple in the North, mainly in the form of chapatis (or roti) because they are often seared over a flame. In the South they make *dosa*, a pancake-like bread, predominantly of a rice and black lentil batter fermented overnight, one of my favourite breakfasts with a vegetable stuffing and shallow fried in ghee. Poppadoms are thin, crisp flatbreads typically made from black lentil flour, chickpeas and rice, with a surprisingly good C:F ratio of under 4, and plenty of iron and protein. In most curry houses in the UK the dough is now deep-fried which reduces their health appeal, but they can also be roasted or microwaved. I like naan bread as an alternative to rice, which has a widespread Middle Eastern and Asian origin, the name coming from the Persian for bread. It's a leavened fluffy aromatic flatbread made traditionally from a mixture of stone-ground wheat and plain flour. Unlike poppadoms, it is low in fibre (ratio 15:1) and so probably not better for me than basmati rice. They are ideally baked in large clay tandoor ovens traditionally made from cow dung to add some extra flavour and presumably microbes.

The Italian equivalent of naan is focaccia which was probably eaten in Roman times, and is a reason I love going to Liguria where they rightly claim to make the best. It is a simple mix of white flour, olive oil, water, salt and yeast cooked in a special oven, with a topping like rosemary or onions. Sadly, it has relatively little fibre (ratio 20:1), although being very optimistic, the olive oil and onions may help. Many countries have equivalents, some as staples, like *injera* in Ethiopia, a sour, spongy flatbread made traditionally from ancient teff grains. Bread was largely unknown in China until late 1200 CE when it was introduced by Arab traders. Since Chinese kitchens originally lacked conventional ovens, steaming was used to cook small, soft, leavened *mantou* or bao buns, made with a yeasted refined wheat flour dough (17:1) that is sugared and steamed in large trays.

The bagel (16:1) is not dissimilar to the bao. The Chinese version is baked over hot coals while the more famous European Jewish bagel (from *beygel*, Yiddish for bracelet) found fame in the US in the early 1900s. This is made mainly with strong gluten wheat flour and some-times rye, and either traditionally boiled or steamed for a few minutes then baked to produce a chewy, shiny crust. Bagels are sometimes thought of as a 'higher-protein' option, but at 10g vs 9g/100g of ordinary bread, you're better off choosing your favourite bread for flavour, not protein content.

Dubbed the 'anti-sourdough' is *shokupan*, or Japanese milk bread. Made with butter, milk or cream plus standard bread flour, this fluffy, slightly sweet bread has more fat content than other breads and a consistency which makes it dangerously easy to devour. It also looks exceptionally good in social media posts. The Australians started the trend, closely followed by London's elegant celebrity bakery Arôme which sells out their version by the afternoon every day despite an eye-watering price tag. With virtually no fibre, we can assume this bread has a very poor C:F but perhaps the added fats help delay gastric emptying and associated blood glucose spikes. Feel free to check your glucose and do a taste test, all in the name of science of course.

Pastries and biscuits

With a certain amount of added fat and sometimes sugar, bread becomes pastry, with little wholegrain or fibre to counteract the fat and sugar content. Cakes are generally considered large versions of pastry, usually with eggs. Pancakes are popular in many countries, but vary enormously. In the UK and France they are usually unleav-ened flour mixed with eggs, milk and butter, but in Canada and the US, the dough is often leavened and thicker. Brioche is on the fron-tier between bread and pastry, but a croissant crosses the line as a pastry, as it is made from laminated strips of leavened puff pastry and contains around 25 per cent fat. I love good flaky croissants and detest bad oily frozen imitations. Surprisingly, the croissant is actually an Austrian invention, brought to Paris for a show in 1889 and evolved with the import of the steam oven that helped make baguettes. The layers of fatty pastry are made by adding milk and butter to flour and in cheap versions, margarine. In blind tastings, artisan croissants always win over supermarket versions, as do those made with Normandy butter. Although in theory all that fat should blunt the speed of sugar uptake, my blood sugars annoyingly peak even after a mini croissant, but it does have a C:F ratio of 20:1.

Doughnuts (50:1), another US icon adopted from the Dutch, are full of fat, sugar and eggs and deep-fried in oil, with very little fibre. Around two-thirds of Americans eat doughnuts regularly and together swallow about ten billion per year. The role of the hole is not to wear as a necklace but to speed up cooking time. Doughnut variants in all shapes have appeared in multiple food cultures around the world and are often called fritters.

While cakes are usually reserved for celebrations, the pastry has become a major daily snack food. In English-speaking countries around 22 per cent of our calories come from snacks between meals. Some of these will be sugary drinks, chocolate and crisps, but pastries and biscuits are an important extra source. While in countries like France, Italy and Spain, bakeries just sell bread, in the UK, they sell sandwiches, doughnuts and grain-based snacks. These include some strange but popular highly processed foods like sausage rolls, flapjacks, shortcakes and ginger nuts.

Cakes and biscuits are a British cultural inheritance that came with tea time, which lives on through an amazing array of products. I still have a soft spot for the orange-filled sponge Jaffa cakes that are quite unique, as they are now defined as cakes after a legal case. In the UK a biscuit is defined as something that is not a sponge and goes soft when stale, while a cake starts off moist and, like a Jaffa cake, goes hard when stale. No tax is charged on either unless the biscuit is coated in chocolate, when it becomes 'decadent'. If proper chocolate is used this may be the only healthy part of a shop-bought biscuit or 'cake': the other thirty ingredients in Jaffa Cakes don't inspire confidence, although because of the plain flour we do get some vitamin additives.

The UK's favourite biscuit is still the chocolate digestive, which despite its name and hundred-year history has no proven digestive qualities with a C:F ratio of 27:1 and an impressive 84 calories each. Surveys show over 90 per cent of Britons eat at least one biscuit daily, mostly sweet, and a third of people always eat one with their tea or coffee. Britons eat an average of 96 packets a year, which doesn't suggest we are yet cutting back on sugar, but low-fat biscuits are now more popular. But these have not been proven to help weight loss or heart disease and may be counterproductive, due to the removal of natural fat that generally dampens down the glucose blood peaks and replacement with many more chemicals.

*

Bread, not biscuits, is one of the oldest human foods and a great source of proteins, fibre and nutrients like iron and calcium. The real difference between breads doesn't lie in white vs brown or wholemeal vs seeded. Real bread made with wholegrain flour, water and yeast isn't the issue, but ultra-processed flour products with 20+ ingredients masquerading as bread could be. Be selective but curious in your bread habits and avoid the daily sandwich rut. Despite the adverse PR, for the majority of us, when eaten in moderation the humble wholegrain loaf has no adverse effects on health, and the whole grains may be beneficial. It can be hard to identify the healthiest breads, but the label and fibre ratio can be helpful. Slow-fermented sourdoughs last longer naturally, and are worth trying, even if you are sensitive to gluten. Buying artisanal slow-fermented sourdough from traditional bakers is a wonderful investment and is more affordable than, say, a daily bottle of wine. Bread is a good investment and making your own is even better. Making bread at home is not difficult, but it does require patience and some forward planning. Life is too short to reject one of the great and ancient pleasures in life – the smell and texture of freshly baked bread.

Five facts and tips about breads

1. Bread is a good source of fibre and protein but can cause sugar spikes.
2. Many bakeries and supermarkets now reheat frozen loaves up to a year old.
3. Choose rye, wholegrain and mixed-flour breads with added seeds for fibre and variety.
4. When buying bread, pick a low C:F ratio and a simple ingredients list.
5. Where possible, make your own or buy slow-fermented sourdough bread.

19. Fungi and mushrooms

Mushrooms are neither plants nor animals, although on a chemical rather than evolutionary basis, like moulds and yeast they are closer to an animal than a plant, consuming food rather than using photosynthesis for energy. Fungi are often called the 'Forgotten Kingdom', as while they surround us in the air and the soil, we can't see or feel them, and take their vital recycling role in the planet and in our nutrition for granted. Like bacteria, not all fungi are benevolent, as we have seen in their destructive effect on our global monocultures of bananas, coffee, wheat and other cereals. But they are one of the few species that may benefit from global warming; I would bet on mushrooms outliving humans.

A mushroom is the fruit of a fungus, full of spores that get their nutrition from substances like sawdust, grain, straw or wood chips rather than the soil, before being pushed above ground by a vast network of underground filaments. Like humans, mushrooms are parasites and can't make energy from the sun; they need to steal it from other plants or animals. Also like humans, they have evolved to live in all the continents in a wide variety of climates and may have evolved along with some insects to feed on animal dung. But though they are flexible, mushrooms do prefer to live in dark, damp and humid locations like the forest floor, feeding on decaying plants and animals. There are hundreds of thousands of species, of which maybe only a thousand are edible and less than twenty are cultivable, usually in big vats of compost.

Mushrooms have a rich umami meaty flavour due to taste enhancers like glutamates and guanosine (GMP), while their unique raw smell comes from octenol alcohol, produced from fats when damaged or eaten by insects. Mushrooms protect themselves with strong defensive chemicals that deter foraging animals and can frequently kill the short-sighted or greedy human, so are packed with polyphenols, along with other unique chemicals. They boast 25 per cent or more protein content and over 90 per cent water that needs to be eliminated before the full flavours and nutrients emerge. Unlike many plants, they retain virtually all their nutrients after cooking or drying. Dried mushrooms keep for a long time and some have even more flavour when re-hydrated in warm water and cooked, like shiitake which produces a special chemical, methionine. Mushrooms also keep their shape on heating, as the cells are surrounded by chitin, a strong structural carbohydrate that they share with insects and shellfish, not plants.

As so many mushrooms are toxic, it is a good general rule to cook them. This helps to liberate many new chemical flavours. Morels are highly prized and toxic if raw, although for excitement the Finns like to eat them just slightly boiled, like eating Fugu fish, in a form of Russian roulette. Mushrooms have so much stored water they can be fried without oil. When you buy them fresh they often still continue growing for a few days, but it's best to use them quickly to maximise the flavours, though they can be kept in the fridge for several days, loosely wrapped in paper or an absorbent cloth or tea towel.

Mushrooms as health food

Mushrooms are a nutritious food owing to their content, which includes selenium, vitamin D, glutathione and ergothioneine. These nutrients help mitigate oxidative stress and could play a role in decreasing the risk of chronic conditions, such as cancer, heart disease and dementia. But importantly they also offer a strong natural umami flavour and make a delicious addition to most meals. After water evaporates in cooking, the remaining mushroom contains sugars, fibre and protein plus a range of B vitamins and, depending on the variety, around a quarter of our daily needs for vitamin D. Like humans, mushrooms have the ability to make vitamin D from sunshine which acts like an enzyme on their skin to convert the stored steroid called ergosterol to the active vitamin. This is now being exploited by exposing mushrooms to natural or artificial UV rays just before harvesting. Just two portions of these super sun-tanned fungi provide a week's supply of vitamin D. The vitamin D survives freezing or drying and is a much better option than the daily supplement pill I have argued strongly against.[1] Mushrooms are also claimed to produce animal-like vitamin B12 which could be useful for vegetarians, but many species produce none. Even if you ate shiitake mushrooms daily, which has one of the highest levels, you would soon tire of the minimum three portions a day required to reach your normal B12 levels. In fact, the addition of a single mushroom serving to our diet would increase intakes of fibre, vitamin D, choline and several key micronutrients without having any impact on energy.

ET come home

Mushrooms uniquely produce very high amounts of an amino acid called ergothioneine (ET) that we can only get from food, which acts as an antioxidant and appears to have important anti-inflammatory mechanisms for humans. In a smart bit of academic marketing it has now been dubbed the 'longevity vitamin'. Except for a few mushrooms like the ones that resemble human ears, most have high ET levels but the most potent is the boletus variety (cèpes in France and porcini in Italy), followed by oyster and shiitake mushrooms. Losses of ET can occur during boiling of some varieties, although both polyphenols and ET are retained in the broth.

Mushrooms are by far the leading dietary source of ET; the only other plants to produce it (in much lower amounts) are asparagus and garlic, most likely via a cosy arrangement with the fungi that is allowed to feed off their roots. Humans have evolved a very specific transporter to move this ET chemical into the body to the sites needing repair, such as injured tissue or those dealing with waste products like the liver and kidneys. It is found in the blood, semen, spinal fluid and even in breast milk. A few cases of deficiency have been reported, especially in patients with dementia and Parkinson's disease. There are few good epidemiological studies, but one followed 13,000 elderly subjects with high rates of dementia for nearly six years. They found regular mushroom eaters (more than three portions a week) had their chance of developing dementia reduced by a fifth.[2] ET probably has as much right to be called a vitamin as vitamin D, a misnamed steroid that we can synthesise from sunlight.

ET has already been exploited commercially and is deemed a safe supplement in many countries. But cancer cells may produce it to protect themselves against damage and ageing, and some microbes also produce it; in particular, the mycobacteria that cause tuberculosis use it as a defence against other cells trying to stop it spreading.[3,4] This illustrates the double-edged sword aspect of antioxidants, which can sometimes overwhelm a host or provoke a bigger damaging response in return. The ET supplements sold commercially have a large number of animal and test-tube experiments to back them up, but as usual, there are no good randomised-controlled trials in humans. Because of this we don't know if it is really the main active ingredient, so until then it is probably better to eat the whole mushroom.

Mushrooms have been used medicinally for over a thousand years in Asia because of their unique chemicals for a wide variety of conditions. There are over 300 medicinal mushroom types, and each has a slightly different composition of micronutrients, phytochemicals and complex carbohydrates which may be used for many conditions. In addition all fungi can produce a wide range of useful chemicals such as penicillin and cyclosporin that act on humans. The mushroom polysaccharides (carbohydrates) and terpenoids (a group of bioactives often overshadowed by the polyphenol group) have shown early promise in diabetes prevention.[5] While so far there is no convincing modern trial evidence that fungal therapy is effective for common diseases, as is often the case, lab studies often suggest excellent anti-cancer potential as do epidemiologic studies.[6,7] A study in over 36,000 Japanese men showed an inverse relationship between mushroom consumption and new prostate cancer, as did a meta-analysis of breast cancer.[8]

Nearly all mushrooms tested have some effects on animal gut microbes and some of the Asian varieties that look and feel (and possibly taste) like old man's ears, have special complex carbohydrates that may be prebiotics.[9] The range of edible or microbiome-accessible carbs (MACs) that microbes can feed off is huge compared to most plants. The list includes chitin, glucans, hemi-cellulose, GOS, FOS, mannans and xylans that can help reduce blood lipids and improve our gut microbes with anti-carcinogenic effects.

There are plenty of test-tube studies but only a few showing changes in animal microbes. One study gave common white button mushrooms to mice and found it improved their gut diversity and sped up their recovery from infection, probably by sending out pro-inflammatory signals to stimulate the immune system.[10] More recently, a well-performed study fed *Ganoderma* (reishi) mushrooms to lab mice which improved microbial diversity and reduced weight gain.[11] They were then able to transplant the poo from these animals into other mice raised on normal diets and got the same beneficial effect. They showed this was probably due to the prebiotic effect of the complex carbs on the microbes. Another independent study in mice used a mushroom extract containing the chitin cell wall and found it had similar beneficial effects on diversity and, via its immune action, reduced infections.[12]

While we still need some good human data, all this points to mushrooms of any variety being a great prebiotic fertiliser, with considerable variety in composition between the species. Several species are now being used commercially to improve health, growth and milk production of domesticated animals like poultry and cows. Another new key area is fungal (or myco-) therapy to help boost the immune systems of patients undergoing chemotherapy for cancer, especially for newer expensive immunotherapies where the gut microbes play a crucial role.[14] Most human studies looked at two types, reishi (long known as the 'mushroom of immortality') and maitake mushrooms, and their effects via gut microbes on lung and breast cancer cells in the lab are, as usual, promising.[13,14] An independent Cochrane review looked at five randomised trials for the reishi mushroom and cancer. Surprisingly, they concluded that though the study quality was patchy, there was reasonable summary evidence of a 50 per cent improvement in clinical response to supplementary reishi treatment and some evidence it helped stimulate the immune system. They suggested that while we await further data, reishi mushrooms should be considered as therapy, and can be safely used in addition to, but not as an alternative to, chemotherapy.[15]

The benefits of mushrooms have now been commercialised through dietary supplements and recently also in the way of latte powders. From reishi and chaga to turkey tail and lion's mane latte, these offer a powerful antioxidant hit, with unproven claims of 'adaptogenic' properties. But lab studies, animal models and some small human studies show that turkey tail (*Trametes versicolor*) mushrooms could have a beneficial immunomodulatory effect for some patients receiving cancer treatment, though this still needs more trials in humans.[16,17]

A rising star is cordyceps. Although not technically a mushroom, it grows at altitudes of 3,800m above sea level in the cold and grassy meadows of the Himalayan mountains, and originates from an insect larval host on which the fungus feeds. As the fungus matures, it eats more than 90 per cent of the infected insect, effectively mummifying the host. Cordyceps has been used for centuries by local practitioners to treat various diseases as well as to enhance sexual potency and desire.[18] Supplementation (short- and long-term) can apparently lead to greater exercise performance and recovery by helping the body utilise oxygen more efficiently and enhance blood flow, and even improve fatigue in the elderly.[19] I bought some of these dried worm-like creatures while on a trip to Bhutan and tried half a gram as a mild, not unpleasant tea. Despite the expense, I've yet to experience all the promised benefits, but then I'm not rich enough to be drinking it daily.

Magic mushrooms

In many countries, hallucinogenic mushrooms are highly sought after, though often illegal. Several varieties produce a chemical called psilocybin that affects the serotonin pathways in the brain. This is the crude basis of many more dangerous 'recreational' drugs sold in clubs like MDMA (ecstasy) and a growing range of others. These psychedelic mushrooms grow all round the world, though many are found in Mexico where Aztecs used to enjoy it in ritual ceremonies. Its effects were first reported in modern times by a family picnicking in Green Park in London in 1799 who, after picking some to eat, started giggling uncontrollably and became delusional.

A clinically supervised study from the prestigious Johns Hopkins Hospital in Baltimore in 2011, which managed to get through rigorous ethics boards, gave careful amounts of the psilocybin or a placebo to eighteen volunteers on five occasions and monitored responses in very controlled conditions over eight hours. Twelve months later, a third reported this to be the most important spiritual and mystical experience of their lives; another third said it was in the top five experiences, and the remaining third said it made them acutely anxious, although this wore off.[20] In a more recent randomised study from the same research group, one week of psilocybin-assisted psychotherapy reduced symptoms in patients with major depressive disorder, so much so that 58 per cent were no longer clinically depressed – a rate normally achieved after many weeks of intense therapy.[21] A randomised trial in twenty-nine cancer patients with anxiety and depression, carried out by a research group at NYU School of Medicine, showed psilocybin combined with psychotherapy improved mood, and its efficacy was related to the strength of their mystical experiences.[22] For the fifteen patients who were still alive four to five years later, between 60–80 per cent of them had continued significant reductions in anxiety and depression.[23] They overwhelmingly (71–100 per cent) attributed positive life changes to the psilocybin-assisted therapy and rated it one of the most meaningful and spiritual experiences of their lives.

Other small studies have suggested it also works for drug and alcohol addictions, attention and obsessive disorders. A pilot study using MRI brain scans of seventeen people showed that it reduces blood flow to the brain's emotional and fear centres.[24] A bigger but still relatively small placebo-controlled study of fifty-nine UK patients with depression showed equivalent effects to antidepressants over six months (although 'tripping' is a bit of a giveaway in a placebo study).[25] This suggests that psilocybin probably acts like a 'reboot' for the brain and is now being taken seriously as a non-addictive drug with minimal side-effects by commercial companies, but will require very close monitoring as part of supervised therapy – so don't try this at home. The laws around magic mushrooms are variable and confusing, and it is possible to get psilocybin-infused chocolate in some countries, which should come with a health warning.

Truffles

Another related fungus that produces edible fruits is the truffle, which can grow as big as a fist but stays buried just underground. Like mushrooms, truffles are parasitic, but are more picky and prefer the roots of oaks, beech or hazelnut trees. They form complex networks underground and attract soil microbes to help them produce smelly chemicals. They reproduce by enticing animals like deer, rabbits and insects with their complex and powerful aromas to dig beneath the earth to find, then eat their spores and spread them in their dung. As humans discovered, pigs have an innate ability to track down truffles. Piedmont in Northern Italy and Périgord in France have the best truffle sites, which are often kept secret and can cause family feuds; they are often considered worth dying for. The best truffles can easily raise £5–10,000 per kg and rare large truffles are highly sought after, especially by Asian millionaires; at auction one paid £165,000 for a monster white truffle from Pisa weighing 1.5kg.

There are hundreds of varieties but two main types, white and black, each with a distinctive set of chemical aromas to attract animals. The white has a strong flavour due to sulphur chemicals that can give it an onion or garlic flavour and is often best served raw and thinly shaved on dishes like risotto or pasta. The black truffle is more subtle in flavour with many different alcohol and ester derivatives, and the best come in early winter and are often lightly cooked. They lose their aromas quickly, so store them airtight in the fridge with some olive oil, bread or rice to absorb moisture. As with all foods, there are health claims of its medicinal properties, but at those prices you can understand that no large clinical trials have been performed. But if anyone wants to sponsor me to check the effects of winter truffles on my gut microbes for a month, do let me know.

With an expensive ingredient and a variable supply chain, you won't be surprised that fraud is common. Chinese black truffles are plentiful and cost a tenth of the French or Italian ones, and are hard to distinguish without genetic testing (yes, someone has now sequenced the main truffles). France now legally imports about 40 tons of Chinese truffles, which have less flavour but massively increase profit margins. More worrying is that European truffle planters are being sold tough Chinese spores instead of local French or Italian varieties, which could permanently wipe out the delicate original tubers in the forests. Many people turn to truffle oils as a cheaper alternative, but many are made with synthetic versions of the chemicals in the actual truffle, at considerable mark-up. Sadly the real truffle aroma doesn't survive long even if preserved in olive oil, so has to be eaten rapidly and seasonally, which makes it fun.

Quorn

Quorn is another source of protein that most people think of as a friendly mushroom-like plant, perfect for vegetarians. It is a mould, meaning it's a type of fungus, but its origins were kept mysterious. In fact, it was probably the first meat substitute, a mycoprotein grown in a lab in the 1970s by a collaboration between a giant UK food company Rank-Hovis-McDougall and ICI, and named after a local village called Quorn. The scientists picked the *Fusarium venenatum* mould discovered in English soil, as it had a very high protein content and tendrils (hyphae) that resembled the size and texture of meat fibres. They grow it in vast quantities in 230-tonne vats of broth and usually mixed with dried egg whites or potato starch (for vegans) to bind it. Quorn was launched in 1985 and briefly used by McDonald's as a veggie burger. It was a big hit in the UK and several other countries in many meat alternative products like mince, burgers and sausages. It ran into problems in the US, however, where authorities and the sensitive American Mushroom Society objected to it being falsely marketed as a type of mushroom.

Approved nutrition claims by the European Commission for mycoprotein products include the usual meaningless 'high in protein', 'low in fat', 'low in saturated fat' and 'high in fibre', and some positive health effects were seen when meat was substituted for mycoprotein. However, to make the mould edible for the hundred plus products it is used for (including fake goat's cheese, meat-free turkey, steak and chicken tikka), a large number of other additives such as flavourings and firming agents are needed. Because most people are ignorant of what Quorn is, there have been a few severe allergic reactions to it. The mould market is growing and as the original patents and exclusivity expire, other fungal species are also being cultivated in giant vats, some of which I sampled as passable burgers at the annual Frankfurt Food Fair. They are generally served with a generous amount of spices and relishes, and while they were obiously not meat they tasted better than bland Quorn. I do know some people who are big Quorn fans, especially to make chilli sin carne and vegetarian Bolognese, and they tell me the secret is always a good slow-cooked tomato sauce base and plenty of spices. This is a good way to increase plant variety anyway so I think it definitely has potential, just not as a direct replacement to firm textures like burgers or chicken fillets.

A growing market

At present, mushroom demand outweighs supply. The global mushroom market size was valued at $46.1 billion in 2020 and is expected to grow at around 10 per cent annually, mainly as a meat protein replacement. Mushrooms are also sustainable: most cultivated mushrooms (half of the world's supply) are grown on low-quality waste streams, transforming them to a high-quality food product. The mushroom's own waste product can then be used as compost to grow other foods, making mushrooms a great contender for a sustainable, affordable contributor to a truly circular economy. Another recent use is as vegan leather, with fashionable designers charging thousands for beautifully manufactured mushroom leather handbags as desirable as the ones made from dead cow skin.

Five fun fungi facts

1. Mushrooms are a rich source of chemicals which play an important role in protecting human immune cells against diseases, such as cancer.
2. Mushrooms and fungi should be a larger component of our diet, providing vitamin D, protein and fibre and no downside.
3. Magic mushrooms appear as effective as antidepressant drugs.
4. Truffles are a rare fungal treat that are best eaten fresh in thin shavings full of complex aromas.
5. Replacing 30 per cent of traditional burger meat with mushrooms or fungi would be the equivalent of taking 2 million cars off the road.

20. Meat

As I ate the tender fatty belly of the porcupine that had been crudely barbecued on the fire I reflected on the complex relationship of humans to animal meat. I had just returned from a hunting party with the Tanzanian Hadza tribe of hunter-gatherers who spent two hours chasing the poor porcupines through tunnels with spears. As well as munching lots of plants and berries that week, I had eaten a different wild animal every day, including several birds and a strange furry animal that looked like a large squirrel with elephant feet called a hyrax. Why do we like red meat and prize it so highly? Are we just hard-wired to love flesh as genetic descendants of our forebears who lived like scavenger hyenas for a million years before we discovered fire? Or because it is the key food item that allowed us the time to grow bigger brains, travel and cross continents? Only recently have most of us had the choice to avoid meat if we want to. Unlike most plants, as soon as flesh is cut, the nutrients and protein building blocks, amino acids and salt are liberated and tickle our taste buds with a unique umami flavour. Most of us prefer cooked to raw meat, which has less taste; when I was offered the raw porcupine heart I politely declined.

Unlike the Hadza who eat several hundred animal species, in the West we only eat a tiny fraction of the thousands of edible species on the planet. We eat mainly just three of the 6,800 mammals for red meat: pig, cow and sheep; only two types of bird, chickens and turkeys; and less than twenty fish from thousands that are edible. We used to eat every edible part of an animal – from cow's tongue to pig's trotters, chicken livers and lamb's hearts; nothing would go to waste with the organ meats often prized for their high levels of vitamin A and iron. Beef liver, for example, has around thirty times more vitamin B12 than lean mince. Nowadays the West sends 99 per cent of offal meat to make pet food, apart from a few speciality dishes such as devilled kidneys or *'fegatini alla Veneziana'* (liver with onions, sage and butter) or the slightly odorous French classic, andouillette sausages (intestines).

As the number of domesticated animals has mushroomed, even in my lifetime I have seen a dramatic 66 per cent reduction in the number of wild animals on the planet. This super-selection came about from our domestication of wild animals ten thousand years ago, which was thought to be a mixture of chance and the docile personality traits of the animals. As these chosen animals multiplied, they became less exotic and more edible and this then grew into a breeding and farming business as the animals became dependent on their captors. The killing of animals is a key component in all the major religions, focusing on the moral implications, respect and avoiding unnecessary violence. Although we have forgotten these principles, meat still plays a huge significance in our cultures. But 3,000 years later with nearly 9 billion mouths to feed and with us eating our body weight in meat each year, it is no longer a rare ritual, and as discussed (see page 80), we must rapidly change our views and habits on animal protein.

Caring for animals

The Jews and Muslims have very similar rules about the animal not suffering, the ritual blessing and the method of death (swiftly dispatched with a knife to the neck). Some Muslims disagree about whether the animal should be stunned a few seconds before the throat is cut with a knife and the exact timing of the blessing to enable the animal to hear it before being killed, emphasising the sanctity of life and death. All these rituals make us feel less guilty about killing other beings for food. The UK still allows a few million animals to be legally killed 'halal' without stunning (or shechita for the orthodox Jewish market), though many other countries do not. Halal meat with the compromise stun beforehand is the way most beef and lamb is now killed in the UK, usually with a recording, rather than a cleric repeating the prayer in the abattoir.

Unsurprisingly, the method of slaughter is not on the label, nor the fact that most animals now travel hundreds of miles to the few remaining slaughterhouses in the UK and for up to twenty-eight hours in the USA, adding to their stress. Australia still ships around 2 million large animals to the Middle East to be slaughtered each year in terrible conditions with a death rate of one in fifty. Vegan and anti-cruelty movements have recently used these images of captive animals and slaughterhouses to great effect via documentaries and social media to expose appalling conditions, previously kept behind closed doors.

The UK has one of the highest levels of non-meat eaters: about one in six are vegetarian, and about one in fifty reports being vegan – four times higher than France and about eight times higher than the meat-loving US. Most self-defining vegetarians state three reasons for avoiding meat: animal welfare, health benefits and environmental concerns. Vegetarianism has only recently become more mainstream, as we realise that we are eating twice as much protein as we need. At current rates, the average Westerner over their lifetime will have con-tributed to the deaths of over 1,785 chickens, five whole cows, twenty-five pigs and twenty sheep, not accounting for those that died before making the plate.[1] We all like to see wild animals in their habitat but animals bred for food now outnumber them by around fifteen to one. Most ethical concerns focus on the needless suffering of animals kept in cramped cages or pens with no social interaction, respect or dignity for all of their increasingly short lives.

Is meat unhealthy?

Many people avoid meat or sometimes red meat for health reasons. This was the original reason I stopped eating it. In the Victorian era, meat eating was supposed to confer power, strength and manli-ness. But nowadays overeating meat is commonly believed to lead to gout, heart disease and cancer. But meat (and seafood) is only a minor factor in increasing risk of gout, much less than other factors like obesity, genes and drinking alcohol.[2] Even the link with heart disease is unclear. Studies of over a million people, including 122,000 health professionals and 530,000 from the US population combined with multi-country studies of 450,000 people from Europe, have shown a modest increased risk of regular red meat-eating on mortality and heart disease.[3,4] Using a daily measure of meat as the yardstick, the increased risk per extra meat portion was around 10–15 per cent, increasing to 30 per cent with processed meats. There was a modest increased risk of cancer by around 15 per cent.

Based on this data a decade ago, reducing European meat intakes by a half, or US levels by only a third, would reduce premature deaths by around 8 per cent. But the associations with heart disease nearly disappear when you exclude Americans who eat lower-quality meat, and are non-existent when you include 300,000 Asians (from Japan, China and Korea) or studies of 134,000 people from poorer countries or all studies together.[5,6,7] The data suggests that quality, not just quantity of meat, is important, and what else you put on the plate. Studies show Americans eat 50 per cent of their meat outside the home, and that meat eating is generally higher in poorer groups with less healthy habits. Most (but not all) studies have shown slightly reduced risks of 5–7 per cent with eating white meat like chicken or fish, although the large prospective UK Biobank study of over 422,000 people found no differences between white or red meat.[8] A clinical trial feeding beef or chicken to volunteers for four weeks found no differences in blood fat levels that could explain the epidemiology, leaving many experts uncertain as to the benefits of white flesh.[9]

Eight placebo controlled clinical trials have tested a compound called conjugated linoleic acid (CLA) to help treat obesity and a recent meta-analysis showed it has a modest effect of 1kg weight loss over twelve weeks in women who are overweight or obese, with other studies showing promise in reducing cancer and cardiovascular health risk.[10] CLA is naturally found in high levels in grass-fed animals, which may be another reason to eat occasional, high-quality, forage-fed and organic meat instead of just buying CLA supplements.

Other studies have been overlooked. These include the eleven-year colon cancer prevention study of 2,000 people and the 24,000 women in an eight-year cancer prevention trial of low-fat diets.[11] These participants, as part of other diet changes, reduced their meat intakes by around 20 per cent. Both studies found no decrease in cancers or mortality as you might have expected in those giving up red meat.[12] So based on the current limited data, there is a slight increased risk of heart disease from eating red meat (though less than previously thought), which increases the more portions you eat; but no clear risk from eating white meat. The risks increase more significantly and consistently for eating all kinds of lower-quality processed meats.

It is worth knowing more about the animal flesh we crave. Meat is made up of water, protein and fat, plus a few carbs, iron, zinc and B vitamins. The biggest difference in meat composition is the lifestyle of the animals. Animals that eat plants outdoors and have plenty of space to move and socialise with their peers have higher levels of omega-3 fats and lower levels of pro-inflammatory chemicals.

We generally eat meat from warm-blooded land animals and divide these up into red and white meat, although these distinctions are somewhat arbitrary. Red flesh contains higher amounts of iron and myoglobin pigments and is made up of the key long distance muscles, with extra nutrients and flavour, but it is tougher to eat. For most people white meat includes poultry, veal and pork, and poultry can include duck which has dark red meat. White flesh has less myoglobin and fewer nutrients and is more tender but less flavourful. Active humans are mainly made up of red muscle, which help us run marathons; pigs, in contrast, don't run far and are mainly white muscle, and chickens, as they sometimes cross roads, are a mixture of both, with their dark legs in constant use, while their white breasts or wings are hardly used at all.

You may be able to eat plenty of meat without problems if the particular microbes in your gut are the right species and can break down the chemicals in meat harmlessly. A Cleveland group discovered that some gut microbes converted a harmless chemical in meat called trimethylamine to a nasty one, TMAO, which causes arteries to clog up with plaque and speeds up blood clots (see page 51).[13] Altering mice gut microbes via diet or antibiotics could reverse these changes. Humans with high TMAO levels had three times the risk of heart disease, and this has been replicated now in many other studies, showing once again that our individual responses to meat through our unique gut microbes might be the key to understanding the sometimes contradictory epidemiological findings. When vegans were persuaded to eat meat their TMAO levels did not change much. This was because they did not have enough resident microbes which could process the original waste products. This suggests we should be wary of too much protein, but having the occasional piece of unprocessed meat may be perfectly healthy, if we leave most of the room in our diets for plants.

Although our ancestors preferred the fattier cuts of meat, since the 1970s we have been indoctrinated into believing these are bad for us due to scare stories about links between saturated fat and heart disease. The latest global research has largely disproved this simplistic story (see page 299), but while there is no consensus yet on eating fatty meat, we do know eating lots of red meat is not good for you. Fat cells are a useful store for all the nutrients and flavours of the plants the animals have been feeding on during their lives. Although there is still fat in lean cuts of meat, the fattier the meat the more your mouth retains some aroma volatiles, particularly with smoked or barbecue meats. Fat also improves the 'mouthfeel' of meat and stops it tasting dry. This is why there is a different sensation when you chew a chicken breast, which is harder to swallow than a chicken leg. Animals are now being killed much younger than before; they are generally leaner with fat that has little chance to absorb nutrients and flavours. In these young animals, the lean meat never gets tough, but with cattle bred for speed of growth, the muscles, although tender, have no time to develop any complexity or absorb any flavour.

In the past, most meat was aged after being killed, allowing time before eating for the enzymes to tenderise and improve the flavour. Beef can safely be aged for up to a month; a week or two for more fatty meats like lamb or pork. Now, except for gourmets buying fifteen-year-old hibernated French (Polmard) steaks for $3,000 each, ageing meat is forgotten, with the emphasis on speed, tenderness and cost.

Pork

The animal that is unfortunate enough to be the world's favourite for eating is the domestic pig, despite it being banned on religious grounds by first Jews and then Muslims. The most consistently popular British lunch of the last decade was the ham sandwich, and nearly every country has its own versions of cooked or cured pork meat. Pig meat has changed radically in the last century as the traditional English pig was crossed with the Chinese pig to produce more piglets and more meat. But in just the last thirty years, because of anti-fat fears, consumer demands and highly selective breeding, we have globally focused on just one of thousands of types of pig – the Large White variety. This pig is about 30 per cent leaner and therefore drier, paler and with less flavour, but is docile and produces many litters. Most are raised in industrial barns and fattened on grain with little to no access to exercise or sunlight. In Europe, Denmark is one of the largest producers and supplies most of the UK's ham and bacon from massive factory farms where pigs are kept in sterile but small pens, living a miserable, dull captive existence before taking the conveyor belt to the abattoir.

The most efficient factories will make their sows produce over twenty-five piglets per year, never leaving their metal crates. The piglets are weaned from their mother at three to four weeks, so the sow can rapidly get pregnant again. Pig farming in the UK is on a much smaller scale with a high percentage of organic farms, where pigs spend time outdoors, and the piglets are weaned later and are healthier. But the meat is more expensive and harder to sell to a cost-conscious public who ignore the conditions of the mega-scale production lines. In the US, around 80 per cent of pork comes from these large multi-crate facilities with over 5,000 inmates that also have a huge environmental impact on surrounding areas due to the waste cesspools used for pig excrement.

In the past every Chinese family had a pig in their backyard; now modern China is the world's largest producer with over 700 million pigs, even though we lost about half of those and about a quarter of the world's pigs in 2019/20 to a painful nasty death from African swine flu, caused in part because of their genetic similarity and lack of immunity. Asian countries now use hi-tech methods to improve the yields of the millions of sows in massive facilities. Farming and feed corporations in China have linked up with tech giant Alibaba to use CCTV cameras linked to supercomputers to collect data on every aspect of feeding and health of over 10 million animals, using heat sensors, Fitbit exercise tracking and voice recognition systems to hear the sound of squealing piglets being squashed by their mothers. The data is being fed into artificial intelligence (AI) programs to predict the best methods to improve fertility and health of the sows and the piglets.[14] Even an improvement of 1 per cent in piglet mortality (which often runs at 30 per cent) is worth hundreds of millions of pounds to the producers. Despite these massive endeavours, pork is about to lose its long-standing status as the world's most popular meat, to be replaced by a scrawny upstart two-legged animal that only became popular to eat in the 1950s.

Poultry

We now grow and eat an astonishing 60 billion birds per year, compared to less than a few hundred million in 1970. Chicken used to be a rare treat on a Sunday when I was a child, now people can eat it every day. Consumption has escalated in virtually all countries in fifty years, the US increasing fivefold, and the UK (starting at lower levels) over twentyfold. A whole chicken now costs just over £3 per bird in most supermarkets, which is cheaper than a pint of beer. Over 2 million chickens are eaten daily in the UK alone. This is only possible because of intensive farming run by a network of a few global companies led by Brazil, China and the US that pay farmers a small percentage of the selling price per animal. A hen is now grown to adult size in thirty-five to forty days at minimal cost, in sheds of 20,000 birds, with artificial heat and light, feeding from drip-feed stations to minimise waste.

When I was a student I worked for a few days on a farm, where thousands of hens were raised and housed in an enormous hanger. Our job was to go in before daybreak, so light wouldn't frighten them, and pick up three in each hand and put them on trucks for slaughter. The sight, smell and noise of treading through all those birds at dawn is not something I will forget. It was a struggle to walk without crushing one and pick them up, but once hens are upside down they go into a trance. They are kept all their lives in the same dim light and mild temperature with a miniscule space per hen, so they could barely move. A few farms do look after their health and welfare attentively to reduce deaths and fractures, but their lives must be pretty dull, like being stuck endlessly in a crowded tube train, with food and drink on tap.

Hens are slaughtered differently around the world, mostly killed by gassing with carbon dioxide in the UK, and by electrocution in water in the US. In some large farms and production lines, it is possible to go from live chick to packaged meat, without a human hand touching the animal. Most male chicks get discarded in grinders or are gassed. Professional chick sexers can test about thirty per minute with 95 per cent accuracy, and no computer image program has yet got close, although there are some fluorescent genetic tests now available before hatching to prevent four billion culls annually, but it's unclear whether the industry or consumer will pay.[15]

A safety concern with chickens (as well as their eggs) is bacterial contamination, with most surveys showing the majority of mass-produced chickens containing significant amounts of pathogens such as *campylobacter* and *salmonella*, and around a third showing signs that the bugs may be antibiotic resistant.[16] Raw chicken is the main source of contamination, which is why chickens are chlorinated in the US and Australia, but cooking all parts of the meat (internal and external) to above 75°C removes this problem. But many people forget that before it is cooked, by just touching the packaging or leaving it in the fridge for too long, hands and other foods and surfaces can easily be infected: a common cause of the 50 million food-poisoning episodes in the US every year. *Campylobacter* kills around 100 Britons every year.[17] With this background, it is hard to work out why people would want to eat raw chicken, as with beef tartare. But the Japanese eat plenty of raw chicken as *torisashi* cut into strips and eaten like sashimi, or slightly seared on the outside and coated in sesame, but the hens are expensively raised and specially slaughtered and instantly refrigerated and then irradiated to reduce the risk of infection. This is now becoming fashionable in a few brave US restaurants, but my advice is don't try it at home.

Organic chickens are raised without antibiotics, pesticides, chemicals or hormones in their feed and in the US the label means they can't be caged. The term is different in Europe, and only relates to their feed, while free-range chickens spend at least some of their lives outdoors with real sunshine and more variety in their feed. These lucky ones get to live twice as long (over eighty-one days) and can exercise their muscles, which with the extra fat they put on, increases nutrients and flavour, but also sometimes the toughness of their leg muscles. This obviously costs a lot more – around three times the price of caged chickens in most countries – and although the sector is growing, it still accounts for less than a few per cent of the market.

Turkeys are raised in similar ways and can be plumped up in just eighty-four days in time for Christmas and Thanksgiving. The speed at which intensively farmed chicks now grow is phenomenal: equivalent to growing a normal 3kg baby to the size of a 300kg sumo wrestler in only nine weeks. How they manage this feat is quite amazing and involves New Yorkers, genetics and a few magic potions.

Ducks are farmed in similar conditions and often they have no access to water for bathing and swimming and their beaks may be trimmed to reduce the risk of damage to others in close proximity. But at least ducks farmed for human consumption run in the millions as opposed to billions, at least for now.

Beauty contests

The market for eating chickens (known as broilers) grew slowly; they cost a modern equivalent of $30 each in 1940s USA. This all changed in 1948 when a New York grocery chain called A&P combined with the US Department of Agriculture to find the perfect breeding hen that was plump and tasty and didn't need hours in a pot. This was the 'Chicken of Tomorrow' beauty contest in Delaware and there were hundreds of entrants, narrowing down to forty-four finalists. They then sent their eggs to a central hatchery where the chicks were raised identically and the modern chicken was born.

Simultaneously, Thomas Jukes, a talented and controversial British scientist, was experimenting with different minerals, vitamins and feeds to see what would help hens grow. He was a strong critic of creationism, vitamin C quackery and environmentalists. He was also working with antibiotics produced by his company (Lederle) and added a small amount to animal feed. He found that while vitamins helped a bit, antibiotics accelerated growth by 250 per cent.[18] A feeding frenzy of antibiotic use followed in all kinds of meat production, which in the US now accounts for 80 per cent of total antibiotic sales, still behind China and Brazil. Rates are lower in Europe although they vary tenfold with the worst offenders being Cyprus, Spain and Italy. After sixty years it is only recently that any agency thought to look at whether antibiotics fatten up humans as well. Unsurprisingly, they do, although no one is quite sure by how much. Although humans consume only small amounts in meat compared to taking antibiotic medicines, it has had a major impact on antibiotic resistance. As we run out of effective medicines, this is a growing global crisis. Furthermore, the prolific use of antibiotics has led to increasingly crowded conditions in battery farms, and reduced hygiene practices in abattoirs and animal markets. This false sense of protection has resulted in devastating viral infections wiping out huge swathes of animals, and cross-species infection such as with swine flu, avian flu, SARS and, most recently, Covid-19.

Conversely, the French have always thought that their coq au vin tasted better with an older animal rather than a baby. In a bid to stop this tide of cheap tasteless chicken they launched the Label Rouge brand, which sells older heirloom hen breeds raised for taste not rapid growth, and allowed to free range in similar conditions to organic raised hens for over eighty-one days. Label Rouge extends to a wide range of products across France, promoting taste and quality at greater cost. So far shoppers in other less discerning countries like the UK or the USA are less willing to sacrifice their £3 bird and pay four times more for an organic bird that could actually walk.

It is hard to believe the epidemiological evidence that eating lots of chicken can be recommended as healthy. Most of the data came from studies from the 1950s to 80s, when chickens bore little resemblance to the bloated baby broilers of today. If you still decide to buy supermarket chicken, remember the farmer makes a profit of around 25p per bird, so don't expect any taste or great nutrients other than protein, and it is very unlikely to make you live longer. A good-quality outdoor-reared whole chicken as an occasional home-cooked Sunday roast is probably the most sensible and sustainable way to enjoy this meat.

Growth hormones, chlorine and meat

Injected growth hormones are hardly discussed now. The reason they are no longer an issue for chickens is they cost too much. They are still legally used in the US for beef and sheep to bulk them up before selling, but with 'apparently' safe levels for human consumers.[19] European consumers and regulators banned them in 1989, after a series of scandals in Italy in the late 1970s when schoolchildren started growing beards and breasts much earlier than usual. (The cancer-causing hormone stilboestrol was eventually found in locally produced baby foods containing meat.) The clash in food safety culture between Europe and the US over growth hormones led to a minor trade war, and US beef cannot yet be imported into Europe. Similar differences in opinion exist over chlorinating chicken which is routinely done in the US to remove external microbial infections, although the chlorine normally evaporates well before ingestion. Whether these stricter rules will continue for the UK post-Brexit remains to be seen, but it might be worth checking the country of origin when you buy your meat.

Beef

Beef has also changed dramatically over time and a good cut of steak is now a frequent choice, rather than a luxury treat. When working in Belgium in the 1980s I found the local steaks were tender, very pink, plump and, for me, tasteless compared to the tougher and fattier British rump steaks of the time. This I discovered much later was due to modern intensive breeding and use of antibiotics and growth hormones, which made them young, rapid-growing and affordable. The chosen breed (Blanc-bleu Belge) has a mutation in the myostatin gene which gives them 'double muscling' and 20 per cent more muscle. The hormones plus their gene defects gave these strange blue-skinned mutated animals such enormous buttocks that the calves were too large to be delivered normally and died unless born by caesarean section.

Beef is globally changing and going the same way as chicken, with leanness and cheapness being preferred. Most beef cattle are mainly grain fed in large feedlots to keep prices low, with no ageing time to improve flavour. There is a very small but growing premium market for grass-fed, organically raised free-range cows, which most people agree taste better because the extra nutrients from the plants infiltrate into the fat around the muscle creating a polyphenol-rich meat with plenty of flavour. Some recent research has backed this up showing a significantly healthier-looking ratio of types of fat in grass-fed vs grain-fed cattle.[20]

Again, 'organic beef' means different things in different countries: in the US organic means they must be fed organic grains and be antibiotic and hormone free and have some access to pasture and non-grain feed; in Europe organic beef usually means the same, with different regional definitions of 'grass-fed'. But in many countries, organic animals are grain fed for the last few weeks to fatten them up, so if you can, it's always good to know where your meat comes from.

At the other end of the scale, certain luxury beef types command prices beyond most people's reach. Probably the most famous is Japanese kobe beef (Japanese beef is wagyu, and kobe is a special appellation with strict rules). Kobe calves are given names and birth certificates and fed on bottled milk for seven months, followed by special diets for three years (over twice as long as normal) until they reach 750kg. The mixture of genes and pampering produces the characteristic marbled butter-like tender meat, high in nutrients.

They are not disappointingly given beer or massages anymore, though they do get an occasional invigorating body scrub.

The perfect steak

Every country has its debate about how best to cook a steak, with French waiters raising their eyes when English or American tourists ask for steak *'bien cuit'* (well done). But the increasingly lean cuts of meat are making it harder to cook them with precision, as the fat that used to protect the moisture and slow down the cooking process has disappeared. Cooking steak rare (to 49°C) is now a risky procedure as the fat has no time to melt and mix with the muscle, and the muscle fibres are slippery and don't release moisture. At higher temperatures above 55°C (medium rare), the fat starts to melt and impart flavour and the fibres are firmer and release moisture. When steak is well done (at 71°C), up to 20 per cent of the moisture is lost, the red colour is also lost as it turns grey, dry, and in my opinion tasteless. The red colour of meat is not mainly from blood but due to a pigment (myoglobin) in the muscle which changes on cutting and exposure to air to a bright red pigment, oxyhaemoglobin. This pigment is destroyed on overheating and the meat turns grey. There is no clear evidence of nutritional benefits of over- or undercooking meat, although you lose some of the vitamins in the fat when you overcook it; conversely, cooking allows you to absorb more protein. Frying meat results in the biggest loss of nutrients with up to 33 per cent of vitamin B12 lost in the flash of a hot pan.[21] Of course, cooking also reduces the risk of contamination with bugs, antibiotics and pesticides, so roasting, grilling or cooking your meat sous vide may be the best way to retain nutrients.

Some prefer their beef raw. Beef carpaccio – thinly sliced dry-cured or raw beef, with olive oil and lemon, often served on a bed of peppery rocket leaves – is popular in Italy, although only invented in Venice in 1950. Steak tartare – raw minced beef with raw egg, onions and cornichons – is popular in Italy, France and Belgium where it is called 'Filet Americain', which is ironic as that's the last place you would want to buy one. A 2015 consumer report sampled 300 US minced raw beef samples and found 80 per cent were contaminated with some potentially dangerous faecal microbes, and one in five has *E.coli* or *staphylococcus* that cause some of the 48 million annual cases of food poisoning. Rates were much higher in cheap feedlot cattle compared to organic or grass-fed animals which had avoided anti-biotics and hormones.[22] Bear in mind that beef is less contaminated with microbes than chicken or pork, so is considered safe in most countries to eat bloody and raw on the inside, although many restaurant chains worry about being sued.

Lamb and other animals

Lamb is a finer and more tender meat and has a special taste and farm-yard flavour due to release of a chemical called skatole (its name unfortunately comes from it being first discovered in human poo, hence scatologic). Sales of lamb are declining in many parts of the world as they are not part of the main fast-food or UPF industry. Another reason is the perceived fattiness of lamb as opposed to lean cuts of beef. On average lamb is slightly fattier, but as they are mostly grass fed, unlike most beef, the fats are better integrated and proteins are probably more nutritious. Lamb is also very rare in the US and has never been popular, probably because sheep don't like living in giant feedlots. China is the biggest lamb producer, followed by Australia, and little New Zealand now has six times more sheep than humans (down from twenty to one in 1982). Kiwi sheep usually live outside all year round, eating the well-watered grass, in a sustainable and comfortable existence until they get to four months and get the chop. If buying lamb, you may want to ask about its birthday. It will usually taste better if the lamb was raised outdoors, and if they spent their first two months in mid-winter, as this was usually inside in a barn. Lamb over a year old is called mutton, which has a very special flavour and was very popular (especially with my Australian mother), but needs time to cook, and with the modern generation unused to strong-tasting meat, is now increasingly hard to find.

Goat has been eaten across Southern Europe and North Africa for centuries, and was the most common religious sacrifice, hence the term scapegoat, and is still popular in certain cultures in stews, but as they don't like being enclosed they have largely escaped the horrors of mass production and herds are mainly used for milk and cheese, although goat curry is delicious and popular in Jamaican cuisine.

I was about sixteen when I first tasted horse meat. I only found out later, but while on holiday with a French family, if you ordered '*un burger*' and did not specify the animal, it had a good chance of being dead horse rather than beef. Later in Brussels I found restaurants and butchers who discreetly specialised in horse meat, which many locals preferred, particularly as a leaner form of raw steak tartare, which is also popular in Japan and many other countries. On a trip to a Kazakhstan food market, horse meat was the main flesh on offer and came in all forms and prices. Compared to beef, though slightly tougher, horse meat has much greater depth of flavour and with less fat, calories and risk of worms, is possibly healthier. Donkey was a popular French dish before World War Two and apparently the meat got less tough with ageing and is still found in some Italian salamis and sausages from Arles.

Most English-speaking countries have cultural taboos against eating horses, donkeys and other pets (as do Muslims and Jews), probably stemming from the working bond between them, just as some other countries have with camels. The Italians are still probably the biggest horse eaters in Europe, but as well as the French, Dutch, Germans and Scandinavians also partake. Horse meat consumption is slowly reducing in Europe and much is exported or used for dog food.

Rabbits and hares are a surprisingly tasty meat, especially in a traditional stew. The meat can be tough and has a strong flavour so cooking requires preparation and time. Ironically, rabbit and hare are perfectly sustainable and reproduce and grow so quickly, they don't really need intensive farming. Their meat is haem-iron rich, naturally lean and unlikely to be contaminated with dangerous pathogens. Unfortunately, bunnies are seen as too cute to eat, and instead they are hunted for sport or culled to keep numbers low.

Game meats, wild animal meats and other 'speciality' meats have a market and there are some passionate individuals trying to expand

our meat repertoire with foods such as ostrich, alligator and kanga-
roo. The biggest issue with wild meats, however, comes from human
populations encroaching on wild animal habitats and consuming
bush and other meats that have resulted in terrifying epidemics such
as Ebola and pandemics such as Covid-19. The more we continue to
steal space from animals, the more frequent these events become.

Reducing our meat intakes

As the data suggests, mortality is slightly increased in heavy red meat
eaters, and definitely higher in processed meat eaters, so it is sensible
to assume we are eating too much for our own good, either because
of something in meat itself, or because meat eaters generally eat less
of a variety of healthy vegetables. We have become so seduced by the
supermarkets and fast-food chains with their ultra-low-price mass-
produced meat that we now eat it daily, with little if any preparation
or thought and often no visual association with the animal it comes
from. In doing so we have forgotten how to eat a wider variety of
animals and different cuts of flesh and organs filled with nutrients.

As we saw in chapter 10, there is a growing market for alternative
meat. The UK chain Greggs introduced the vegan sausage roll as a
PR gimmick and it is now their biggest seller. The interest in using
insect protein (fed on food waste) to replace other animal-derived
proteins has shown that they provide high-quality protein with complete amino acid profiles which support muscle growth, and in a
completely sustainable way.[23]

We currently get about 20 per cent of our energy needs from animal protein, which is at least five times more than our ancestors. If
we are serious about sustainability, we can easily swap this protein for
legumes, nuts or insects. Around two billion people on the planet
exist without eating meat, so it is clearly not essential. Switching
from daily carnivores to weekly omnivores, and paying more for
higher-quality meat, may be a healthy option that will buy us some
more time. An even better case can be made for giving up low-quality
processed meats entirely.

Five meaty facts

1. There is little evidence that occasional good-quality meat consumption is associated with poor health outcomes.
2. On the other hand, cheap processed meat products are definitely bad for our health.
3. Reducing meat intakes, especially beef and lamb, can have major impacts on global warming and on your health if replaced with diverse vegetables.
4. Meat as we know it now has changed drastically since the mid-twentieth century. Modern intensive farming practices do not produce healthy, nutritious or ethical animal meat.
5. Meat alternatives and lab-based meats are part of our future.

21. Processed meats

Our ancestors invented what we now call meat processing as a way to preserve and enjoy all parts of an animal when meat was a very occasional treat. Certain cuts and leftover meat would be covered in salt, wrapped and left to dry in specific conditions where microbes, the salt and the air would allow the flesh to dry and be safe to eat for months to come before the next animal was killed – think freshly sliced jamon off the bone and dried salamis in mouldy white skins.

The WHO defines processed meat as 'having been cured, smoked or similarly treated to enhance preservation and/or flavour'. Man has been 'processing' meat by stripping cheap meat from the carcass, boiling it up and reconstructing it to have a new shape, with ingredients added to make them stick together and last for long periods as in sausages and haggis for centuries. Salt (sodium chloride) has been used on meat for thousands of years as a preservative, as has drying meat with heat to produce jerky, biltong or bresaola. Both salt and drying deprive microbes of moisture to feed on, but the salt also tenderises the meat and makes it translucent, and deters most microbes from hanging around.

By the Middle Ages an impurity in sea salt was found that improved meat even more. This was called saltpetre (a collective term for sodium and potassium nitrate mixtures), which was transformed by friendly bacteria into the active chemical sodium nitrite. The nitrite forms nitric oxide that binds to the iron in meat and so prevents the breakdown of fats (and the rancid smells). Combining with ripening *staphylococcal* bacteria on the meat surface, the newly formed nitric oxide keeps the muscle pigments a vibrant red or pink colour rather than an unappealing grey. So the combination of salt and nitrites has been used naturally for centuries in artisan meats; well before anyone worried about the potential risks of nitrosamines that are also produced when nitrites mix with other proteins (see page 38). Once these links between nitrites and microbes were discovered and understood, a leg of pork could be cured with salt for many months, with the help of microbes transforming bland flesh into an amazing complex array of fruity, smoky and savoury flavours and aromas.

Today the wonderful Jamon Iberico de Belota is cured for over eighteen months using ancient drying methods. Special black-footed pigs (*pata negra*) are weaned on a luxury diet and are free to roam eating acorns, chestnuts, roots and olives. Prosciutto di Parma is often made from older pigs fed on grain and whey from parmesan cheese. This small village pursuit has become big business, selling nine million ham legs a year and standards have slipped, with concerns over the distressing conditions the pigs are kept in. San Daniele ham is more delicate and its production is protected (DOP), meaning the pigs are a bit happier living and dying in the beautiful mountains of San Daniele, but it is harder to find. Nitrites are actually not essential to processing, and the top-end Italian Parma and San Daniele hams actually have little natural nitrites in them and are safe to eat. They have a different flavour and an even rosier colour than nitrite-rich Spanish and French hams, which also have their own unique flavours.

In artisan salamis, scraps of the less appealing parts of the meat (usually pork) are first chopped up and mixed with spices, seasoning and salt, then rolled up and put into a (cleaned) stretched animal's intestine (pork, sheep or ox depending on size) and allowed to dry in a special warm and airy space for several weeks, where the lack of moisture and salt will drive out unwanted microbes and encourage lactic acid-producing microbes. The kitchen where the sausages are prepared will naturally contain all the microbes needed to kick-start the process. After a few weeks, these microbes take over and become a stable community, breaking down and tenderising the meat and fat to provide a unique set of flavours. The drying and ripening process continues for a minimum of six weeks and often, for the higher-quality salamis, many months. The skin of the salami becomes colonised with a white fungal mould that adds further flavour and protection. Once in this stable state, the salami can last months or years. The microbes in each salami can vary enormously, and like cheese they all thrive in the acidic environment, although the actual bacteria, yeast and mould species (commonly penicillium) are different.

Modern processed meats

Newer techniques emerged from a need to preserve meat before fridges and times of hardship such as wartime with corned beef, spam or mortadella/bologna. And whilst artisanal slow-cured meats still exist, there is a new type of processed meat that replaces time and patience with many chemicals which, by now you'll know, is not a good idea for long-term health.

As mentioned earlier (see page 35), processed foods are designed to give a very consistent mouthfeel experience thanks to the destruction of the food matrix. People report that the smooth, non-chewy texture of a McDonald's cheeseburger is what makes it so delicious – and so much easier to eat two or three in one go. The same low-quality, highly processed meat can be found in 'readymade' shepherd's pies, lasagne, meat pizza toppings and other convenience foods. As we've seen, processed and pre-made food can contain some surprises (see page 34). Horse meat in burgers, pork meat in lamb curries and minced rats in special fried rice are all examples of real meat fraud which is worth millions and will likely continue when there's money to be made and long complex food webs.

In mass-produced salamis, saltpetre is now replaced by the active ingredient sulphite. Even within a distinct type of salami, industrial methods that use less salt encourage a very different community of bacteria and yeast to grow compared to the same salami made from traditional artisan methods.[1] The cheaper the product, the less time is taken; the expensive fermentation and drying step is sped up using a combination of higher temperatures, commercial bacterial and yeast starter cultures, and many more additives are needed to preserve it.[2] Cheap salamis are essentially ground-up meat and bits reconstituted to look like slices of traditional salami, lacking the more complex taste and texture of the purer simpler form. Real salami's only similarity to the plastic-wrapped 'salami' slices in the economy section of supermarkets is that they both contain pig DNA. An industrial salami can be made ready for eating in a few days, but remains sour and lacks any complexity, needing flavourings and powerful spices to disguise its shortcomings.

Bacon

The Brits alone eat 159 million kilos of bacon a year, and the smell of sizzling bacon is a real test of will, being made up of hundreds of volatile chemicals that make us hungrier. Bacon comes in many forms and names depending on the country and can be smoked or unsmoked. Most American bacon is what Brits call smoked streaky, with fatty streaks from the belly, while British back bacon is leaner from the loin or shoulder and can't be called bacon in the US. Most bacon is cured first by adding salt and nitrites and sometimes sugar, then undergoes various degrees of hot or cold smoking which combine on cooking to produce the multiple aromas. High-quality bacon is cured over several weeks or months and has pork, salt, nitrites and sugar as sole ingredients, but is only a tiny percentage of the market. Manufacturers use many tricks to produce cheaper copies including additional flavourings and colouring to recreate the authentic smoked bacon experience.

Cheaper industrial bacon is made in just a few days by dramatically speeding up the process, pumping the meat with water and adding salt and nitrites using micro-injections. Extra additives and preservatives such as ascorbic or citric acid to extend shelf-life are also needed, and phosphate and hydrocolloids like carrageenan or agar to retain water and give it a plump feel. Dried collagen protein is cheaper to substitute than meat protein and adds texture. Poor-quality bacon, which is often four times cheaper, is easy to spot: it will exude a milky moisture in the frying pan from the undissolved phosphate and extra water, which to some people tastes soapy. It will also have many extra ingredients, including ascorbates or erythorbate (used as a colour fixative) that tell you it was probably brine injected rather than cured traditionally – though this fact is strangely omitted on the label.

Some new 'healthy' bacon claims to be uncured to avoid the deadly nitrites; but if it's not cured, it is still pork and not bacon. Non-nitrate methods take longer and (as in Parma ham), have fewer ingredients, and may turn out in time to be healthier. Blind taste tests, as in other fields, can be counter-intuitive, and annoyingly show that some people prefer cheaper varieties. Your bacon preference will depend on your views on the health risks of nitrites, nitrosamines and other unknown chemicals, your genetic attraction to the cooked aroma, religion and views on animal welfare. Eating bacon is a very personal and individual choice.

Similarly, people who are used to eating reconstituted cooked ham or luncheon meat may not enjoy whole cooked and freshly sliced ham, which in comparison has much more texture, flavour and inconsistent mouthfeel.

Sausages

The British love their sausages. Over 85 per cent of Britons eat sausages at least monthly, and twice as many sausages as burgers are sold daily. Apart from ancient haggis, traditionally British sausages used to be 100 per cent raw meat, like French versions, until the mid-nineteenth century when cereals such as breadcrumbs were added. The key skill for each regional sausage-maker was picking the right meat and combination of spices (other than ubiquitous black pepper), as there is no fermentation or ripening process. Although high-quality products have over 90 per cent meat in them, with just added salt, sulphites, and bread or cereals, cheap supermarket versions have over twenty ingredients with around 50 per cent meat, with plenty of water and a whole range of chemicals to stop it leaching out. The skin of a cheap industrial sausage is usually made using synthetic cellulose derived from wood or cotton, or collagen from cattle hide, or sometimes polyethylene plastic, which needs to be peeled before eating. The high water content causes the sausages to aggressively spit in the pan, giving them the name 'bangers', so many people stab them while in the pan. If you have good-quality sausages, puncturing them will just lose flavour and moisture.

Cheap pork sausage meat is now a major source of human infection with a newly discovered virus called hepatitis E, which is only common in animals reared in cramped conditions. Globally, the WHO estimates there are 20 million infections with 3.3 million symptomatic cases and 44,000 deaths accounting for a 3.3 per cent mortality rate, which is higher than another well-known global virus causing headlines today, and most doctors (including myself) had not encountered it until recently.[3] While most infections are harmless and go unnoticed, they can cause rare but severe illnesses, such as liver failure, or arthritis. A medical colleague was infected recently and suffered from a rare neurological condition called Guillain-Barré that left him weak and unable to walk, forcing him to retire. This newly discovered virus was strange because the particular strain was very rare in the UK and not found in British pigs or meat. It was eventually traced to pork products from the Netherlands and Germany that were used for the sausages.

Chicken nuggets

Processed chicken started to take on the burger as a fast-food staple, thanks to companies like Kentucky Fried Chicken (KFC) founded by Colonel Harland Sanders who served pressure-cooker-fried (as opposed to deep-fried) chicken pieces in paper buckets. By 1963 they were the largest fast food company in the US, and are now a multinational corporation owned by PepsiCo. In 1981 the revolutionary Chicken McNugget appeared. The meat from our traditional Sunday roast became a cheap snack, and with consumers wanting more every year, the supply chain has struggled to keep up. The McDonald's concept was simple: deep-fry a boneless chicken and flash freeze it for reheating. A team of chemists came up with these 'not-so-simple' ingredients:

White boneless chicken, water, salt, seasoning (yeast extract, salt, wheat starch, natural flavoring, safflower oil, lemon juice solids, dextrose, citric), sodium phosphates. Battered and breaded with water, enriched flour (bleached wheat flour, niacin, reduced iron, thiamine mononitrate, riboflavin, folic acid), yellow corn flour, bleached wheat flour, salt, leavening (baking soda, sodium acid pyrophosphate, sodium aluminum phosphate, monocalcium phosphate, calcium lactate), spices, wheat starch, dextrose, corn starch. Prepared in vegetable oil (canola oil, corn oil, soybean oil, hydrogenated soybean oil) with citric acid as a preservative.

No one claims nuggets are good for you, and despite some cheap supermarket varieties having less than 50 per cent meat in them, they have a cult following as a comfort food and, unfortunately, children's food. This chicken is mechanically scraped off the bone with high-powered hoses and then essentially glued back together to resemble a piece of chicken. Some brands sell ultra-processed reconstituted and artificially flavoured chicken products as 'roo per cent chicken', which fools some shoppers into thinking their cheap texture-less chicken supper is actually quite wholesome whereas it is likely to have added, as a minimum, phosphates, potato starch and vegetable oils. It's not wholesome and like other highly processed foods, not associated with good health outcomes when consumed regularly.

Meat and cancer

At the end of 2015 an international committee of twenty-two scientists from a group called IARC produced a WHO badged report about red and processed meats that upset a lot of people. It said that all the evidence pointed to processed meat being a definite carcinogen, citing an 18 per cent increase in colon (bowel) cancer in people eating an equivalent of two rashers of bacon a day.[4] The group badged the chemicals in red and processed meats in the same category as cigarettes. Of course context as usual was missing. The cancer risk equivalent to daily smoking was eating around 100 rashers of bacon every day, or that smoking three cigarettes *a year* equated to the average cancer risk of an Italian meat eater.[5] So the 'bacon causes cancer' headlines should be taken with a large pinch of salt . . . But taking all the evidence together, it still suggests risks of increased mortality by eating heavily processed meats too often and when we choose our bacon, it's worth looking out for the better-quality option.

If we accept regular heavily processed foods and meats are bad for you, the conventional wisdom suggests this is mainly due to the extra amounts of fat and sugar. This now seems unlikely. The cheaper the product, the more chemicals and additives it contains. While an artisan product has four to five ingredients, a cheap one with proportionally less meat will have around twenty, including emulsifiers and two or more preservatives. These products are not officially regarded as dangerous based on the traditional safety tests on lab animals, but increasingly new studies show they can be harmful to our gut microbes, and so to us.

Common emulsifiers are detergent-like chemicals used to bind meat and sauces together in most processed foods, and they pass through the gut undigested. They are not friendly to our gut microbes as they prevent them communicating with each other and with the mucous layer of the gut that contains most of our immune cells. This leads them to produce abnormal chemicals causing metabolic problems such as obesity and diabetes and allowing nasty microbes to flourish.[6] Mouse studies have also shown that common emulsifiers like CMC and P80 cause low-level inflammation and long-term irritation of the gut lining, leading to increased risk of colon cancers.[7] None of these changes are massive or distinct in humans, but over time regular intakes of these substances in processed food could cause long-term shifts in our microbes that can account for the extra risk of heart disease and possibly cancer seen in epidemiology studies. Our gut microbes have a big influence on the pro-inflammatory chemical TMAO (see page 51), a natural by-product of L-carnitine digestion associated with a host of unpleasant diseases, largely dependent on our microbiome. Once again, the clear message is that eating a small quantity of quality meat with plenty of plants and fermented foods is the healthy approach.

Pet food, gummy bears and foie gras

Other highly processed meat products which are often ignored include pet food, gummy bears and foie gras. Though popular with different age groups and species, the production of these three foods has a very negative impact on the animals they derive from. Gelatine is extracted from cow and pig bones by boiling, drying and washing with a strong acid base to extract collagen. The result is the bounce in our gummy sweets and the wobble in our jelly, unless you opt for the 'veggie' version. The skincare collagen industry is also booming; offering brighter bouncier skin with collagen powders and pills, with little mention of the cow bones used to make it. Both pet food and collagen are discreet by-products of the meat and leather industry. Dogs can live without meat products so with some thought you could try to make your dog a reluctant vegetarian, but your cat won't survive the same experiment.

Foie gras is to many the epitome of unhealthy and cruel food traditions. Ducks and geese are overfed by 'gavage' (aka force feeding), in small-housed conditions for a miserable lifespan of 100 days, so their livers accumulate hugely unnatural amounts of fat and grow around ten times their natural size, to be served as a delicacy. Its popularity is declining in many countries, where a growing number have banned either production or imports. But in France they still love it and many farmers claim the ducks and geese enjoy the extra food.

Chewing the fat on processed meats

1. Regular processed-meat consumption is associated with increased heart disease and probably cancer.
2. Not all processed meats are the same; traditional methods are less likely to be harmful compared to modern fast methods using chemicals, emulsifiers and artificial flavours.
3. Ready meals, frozen nuggets and other meat products are made with poor-quality ultra processed meat.
4. Nitrites are not the main chemical to worry about: a cocktail of chemicals is what we need to avoid.
5. Beware buying '100% natural chicken breast': if it doesn't look like a part of the original animal, it's probably processed.

22. Fish

Why do we see fish meat as so different to mammal meat? Is it because it is hard to interact with fish and we don't raise them in the way we do mammals? Few religions have strict rules prohibiting fish, although Judaism bans some bottom-feeding (scavenger) fish, and shellfish as an afterthought. Fish are made of the same stuff as us, they bleed, have organs and four vestigial limbs and two eyes. They have a mixture of red and white muscle also made up of the same protein myosin as land animals, although it has a slightly different structure which we only really notice when it breaks down faster on heating, so is easily overcooked, at least in most British restaurants.

Many still eat fish and not meat for different reasons; including it being much healthier, or that fish don't feel pain, or it being sustainable if you are careful. These reasons are all becoming harder to justify. The traditional idea that fish feel no pain or stress when hooked or netted looks increasingly unlikely. Most experts now agree that fish have pain receptors (nociceptors) and react similarly to other small mammals in experimental conditions.[1] The Japanese believe fish feel pain and ensure that the finest tuna are killed instantly via a sharp spike into the brain and then the spinal cord (*ikejime* technique) to prevent unnecessary stress which they say devalues the meat. Most other countries' fishermen don't consider it, although most would dispatch a mouse or chicken more humanely. Crustaceans like lobsters and crabs certainly feel pain and several countries such as Switzerland have rules stating they must be killed or chilled in the freezer before they are boiled alive (Geneva Convention for Lobsters). While other shellfish such as mussels and oysters probably can't feel pain, squid and octopus (one of the most intelligent sea creatures) definitely do.

Recent evidence suggests that eating fish could be sustainable, but only if everyone worked together to preserve some key areas of marine coastline. This would increase biodiversity, improve the long-term yield and crucially secure all-important marine carbon stocks which suck carbon out of our overheated atmosphere, but currently only around 3–5 per cent of our seas are protected this way. In the meantime, eating fish can't be considered as a more environmentally friendly option than eating meat.[2]

Fish is supposedly good for us: it is lower in 'deadly' saturated fat than red meat, and has more of the healthy omega oils and vitamins like the 'sunshine' vitamin D. For several decades we have been preaching that fish is crucial for good brain development, helping children's education and avoiding heart disease. The current dietary recommendations in the UK, US and most countries say we should all eat two to three portions of fish per week. But telling people to eat two servings of fish every week is now equivalent to saying they should all drive two petrol cars. These targets are currently unachievable even with current stocks, and will be even more unrealistic as populations grow. Recent trips to restaurants in Greece and its idyllic islands bring home how bad the problem is. I found kitchen freezers full of frozen calamari and farmed prawns from Thailand, as the supply in the Med has largely run out and fishing boats are used mainly for tourist rides to another Blue Grotto.

Less than seventy years ago no one would have believed we might one day run out of fish. It was still common to see shoals of Atlantic fish miles wide and hundreds of metres deep, each producing thousands of eggs each that would ensure an everlasting supply. Yet since 1970, population growth has been outstripping fish production.

Europe now imports over 50 per cent of its fish and the US over 90 per cent, mainly from Asia. But these fish exporters won't be able to do that for much longer, as 90 per cent of the world's fish are now under threat of extinction. A third of our fish species are officially overfished and the other two-thirds are at capacity, and these figures ignore the 10–20 per cent of illegal catches. Billions of fish are killed inadvertently as collateral damage from industrial fishing using massive nets. Furthermore our own strict rules, preferences and supermarket demands mean that up to half of all fish caught and killed are thrown away.

Industrial-scale fishing with massive nets is destroying the ecological structure of the seabed, akin to deforestation on land. Atlantic salmon are no longer returning to Irish and Scottish rivers and are an endangered species. The British National dish used to be fish (fried in batter) and chips until overfishing of the previously plentiful cod and haddock stocks took their toll on supply and prices rocketed. The very British chicken tikka masala has now replaced it in popularity.

Fish farming

Most people don't realise that the majority of fish we now eat are farmed, but farmed fish overtook wild fish back in 2009, and continues to grow. Most of our salmon, trout, carp, tilapia, catfish, sea bass, sea bream, hake, prawns and shrimps are now produced this way, and the list is growing each year as the wild versions become rarer and more expensive. Cod is now being farmed despite it being a tough animal to cage; even the solitary octopus is being farmed in trials as it has become so expensive. But the more we farm fish the more we endanger the wild species, not just from rogue fish escaping and terrorising the locals, but from their carnivorous habits. Much of the fish feed comes ironically from killing other smaller fish like anchovies and sardines to add extra omega-3. As well as the ground-up smaller fish, they are fed fish oil, soy, GM yeast, chicken fat and sometimes ground-up feathers. To make farmed salmon look more like the wild pink salmon that naturally feed off shrimps, algae and krill, they are fed a pigment (astaxanthin), a synthetic version of the natural marine carotenoid that is sold as an antioxidant health supplement.

Aquaculture is under pressure to be more sustainable. In 2015 it took 1.3kg of wild fish to feed 1kg of farmed fish like salmon: a continuous 30 per cent net loss of fish. Activists claim the ratio is in reality more like 2.5kg to 1kg and point out that the 460,000 tonnes of fish food used in Scottish farms is equivalent to the whole UK population intake of fish in a year.[3] Fish farmers claim this is no worse than the ratios for pork (2.8kg) and industrial chicken farming (1.8kg).

Fish farms in countries like Norway and Scotland (also owned by Norwegians) say they are progressively trying to use less wild marine feed to reduce these negative ratios that will swiftly cripple our ocean ecosystems, but using land crops has similar problems. Other fish farms are less bothered as long as they are profitable.

As well as using up our natural resources, some intensively farmed fish should come with a health warning. Less well-monitored countries routinely use high levels of antibiotics to help growth and reduce infections in farmed salmon. Chile alone used 300,000kg of antibiotics in 2014 causing massive problems of microbial and antibiotic resistance, also affecting humans. A 2014 US study looked at antibiotic levels in twenty-seven fish samples from eleven countries, bought in Californian and Arizonan shops, including shrimp, tilapia, salmon, trout and catfish. Antibiotics were detected in 75 per cent of samples, including those labelled 'antibiotic free'. All levels were within the US legal limit, but as we have seen in mouse experiments these could still have an effect on human gut microbes, increasing obesity and allergy.[4,5]

Most reputable fish farms have stopped using antibiotics routinely, but a 2017 study has shown industrial fish feed could still be a hidden problem. Five mass-produced fishmeal products were tested from around the world and found to contain not only considerable levels of antibiotics but hundreds of antibiotic-resistant genes. The team showed that these antibiotics and genes can transfer from the feed to the fish and from there to humans.[6] This is because countries like Russia, China and Peru still use antibiotics to grow small fish for cheap fishmeal, and although the microbes are usually killed, their antibiotic-resistant genes can be transferred after death to other microbes. The sheer scale of farmed fish can also pose problems: 300,000 pacific salmon escaped recently from faulty cages in Puget Sound. As you can imagine this was a shock to the local fish, competing for the same resources, seeing swarms of dirty, lice-infested, disease- and antibiotic-ridden, hungry inmates invading your peaceful world.

Having millions of fish swimming in large cages in the sea may seem semi-natural until you think about getting rid of all that fish poo and chemical and antibiotic waste. To put this in some context, there are plans for Scotland to build the world's biggest fish farm which would produce more toxic and faecal waste than produced by the 600,000 humans of the city of Glasgow.

How fresh is your fish

I remember taking my children to fish trout from a farm, and they were gleefully pulling out a fish every five minutes (which I had to pay for), but these brown trout tasted dull and greasy. Farmed fish vary depending on conditions and the species, and taste-wise are not all bad. My local fishmonger says that most farmed sea bass are pretty good and consistent in taste, as the ocean-caught ones can be highly variable depending on what they have been eating, though the best wild line-caught sea bass always taste superior, as they will be less stressed and bruised than those brought up in a net. The quality comes at a price, which can be fivefold.

You should always try to smell the fish in a shop; it should smell mildly fishy when raw, with no sulphur or fruitiness. Freshly caught fish can also smell grassy or of herbs as they share similar unsaturated fats to plants. Fish and shellfish keep much longer if stored close to 0°C, and can be stored in a refrigerator surrounded by ice. Ocean fish usually smell and taste stronger than freshwater fish because they have an even greater concentration of amino acids than meat and many, like glutamate, provide a strong savoury flavour. Some fish – the shark, ray, cod and pollock families – have particularly high levels of TMA, an amine chemical synonymous with 'fishiness'. As we discussed earlier with animal meat (see page 246), microbes transform TMA to and from its oxidised form TMAO with different effects. In humans, people with high TMAO levels have higher risk of heart disease, but in live fish, it seems to be a healthy sign; in dead fish, the more TMAO is converted by microbes to TMA, the more putrid the smell of the fish. Acid in lemon or vinegar can reduce this decaying process, but we still don't know if these fishy chemicals have harmful effects in humans, other than just on our noses.

Salmon

Salmon today is the aquatic equivalent of chicken, officially the most popular fish eaten in the UK, and number two in the US. Atlantic salmon used to be caught wild in rivers and more often the sea in vast numbers during their 5,000-mile journey. Many local industries that survived on fishing and smoking have now gone extinct. Only thirty years ago, smoked salmon was a super luxury food, which many people couldn't afford, but now is sold at many corner shops like cheap ham. The reason for the plummeting cost is the threefold increase in production due to industrial farming on an enormous scale in the seas around Scotland, Norway, Canada and Chile, run by Norwegian or multinational companies. The good news is that most people can now afford to eat this fish regularly. Again, the bad news is this comes at a cost.

As the salmon are bred to above all eat and grow fast, they no longer resemble their wild cousins. They are caged close together swimming in circles, with lights controlling the seasons; infections are common and spread rapidly, causing many less regulated countries to use tonnes of antibiotics routinely. A previously rare parasite called the salmon louse has become a major pest, and has overrun an estimated 50 per cent of the 250 Scottish farms and many others worldwide. Lice can kill and severely injure the fish and currently are killing one in five, costing the industry over £1 billion a year. Control is difficult, as the lice are becoming resistant to all the antibiotics and pesticides thrown at them, so companies are now using hundreds of thousands of tonnes of hydrogen peroxide chemicals to control them, at considerable cost both financially and to the fish.

Moving the fish to colder deeper water with more space is not yet economical, but the Norwegian fish companies are now investing in giant offshore oilrig-like structures to house the fish. Keeping lice numbers down is the aim; legally the industry allows less than one louse per fish, but the average salmon in UK supermarkets now has over three and sometimes up to twenty lice, which we usually ingest. The industry tells us they are quite safe, as they are usually killed by further chemicals and pesticides, but eating dead lice as extra protein is no great consolation.[7]

The small fry

We are encouraged to eat other smaller oily fish such as mackerel, herring, sardines, anchovies and sprats that have reduced in popularity, and are used mainly as feed in fish farms for larger fish, or for animal feed to supply valuable omega-3 oil to replace pasture grass. There are plenty of mackerel in the Atlantic; sailing in Devon the shoals are so numerous I've seen the fish jumping into the boat without any hooks. Those sights will become a rarity. Mackerel contains more total fat and as much saturated fat (around 4 per cent) as rump steak, with the same protein content. Anchovies are a fish I thought were only used as a pizza topping, until I spent time writing this book in the Costa Brava in the Bay of Roses where I swam most days surrounded by thousands of anchovies that grew bigger over the summer. These are a local delicacy grilled fresh with olive oil and lemon, or marinated and canned. Sardines can be similarly nutritious and delicious as an alternative to tinned tuna. In other parts of the world these smaller oil-rich fish are becoming endangered, as industrial fishing hoovers them up for use as animal feed, destroying much of the seabed in the process. This has risks for our planet, as many regard these fish as keystone species as they eat plankton.

Plankton is the water equivalent of grass and converts sunshine into energy (and omega-3 oils). To enter our food chain, plankton requires small fish like anchovies to eat it, who then get eaten by larger fish, which we then eat. Small fish often get preserved in tins. The canning process has been discussed elsewhere (see page 68), but is quite safe for most fish, either stored in water, brine or oil. Most sardines and tuna are sold in this way worldwide, with no major loss of nutrients, or extra risks of toxins or contaminants compared to fresh or frozen fish. As the tinned fish lasts over a year, there is much less risk of food waste and a tin of anchovies or mackerel in the cupboard can be a perfect foundation for a tasty meal.

Brain food?

The meta-analyses summarising the many randomised clinical studies have shown no consistent supplement effect on children's brain function, yet omega-3 supplements remain heavily marketed at children in our pharmacies today.[8] I used to vainly try to force my non-fish eating son Tom to take omega-3 to help him at school. (I learned much later that he had been spitting out the fishy capsules and hiding them in a large soggy pile at the back of a kitchen drawer, proving he was more intelligent than me.) The Norwegians are keen to push the benefits of oily fish rather than supplements, but their own trials of 214 preschool kids given either mackerel or herring instead of meat for four months failed to find any improvements in cognition.[9] So unless you are pregnant, the evidence of a protective effect for omega-3 supplements is non-existent, and shouldn't be routinely recommended.

Fish, longevity and health

Even if it were sustainable, should we be eating two portions of fish a week as recommended to make us live longer? *National Geographic* photos of smiling 110-year-olds eating sushi in Southern Japan have distorted our view of the benefits of fish. For years, the type of fat oil produced naturally both by fish and animals eating grass has been cherished, and omega-3 supplements are taken by about 10 per cent of Americans and about one in five Britons, being their commonest supplement. It is widely recommended to prevent heart problems or cancer for people who find it hard to eat their two portions of fish per week. But data is strangely not as good as people think: the latest studies and massive clinical trials did not show any strong benefits.[10]

The benefit of fish eating is hard to determine from epidemiology studies: a large observational study of 500,000 Europeans followed for fifteen years found no overall benefit on mortality, but a suggestion that excessive consumption may actually increase mortality slightly.[11] A recent summary of all the twenty-nine studies performed to date (with all the caveats) showed a very modest 7 per cent reduction in mortality per weekly portion (compared to a 24 per cent for nuts).[12] A 2018 US meta-analysis looking at only the large high-quality studies lasting over a year was even clearer: there was no effect whatsoever of supplements on risk of heart disease or stroke, and they should not be recommended.[13] Independent reviews have found no significant benefits for other common uses such as in treating dementia or cognitive decline, or osteoarthritis.[14,15] For a whole year, fish-loving journalist and marine ecologist Paul Greenberg ate every kind of fish and marine life he could find for virtually every meal, hoping he could show all those nutrients and omega-3s would make him super healthy. After this enormous effort, he saw healthy Japanese or Mediterranean levels of omega-3 in his blood, and expected to be brainier and healthier, but was disappointed.[16] The only change he saw was in his blood pressure, which was in the wrong direction. As a final nail in the proverbial coffin, Cochrane published a statement in 2018 to confirm that the effects of omega-3 supplements has been overhyped and that the nut-derived ALA may be just as efficient in providing benefits.[17]

One group of people do seem to benefit from Omega-3 supplementation, though. A Cochrane review synthesising evidence from seventy randomised, controlled trials of omega-3 fatty acid supplementation during pregnancy showed that it reduced the risk of preterm birth by 11 per cent and early preterm birth (before 34 weeks) by 42 per cent.[18]

So, the evidence for eating whole fish to benefit our health is still weak, although many fish-eating populations look healthy, particularly if combined with a Mediterranean or Asian diet. We can't yet rule out individual differences that provide benefits in some people that could depend on their unique microbes and whether they like fish or not. In 2017, Ana Valdes and Cristina Menni from my team looked at blood levels of fish oils in 850 of our adult twins and found that people with higher omega-3 levels from fish had healthier gut microbes and lower blood pressure.[19] This worked by an indirect mechanism, whereby in people with large numbers of *Lachnospiraceae* microbes, eating fish produced a metabolite (N-carbonyl glutamate, or NCG) in their guts which acts on blood vessels. In the future we may be directly ingesting the actual metabolite that microbes produce, (known as 'postbiotics') and cut out the fish. This mechanism may go some way in explaining the observation of fish-eating nations having more healthy life years.

If we accept that real fish oils like omega-3 may be beneficial for some of us, and supplements fail because they probably lack some other key ingredients, which fish should we eat for health? While wild salmon has very high levels of omega-3, some farmed salmon has even higher levels, as do small oily fish like mackerel, herring and anchovies. At the other end of the scale, scallops, shrimp, cod, haddock and tilapia have low levels, and tuna is intermediate and highly variable, so not a reliable source. The closer the fish are to the source of the original nutrients in plankton, the healthier they are for us, so it is probably better to eat small fish that eat plankton directly rather than eating the fish that feed off them naturally or via artificial feed. This food chain principle is the same for nutrients in all animals, but how do you really know what fish you are eating?

Fishy labels

Labelling fish is a major global problem, and we can be easily fooled. Some fish names are entirely fabricated to sound better to gullible consumers. Pacific rock fish, for example, is a previously discarded fish with no name, and the ugly Patagonian toothfish, which used to be rejected, was a runaway success when rechristened Chilean sea bass in the 1990s. Rebranding is one thing, and if it serves to make discarded fish edible, can be beneficial, but deliberate fraud is different.

As discussed (see page 271), fake fish is big business. A global report of fifty-five countries and 25,000 samples suggested the problem affected one in five fish sold, with 58 per cent of substitutes being cheaper, potentially harmful fish like Asian catfish or escolar. In Italy, 82 per cent of grouper, perch and swordfish sampled were switched for a cheaper, often endangered species; in Belgium and Germany, most bluefin tuna and sole sold was actually something else.[20] In the UK, expensive cod for fish and chips is often replaced by cheaper pollock, and in a Los Angeles survey using DNA testing between 2013 and 2015, half of raw fish in sushi was mislabelled, with snapper and halibut swapped for cheaper flounder, often without the restaurateur's knowledge.[21]

Tuna is a particular problem because of the demand and high prices at the top-end. US surveys reported over 70 per cent of sushi tuna was fake, and the use of 'white tuna' is common in restaurants. The problem is that white tuna doesn't actually exist, and is usually escolar, a cheap fish nicknamed 'ex-lax' for its effects on the gut, that are so bad it is banned in Japan and Italy.[22] A bycatch of tuna fishing are dolphins, who often get thrown back in the water maimed or dead. FSC-certified tuna and dolphin-friendly tuna makes it more likely your tuna sandwich isn't a complete environmental and ethical disaster (though is far from foolproof). Unless you know your fish or sushi restaurant well, and you are worried about mercury, it may be best to skip the tuna. I have swapped my tuna mayo sandwiches for an equally satisfying and nutritionally superior chickpea rye sourdough version. Smash some tinned chickpeas with the back of a fork adding lemon juice, caraway seeds, spring onions, garlic salt and mayo. Add some torn nori sheets for extra flavour. Sliced celery adds some extra crunch.

Raw fish

Raw fish meat is easier to eat than that of land dwelling animals because of the effects of gravity; fish don't need as rigid a structure as they are floating in water and their muscle fibres are softer, with less connective tissue to keep the strands together. This is why fish can easily be overcooked and dry, and a thin fillet can be adequately cooked in a minute.

The Japanese have been eating raw fish in the form of sushi or sashimi for centuries, and the Peruvians and Chileans have been marinating 'ceviche' without major health problems just as long. There are slight risks of ingesting parasites, but the risk is much smaller than with undercooked meat. Sushi was originally used as a way of preserving fish by wrapping it in salt and rice, allowing microbes to ferment and protect it from going rancid, and has slowly evolved to the global business we see today.

Unlike raw meat, it is easier to digest raw seafood safely and extract most of the nutrients. Knowing the best fish to eat and the best cuts to pick are an art in themselves. On a recent trip to the Northern Japanese Island of Hokkaido, I realised how sushi can be taken to a totally new level. We tasted the most delicate mouth-melting fatty tuna that has unfortunately spoilt me forever.

The Japanese pride themselves on knowing the origin of each fish and the wholesaler, so reducing risks of infections, which still occur but are rare. In Japan, there is a heated debate over whether fish should be frozen first, with sushi masters saying it ruins the texture. In Europe and the US this is mandatory as freezing kills off common parasites, such as *anisikid* worms which cause thousands of gastric incidents in Japan each year, due directly to the worm or an allergy to it. Japanese scientists used tasting panels to see if there was a consistent difference between frozen or fresh mackerel and squid sushi (which are commonly infected) using about 300 samples and forty medical students. Most people couldn't detect a difference. The Dutch also traditionally eat raw herring but the EU made it compulsory to freeze it first, presumably not altering its taste, but reducing infections.

Fish fingers

For many of us born after 1955, our first taste of fish is likely to have been Captain (Clarence) Birdseye's Frozen Fish Fingers. The UK, where they really took off, still consumes 1.5 million daily. They are made from large frozen blocks of whitefish, and so well disguised that, according to a 2017 British Nutrition Foundation survey, one in five UK adolescents (in a credit to our education system), believe they are made of chicken. Most fish fingers do contain real fish, although cod is often substituted for pollock or coley (which can taste fine), and are often sold as more exotic, and expensive, fish goujons. As prices have increased, the fish content has dropped and now varies from 50–70 per cent, with breadcrumbs, batter and filling making up the rest, but they are still the commonest form of fish eaten in the UK and are big sellers in Australia where New Zealand hoki is used.

Heavy metals

Yet another problem is heavy-metal contamination of fish. Chemicals like cadmium, lead and particularly mercury, from many different industrial processes using rocks or minerals, leak into rivers and oceans, and into the fish, then into our gut. For most people, the risk from heavy-metal toxicity by eating fish and shellfish may not be a major health concern, but some fish and shellfish contain much higher levels of mercury, a potent neurotoxin that in high levels may harm an unborn baby or young child's developing nervous system. In adults, severe mercury toxicity can also cause accelerated cognitive decline. So, did my hospital canned tuna sandwiches make me healthier or has it hastened dementia? Finland has the highest rates of dementia in the world and they eat a lot of fish compared to most countries, but they also have long dark winters and a very high rate of depression and suicide. This has led to a theory that high mercury levels due to fish eating and industrial exposure have combined with certain nerve toxins (BMAA) produced by deadly blue algae floating on lakes to create 'the perfect storm' to increase dementia. It is a nice headline-grabbing theory but just lacks good data to support it.

Apart from a few extreme publicised cases, the data on the real dangers of fish mercury poisoning is largely circumstantial and as an average fish eater it is hard to know how much to worry, or what types to eat. In general, larger fish like yellowfin tuna, shark, marlin, halibut or swordfish that live a long time and eat lots of other fish, have high levels of mercury, which transfer when eaten to humans. Fancy executive health checks now often include testing for heavy metals, and a friend of mine with high blood levels was told to cut back on tuna and eat smaller fish. But the problem is that these new blood tests are much more sensitive than ten years ago, making us think that heavy metal contamination is increasing, when perhaps we have always had these same results.

The data on risks in humans is patchy and despite over thirty studies implicating many diseases, the results are so far inconclusive.[23] The US FDA decided in 2016 that the potential benefits of eating canned tuna (apparently improving IQ!) for the American population, including pregnant women, far outweighed any risks of mercury toxicity.[24] We also found in our twins that blood levels of lead and cadmium are influenced to some extent by our genes, so levels normally vary between people. While it is wise for pregnant women to avoid eating lots of tuna or marlin sandwiches as the mercury is likely to accumulate in their developing baby, the evidence for harm in the rest of us is still unclear, provided we have a varied diet with only occasional fish suppers. Reducing our intake of long-lived wild fish would undoubtedly help make them more sustainable.

*

If you like eating fish, try to vary the species you consume, and where possible choose fish that are sustainable, preferably small, low in antibiotics and mercury and high in nutrients. Eating more of the fish that we currently kill for fish farms makes more ecological sense and should be healthier. If picking sustainable fish in your area is a tough task labels like the Marine Stewardship Council (MSC) and websites can help inform your choices, though there are some problems with these labels, as we have discussed (see page 278).[25] Thinking more widely about the ocean environment is vitally important. The amount of plastic added to existing waste each year, whether in sealed landfills or strewn across land and sea, could more than double to 380 million tonnes by 2040 if we don't do something. By then,

around 10 million tonnes of this could be in the form of microplastics, which we could end up eating.

While the health benefits of fish have been overstated, if you enjoy
it as I do, simply replacing farmed meat with farmed fish would be a
mistake. Once again, paying more and eating less makes sense for better quality and the environment. Without the promised major health
benefits of fish, we have to think more about enivronmental, ethical
and sustainability concerns.

Five fishy facts

1. Unless you are pregnant or recovering from a heart attack,
   overhyped omega-3 is not a useful supplement.
2. Half the fish we buy is fake, so check the origin and invest in
   good quality.
3. Eating two portions of fish per week is not needed for health
   and is not sustainable.
4. Most fish we buy are farmed fish that use twice as many
   smaller fish to grow so are an environmental and ethical
   disaster. Use accredited labels and websites to help you
   choose wisely.
5. Fish stocks will run out in most parts of the world within
   twenty years if we continue to fish at the current rate.

23. Marine bugs and
other seafood

The marine equivalent of insects are the crustaceans like lobsters, shrimp and crabs. These sea bugs were once deemed as inedible as woodlice and in Maine before the 1870s, lobsters were so numerous that they littered the beaches in huge piles, fed only to servants, or to prisoners as a punishment. There was enormous stigma attached to eating them, which explains many names for forms of lobster or crayfish around the world, such as Moreton Bay Bugs or Balmain Bugs in Australia, which have only recently become a delicacy. Lobsters have become big business, and the big ones fetch big money. As usual, however, the more delicate flavoursome protein comes from the smaller animal. The best lobster flavours also come from the Maillard reaction where sugars and amino acids meet, which can occur at lower temperatures in lobster than with meat, if it is cooked rapidly. Most Maine and European lobsters can't be farmed intensively as they like to eat each other, but increasingly farms in places like Cornwall and Tasmania are learning how to economically grow different, more peaceful species.

Shrimps (often used interchangeably with prawns that are usually larger) are the favourite seafood in the US where the average American eats over 2kg a year and where 99 per cent are low-quality imports from farms in India, China, Vietnam, Thailand and Indonesia. To preserve the colour before packaging, sodium bisulphite is added, and if pre-peeled, as in cheap ham, tripolyphosphate is added to retain water and increase the price. The only way to tell if your shrimps are chemical free is to read the label, and try to buy raw shell-on ones that are less likely to have been tampered with.

In Asia, mangroves are being destroyed at a frightening rate to make way for massive seafood farms with little pesticide or environmental controls. Many farms are abusing their workers, often in servitude as well as the animals: cutting out the eyes of female prawns so they spawn faster, and killing them with chlorine. To raise 1kg of farmed shrimp it takes around 2kg of wild fish feed, salvaged from bottom trawling that destroys everything, including millions of turtles.

Organic farmed prawns are more expensive, around 12 per cent smaller, and they still use fish food, but if strictly controlled should use no chemicals, antibiotics or pesticides and be slightly better for the environment. At the other end of the scale, fresh wild prawns or shrimp from many places in the Mediterranean or the Gulf of Mexico can taste marvellous, although at ten times the price: probably what we should be paying for these rare treats to conserve the seabed.

Molluscs are the general term for animals with a shell, like snails, clams and oysters, or which once had a shell, like slugs, squid and octopus. Scampi and chips is a classic British pub dish and most British people believe that scampi swim happily in the sea. In fact they were created in a food lab as a mix of deep-fried breadcrumbs and unwanted langoustine tails (also called Dublin Bay prawns) in the 1960s. Now the cheaper varieties of this ultra-processed food contain very little, if any, langoustine and are mainly scraps of other white fish like the tasteless Vietnamese pangasius catfish, bound together with a dozen other chemicals, flavourings and dyes and moulded to make them look like real prawns.

Crabs are clever crustaceans that can detect when another crab is sick; unfortunately for the Atlantic Horseshoe species, their blue blood saw them harvested for Covid-19 vaccines as it contains a unique protein to detect bacterial contamination. Crab sticks contain no crab and are just fake, dyed, mashed, malleable farmed white surimi fish with crab flavourings and chemicals.

Scallops are harder to fake and are found across the world in cold waters and if fresh can be eaten raw or fried briefly for a minute each side. Because scallops are often taken from their shell, restaurants often pretend they are from more expensive varieties such as king scallops rather than cheaper Japanese varieties. The main problem with them is that most are gathered by dredging the sea bottom, which as discussed destroys the ecosystem for decades. Although this practice should be widely banned, only Norway has to date done so. The solution is to pay more for diver-caught scallops or source them from increasing numbers of reputable farms such as in Loch Fyne, which are potentially sustainable.

Plastic fish and molluscs

Many common fish we eat are now full of plastic microparticles. In one study, 73 per cent of deep-living (mesopelagic) Atlantic fish, which bigger fish like tuna feed off, had significant levels of plastic, especially sea bass and mackerel.[1] Molluscs like mussels, clams and oysters also ingest microplastic; they are bi-valves, that naturally filter our water and pick up the sediment they can't break down, and unlike fish which we would normally cut open and gut, when we eat them, we also eat their intestines.[2] Just six oysters can contain around fifty plastic particles, and mussels likely contain more. The Spanish eat the greatest volume, but Belgians eat the most molluscs per capita of any country with 'moules frites' (mussels and chips) being the national dish, so may be ingesting 11,000 plastic microparticles per year.

We know virtually nothing of the potential risks of humans accumulating plastic in our intestines, but we do know more how our gut microbes will respond. Research on mice fed microplastics have shown that the microbes change to become more inflammatory and with a poorer immune response.[3] What we don't know is whether the microplastics or even the smaller nano plastics we eat are more harmful than the many plastic fragments already in the air we breathe. One scientist estimated that we breathe the equivalent of a credit card of plastic into our lungs each year; a 2022 report confirmed that in eleven out of thirteen people having surgery, plastic was detected in the deep part of the lungs.[4]

Global warming is controversial if you are a politician, but a harsh reality if you are a mollusc like an oyster or other crustacean. As the oceans absorb more carbon dioxide, the water becomes more acidic and oysters become less fertile. Plankton microbes may be the only long-term survivors, as this reduction in molluscs is bad news for everyone else – they act as efficient cleaning systems for our oceans, which we certainly need more of, rather than single-use plastic.

Casanova health food

Oyster-eating has been common for as long as 20,000 years, according to some archaeological studies of Australian aborigines, and the Romans farmed them on the coasts of Britain, where they became a popular food for the masses. In mid-nineteenth-century London, the fish market sold 500 million oysters a year until gradually stocks became depleted and costs increased. They are a great source of protein and several vitamins, including zinc. French doctors still prescribe oysters as a natural way to replace vitamin deficiency – even in kids. Two to four oysters give you your daily B12 needs, as well as some iron, calcium, zinc and magnesium. They, like other seafoods, are full of (harmless) cholesterol.

It is unclear if our ancestors thought these slippery creatures were just tasty and nutritious, or had extra aphrodisiac properties. In many Latin-based languages the words for shellfish are generally affectionate, if crude, terms for the female genitalia, suggesting the physical resemblance led to the global food association. Casanova reportedly regularly breakfasted on five dozen oysters to improve his performance before his reported 122 amorous conquests, and oyster sales still peak around St Valentines' Day in many countries.

Although scientists have tried and failed to show these aphrodisiac benefits of shellfish, other websites still pronounce as fact the libido-enhancing effects of mussels and oysters, claiming the zinc in oysters can help in the manufacture of testosterone. Zinc is found in soil, but this doesn't make mud an aphrodisiac. These stories show our gullibility and the power of the 'placebo' or, more likely, the actual sensual tactile experience of slurping a slimy creature into your mouth, that possibly lab animals don't experience.

Oysters, clams and mussels are good examples of 'natural' unprocessed food that needs little preparation, and can be eaten raw or simply cooked. Whereas mussels or clams are nearly always steamed for a few minutes, most people prefer raw oysters. This is as close as you can get to tasting the ocean, and if eaten close to the sea you can pick up not only a metallic taste of the local sea minerals, but all kinds of volatile taste and flavour molecules that overlap with those found in cucumbers, mushrooms, or even lemons. The longer after harvesting you wait, even if kept on ice, the more the flavour changes to a fishy aldehyde smell, then the microbes will break down the protein to produce nasty sulphur odours.

Eating oysters can sometimes be risky. Each year the newspapers pick up on some unfortunate individual who actually died, like the 2018 report of a Texan woman who visited Louisiana and ate two dozen Gulf oysters and succumbed to a 'flesh-eating microbe' that attacked the skin on her legs. But she also may have caught the microbe not by eating anything, but by wading in the stagnant water with small cuts on her leg while she was crabbing. Two particular microbes are a real problem: *E.coli*, which causes gut infections and food poisoning, and the *Vibrio vulnificus* bacteria, cousin of the nasty bug that causes cholera. These bacteria often get into the water by faecal contamination with sewage or after storms, the oyster then filters them through its system, increasing the concentrations, causing infection in the person who eats it. There are an estimated 84,000 infections reported annually in the US and around ten deaths on average; the CDC records thirty-five global deaths per year but there is a reported increase of the bacteria even in the UK's waters due to increasing water temperatures which may lead to more infections.[5]

Molluscs are also susceptible to viruses like humans, particularly during epidemics like with the norovirus, and while their primitive immune systems can resist low levels, they can become overwhelmed. In 2009 the famous Michelin three-starred restaurant, The Fat Duck in England had a norovirus outbreak in its popular shellfish dishes causing 500 cases, and had to close temporarily.

To reduce your risks, it is important to know the source of the oysters or mussels, as well as having confidence in the fishmonger or restaurant. The risks are commoner in estuaries and in the US increases with water temperature, especially at over 26°C in warmer months. Most areas are monitored weekly for bacterial levels of *E.coli* and *Vibrio* as well as unusual blooms of algae that can cause sickness. Once harvested oysters are usually purged: kept for two days in fresh seawater tanks and blasted with ultraviolet radiation which kills most bacteria (but not viruses). Connoisseurs believe purging reduces the special ocean flavours of oysters, a bit like pasteurising cheese or milk. Oysters, if clean, can keep in the refrigerator for up to a couple of weeks, but (like mussels) will die if immersed in fresh water and don't do well if frozen.

To reduce risk, many people discard oysters and mussels that are hard to open. The general rule on never eating molluscs that do not open on heating comes from mussels. This is actually a cooking myth started by the great British food writer Jane Grigson in her 1973 *Fish Book*, and the rule spread rapidly around the world. An Australian biologist Nick Ruello challenged this by cooking thirty batches of mussels and found that on average one in nine failed to open on cooking. It transpired that 100 per cent of these reluctant molluscs were fine to eat when opened with more force, with no 'off' taste or sign of infection. He put this down to differences in the muscle structure keeping the shells closed. This powerful myth causes mussels and many other molluscs like clams to be regularly overcooked, or unnecessarily wasted. Another saying is to avoid eating shellfish when there is an 'R' in the month. Although local deviations may apply, this originates not from the risk of infection, but from the reproductive cycle of the oyster and mussel, which use their energy and resources in summer for breeding and so reducing their plump flesh. So unless the seawater gets much too hot, the R rule is nowadays more an individual matter of taste.

The Spanish, French and Italians love raw sea urchins, and they are a sushi delicacy in Japan, but faint-hearted Anglo-Saxons find them too slimy, and in Maine the locals politely call them 'sea whores'. Jellyfish are predators who aren't technically fish and should be called just jellies. In Asian cuisine jellies are a delicacy – often prepared by a highly trained 'Jelly master' who removes any toxins – and can be served dry, salted, or sliced and raw in a vinaigrette or hundreds of other variations. I tried some pickled diced jellies in Shanghai, but my untrained taste buds failed me. I could be wrong but don't think eating jellyfish will save the planet, although with global warming they may well take over the world.

We are less squeamish about eating fish eggs; sturgeon's eggs in particular or caviar. Beluga caviar comes from the Caspian Sea and costs up to $7,000 a kilo, and if it comes from the rare mutated albino sturgeon fish, can fetch over £20,000 per kilo if the eggs are large. These long-lived fish are massive and can grow up to 900kg, making them susceptible to overfishing and pollution. Because of the prices caviar fetches, beluga fish are now an endangered species, leading to bans in many countries. How caviar became a delicacy is unclear, but beluga sturgeon used to be common in European rivers and in the fourteenth century even the English royal family were impressed enough to give it 'royal fish' status, so they could claim any sturgeon caught in English waters as theirs. To extract the precious eggs, the old female sturgeon is first caught and sedated, then her ovaries and the roes are removed. Other farmers use small incisions so that the female can keep producing. The eggs are then washed and salted either in a raw state to retain the delicate flavours and textures, or pasteurised to reduce the complexity but give it greater shelf-life.

Because of the bans, high prices and overfishing, industrial caviar farming has taken over in many countries from Canada to China and Saudi Arabia, producing millions of tons per year. As well as farmed versus wild caviar, there are many cheaper versions, using related or hybrid sturgeons, or those that produce smaller, less shiny eggs, or simply using the roe from cod or salmon. There are also vegan imitations using seaweed. Naturally where prices are high, food fraud is rife, and it is easy to substitute cheap eggs for the real thing. Bulgaria and Romania have access to rare wild caviar from the Black Sea and the Danube river, and all caviar should carry a clear label of origin, wild or farmed, and the species. Of twenty-seven samples tested genetically, only ten were accurately labelled, seven were completely fake, not even containing fish, many were lumpfish, and four contained illegal wild caviar.[6] So buying expensive caviar is a bit like Russian roulette. If you are an average oligarch, and eat a tablespoon of real caviar regularly for breakfast, the good news is you will be getting your daily ration of vitamin B12 and plenty of protein. The bad news is that if it's wild, you will absorb heavy metals like mercury which could make you forget where you left your money.

Fermenting fish

Deliberately infecting fish with microbes is a traditional way to make inedible or toxic fish digestible and long-lasting. The most famous fermented fish is *harkarl* Icelandic fermented shark, supposedly introduced by the Vikings, which is normally inedible because of the high levels of urea and harmful TMAO (see page 51). If you fancy preparing your own to impress the neighbours, simply get some Greenland shark from your fishmonger, ask them to behead and gut it, then place it in a sandy pit in the ground for about three to four months, dig it up, slice it into strips and hang to dry in your shed for another few months. Then simply cut it up into cubes and serve on cocktail sticks. If your guests are after a unique experience, they won't be disappointed. Even Gordon Ramsey had to spit it out, and the hardened chef and food writer the late Anthony Bourdain described it as 'the single worst, most disgusting and terrible tasting thing' of his career. It's the overpowering, rotten smell and ammonia that most people can't stand, although some aficionados can detect pleasant umami and complex nutty notes.

While on a book tour in Sweden, I was given some fermented herring (*surströmming*) to take home, which is prepared much the same way but with brine. What they didn't tell me was that the smell is so overpowering that if you open it inside your house, the stench can last for years. I also could have been arrested or even died. I had taken it as cabin baggage and had the tin exploded in the aircraft, the smell in the confined space would have incapacitated the crew before we plunged to our deaths. Anyway, I made it back alive with my tin that was bulging ominously, and left it safely in the garden. Two years later I had forgotten about it until some builders thought they had damaged the sewers, and after fleeing returned to find the punctured tin under some earth. Pickled herring in vinegar, on the other hand, is quite pleasant as is the less common smoked herring, and they both offer plenty of omega-3 and protein.

Seaweed

One sure way to combat the effects of global warming and dwindling fish stocks is to grow more algae (aka seaweed), although seaweed is usually a mixture of algae and fungi. I learnt recently that some of my Australian ancestors were originally kelp farmers on the Isle of Skye, who sold most of their stock to France in the nineteenth century, before the soap and glass manufacturers they supplied collapsed. Seaweed and algae reduce carbon dioxide and acidification and are a good sustainable supply of nutrients, and like molluscs are as close as it gets to taste the ocean. Only thirty-five countries grow their own seaweed for eating, which is now a growing multi-billion-dollar industry projected to reach $30 billion by 2025. As with land plants they are all constantly eaten by marine life, and have built up a wide range of chemical defences, including chlorine, sulphur, iodine and bromine that provide their smells. It has been a delicacy in Asia since ancient times, and even the sixth-century monk St Columba on the lonely isle of Iona was partial to a seaweed snack providing polyphenols and antioxidants, and iodine to prevent goitre. The Irish have been adding it to porridge and puddings for centuries, and the Welsh to oats to make laverbread. As well as being farmed for food, seaweeds are used to produce sticky 'natural' hydrocolloids as additives in processed foods. They are widely promoted as being healthy based on their ingredients rather than any good human data.[7]

Seaweed comes in four main categories: green algae (e.g. sea lettuce), brown algae (kelp or wakame used in miso), red algae (laver or nori used for sushi) and blue-green algae (spirulina). They are mainly composed of water, but have plenty of protein, fibre, carbohydrates and some saturated fats as well as antioxidant polyphenols and a range of important minerals such as calcium, magnesium, iron, selenium and most of the vitamins (A, B, C, D, E, K). The Japanese, Koreans and Chinese have been cultivating and eating seaweed for centuries, with the Japanese eating over 5kg per person annually.[8] Some of their health and longevity may be due to the fibre and nutrients in the algae. They eat it in many forms; from food wrapping, sushi, in basic dashi sauces or in soups, but like all humans Japanese people only have about twenty natural gut enzymes to break down these complex carbohydrates, so are only able to digest the complex structures of the algae and extract all the nutrients and polyphenols when they become 'infected' with the right gut bugs: a special strain (*B. Plebeius*) with an algae-digesting gene that normally lives in the sea. One day this hopped into their intestines carried on some other algae-eating fish and transferred its genes to its cousins in their gut. It now lives in Japanese colons and waits for its daily dose of seaweed.

While many fish-loving Spaniards living near the coast seem to also have the special microbe gene, most land-dwelling Europeans and Americans have yet to acquire it, but the more we eat seafood and algae the more likely we are to get 'infected'. Recent studies show that there are many other marine bacteria feeding off algae that readily transfer their genes to human gut bugs, thus allowing them to ferment and digest rare foods and 'capture' this new niche market. This is the perfect symbiotic relationship, as the rare microbe gets to populate the gut, and the human can benefit from the nutrients and the extra microbe diversity. So even if we don't like sushi, we should all suck on a piece of seaweed every now and then to reconnect with the oceans and improve our diversity. An alternative is to buy seaweed products which resemble pasta in texture. I make this seaweed pasta together with traditional linguine and sauté the lot with some fresh cherry tomatoes, fresh parsley, lots of EVOO and garlic for a delicious, cruelty-free sea-flavoured meal with a dampened glucose spike thanks to the added fibre.

Some special much-hyped algae-like supplements like spirulina (whose proper name is *Arthrospira*, a cyanobacteria also misleadingly known as 'blue-green algae') are now big business as 'superfoods'. As well as a food supplement added to expensive salads and smoothies, it is used as an anti-ageing cosmetic. Evidence suggests it may play a role in regulating obesity, with spirulina supplementation trials showing they help weight loss in obese individuals. These probiotic bugs were unknown to me, until we found for the first time that they (a close relative of *Arthrospira*) can live in human guts, although they seem to prefer vegetarians. Fifty years ago they were wrongly thought of as algae, but in fact they are ancient photosynthetic bacteria. We owe our existence to them, being the first bugs to produce oxygen and so our breathable atmosphere.

Arthrospira is quite unique in terms of nutrients. Its dry weight is nearly 50 per cent protein, plus it has polyunsaturated fats and con- tains all the essential amino acids, plus B vitamins, trace elements, carotenoids and plenty of easily absorbed iron. Some websites falsely claim it is a source of B12, as it produces a form of the vitamin that humans can't use. It likes to grow in warm alkaline water at around 35°C and needs little feeding, and grows in sunlight or under an LED lamp. It is very economical to grow and uses ten times less water than soybeans to produce the same amount of protein. It has been pro- posed as a cheap solution to famine, as well as the perfect (but expensive) addition to a vegetarian smoothie, and the ideal compan- ion on a space flight. So why don't we all eat it as a daily probiotic supplement? So far all the data on its benefits come from its potential nutrients, test-tube studies or lab animals. The human studies are too small or of such poor quality that they can't yet be relied on.

One study of eighty-seven malnourished kids in Gaza showed that 3g of spirulina supplement was superior to multivitamins over three months, and there are some encouraging small pilot studies in people with HIV.[9] In countries like the US it has been approved as a 'safe' supplement for years, meaning ironically the opposite as there are no regular safety quality checks (unlike pharmaceuticals), and it is easily contaminated with other toxic cyanobacteria (like *microcystis*) that cause illness. Studies in Greece of thirty-one commercial supple- ments showed they contained hundreds of different bacteria that shouldn't be there, and others can contain human pathogens.[10] We would also have to eat a lot of it (probably around 3g daily) to be sure of getting all the nutrients, so while it's probably OK to add it to your smoothie if you can afford it, make sure the source is trust- worthy. As there are much cheaper sources of protein, I wouldn't convert your bath to an algae farm quite yet.

IVS (in-vitro seafood)

An exciting prospect for seafood lovers comes in the form of lab-grown fish meat. Fish meat lends itself especially well to this method, thanks to its ability to grow with little oxygen, low temperatures and using mushroom and crab proteins as a base. The work being done on this at the moment suggests we will be eating ethical, nutritious and environmentally friendly sea protein soon.

*

Seafood is nutritious and can be delicious but the claims and associated price tags of certain products are not backed by science. Oysters won't improve your love life and caviar is a cruel way to harvest fish eggs with a high likelihood of fraud. However, seaweed holds great promise and we can enjoy moules (plus or minus frites) and spaghetti vongole with confidence that they are better for the planet and good for our health.

Five seafood tips

1. Many prawns and other seafood are farmed in non-sustainable ways.
2. Oysters and mussels are a good source of protein and nutrients, sustainable and good for the planet, but not necessarily for your sex life.
3. Farmed fish is used for UPFs, and scampi are not real seafood.
4. Microplastic pollution is harming our fish and probably us humans too.
5. Seaweed is a food of the future with plenty of nutrients.

24. Milk and cream

When I was seventeen, my mother sent me to an acupuncturist and naturopath for my persistent problems with sinusitis and I was prescribed a dairy-free diet because the expert was convinced dairy products 'caused' excess mucus and allergies. I followed his advice diligently for several years but had no change in my symptoms or rates of infection. These dire warnings about milk, yogurt, butter and cheese (and sometimes eggs), made me wary about eating dairy for many years, and I was not alone. Fears of allergy and heart disease have made many people give up cow dairy in favour of goat's milk, or processed soy, rice, oat, coconut and almond milk; switch from butter to margarine; and give up cheese. Since the mid-1970s, milk consumption has more than halved in the UK to just 330ml per person per week, and low prices and the power of supermarkets are putting dairy farms out of business, leading to high rates of suicide among the farming community.[1] In a 2017 survey, one in six British people said they were either already dairy free or considering it. The anti-dairy feeling is strongest in the under-forty-fives, where health concerns are the main worry, followed by animal cruelty and the environment. Of health concerns, the fat and sugar content of dairy were predominant, focusing on weight gain and heart disease. However, while low-fat dairy still dominates the shop shelves, the latest sales trends show the public are polarising into avoiding dairy entirely or re-embracing natural full-fat products like milk, yogurt or butter.

In the current health debates, we forget the reason we originally started drinking milk, this natural emulsion of fat globules in water which, like tiny ball bearings, provide a pleasant, smooth texture on the tongue and palate. Our mother's milk is the ultimate health drink, having evolved over millions of years to have the chemicals and nutrients in the right balance to ensure our growth, protection and survival. Virtually all babies are designed to both like breast milk and be able to digest it. Once animals were domesticated, drinking cow's, sheep's or goat's milk was as close a substitute for breast milk as humans could find.

There were two main obstacles to humans using milk nutrition. The first was that it made us sick. The majority of human adults on the planet originally lacked the lactase gene that makes the enzyme that breaks down the complex sugar lactose into the smaller sugars. Around 8,000 years ago, a gene mutation arose by chance in the lactase gene that kept the enzyme active past childhood and allowed some people to carry on drinking large amounts of milk, just like babies. This particularly helped young children from these mutant families survive fatal infections and grow faster and taller. Soon the extra survival rates and fertility of this group allowed the mutation to dominate North Europeans, where it reached 90 per cent prevalence. This knowledge of milk's genetic background has filtered down to a small group of white supremacists, mainly based in the US who are weaponising milk-drinking as a sign of white power with the slogan 'if you don't drink milk – go home'. Unfortunately, these guys didn't fully read the literature as otherwise they would have realised that the gene is also present in parts of East Africa, and especially the Middle East, where the mutation must also have been useful.

Cow's milk

This is the most consumed dairy product in the world and is now cheaper to buy than bottled water. Most of it is water (87 per cent) and was designed by natural evolution to make calves grow fast in the first year of life with targeted hormones and micronutrients. The rest is made of a mix of carbs, mainly lactose sugar, and the main proteins casein (that makes curds) and whey, and the main fat is saturated fat. It also has most of the major vitamins, amino acids and many nutrients, especially if the cow is grass-fed. For most of the last 8,000 years, regular consumption was only really possible if you lived close to a cattle or dairy farm because unwanted microbes would spoil the milk. This all changed thanks to pasteurisation, invented at the end of the nineteenth century. The heating process doesn't kill off all the microbes, just the most sensitive including many helpful ones, and doesn't preclude others contaminating it later, but it is much safer than raw milk.

While for most of the last century milk was considered good for children, its benefit for adults has been more controversial. From the 1960s and 70s, it was heavily promoted by the government-backed dairy industry as being an essential high-protein natural food for growth and health, that made your skin smooth, your hair shinier, and could cure everything including premenstrual syndrome. Now many believe it is an alien allergen that has fattened us up, and is even dangerous for children. While 65 per cent of the world who lack the lactose gene as adults are intolerant and find it hard to drink a whole glass, some more severe reactions do occur. Milk protein allergy (unlike lactose intolerance) is rare but does exist. This allergy can affect one in fifteen babies and wears off usually by age five, and is easily treated by avoiding milk and milk products.[2] This allergy can be serious but is often over-diagnosed in fussy babies and tired parents, moving them from breastfeeding to more expensive and unhealthier replacement formula options provided by the food industry.

Recently, milk has been implicated by isolated studies and media stories in several modern diseases affecting children and young adults such as eczema, acne, indigestion, IBS and allergies. The reports come from soft observational studies of varying quality, and are unlikely to prove to be causal, though more recent evidence suggests possible mechanisms that explain how large quantities of milk can cause inflammation, unrelated to its fat content.

After the high-fat food cull took hold, many governments encouraged the switch to less tasty skimmed or semi-skimmed milks. With all the negative publicity, milk sales have been slowly falling in most western countries since the 1970s. In contrast, milk drinking is on the increase in non-traditional areas like China and Asia. Many Chinese will only drink warm milk, and some markets sell it in baby bottles to adults in shopping hotspots. This is one factor in increasing heights there, where it may be both a cause and consequence of increasing prosperity.

Milk drinking and height are associated across many populations, with the tallest populations in Europe (the Dutch, closely followed by Scandinavians) being the biggest drinkers. Milk is designed in all animals to help growth, and contains all the essential minerals and vitamins to do this. Milk drinking by children can prevent muscle problems due to protein and vitamin B12 deficiency, and rickets due to vitamin D deficiency.

Mother's milk was never designed by evolution to be drunk beyond the age of three, but because of our gene mutations, drinking all forms of milk may come with both pros and cons in adults. It is widely assumed that it also helps strengthen bones in adults because of the natural calcium and phosphorus (and in many countries, sup-plemented vitamin D). Many governments and doctors recommend adults drink up to a pint a day for bone health. The latest data is clear and simply doesn't support this. A study following over 200,000 women with 3,500 fractures showed no protective effects of milk.[3] Other data from several studies found no clear association with the gene for tolerating milk and fracture rates.[4] We might have guessed this thirty years ago from observational data, as the biggest milk drinkers in Europe, despite being the tallest, have the greatest rates of bone fractures, and the Chinese and Japanese with traditionally low milk intakes have the lowest. Globally, most people get their essential bone nutrients, not from dairy, but from plants, such as leafy greens including kale, cauliflower, broccoli, collard greens, spinach, herbs like basil, most nuts such as almonds, seeds and pastes like tahini, fish bones (mackerel, canned salmon), or meat bones in soups or broth (see table, page 440).

Is milk actually good for us?

Without any obvious benefit to bones in adults, is there any health advantage? The big concern over milk has been heart disease and weight gain, due to the outdated view of animal fats. More recently focus has shifted to milk's ability to increase growth in children regardless of their nutritional status and whether that additional growth is healthy in the long term. The nutrient-sensing pathway that milk activates (mTOR) is clearly useful in early growth but has been linked to cancer, ageing and heart disease mechanisms. Epidemiological studies also recently confirmed a correlation between cow's milk consumption and birthweight, body fat, earlier onset of fertility in girls, growing taller during childhood (as shown by the Dutch), but unfortunately increased acne, type 2 diabetes, several types of cancer, and all-cause mortality.

Current US milk recommendations are supposed to improve calcium levels in the diet but the amounts are based on old unreliable studies in just 155 individuals and there are healthier sources. The context of milk drinking could be important. A study of 138,000 people from twenty-one developing lower-income countries (PURE study) with much lower baseline milk rates, found higher dairy intakes slightly protective for heart disease and overall mortality.[5] But results could easily be biased by associated health habits. To get around these biases, large studies of 1.9 million people used, as a surrogate marker of milk drinking, the genes for breaking down lactose (a method called Mendelian Randomisation) and confirmed the association with obesity, although found lower blood cholesterol levels. When considering the latest evidence, long-term regular consumption of cow's milk does not seem a great idea for most people, and again moderation may be the key.

Low-fat and skimmed milk

Most whole milk is skimmed by industrially spinning it in a large centrifuge, which separates the perfectly balanced liquid into two streams, fatty cream and fat-free milk. The thin milk is then sent to a condenser and spray dried to remove water and make it more concentrated. This is the equivalent process to refining grains: what is left is all the carbs, no fats and far less of the original chemicals and nutrients.

Studies have consistently failed to show any advantage of

swapping to low-fat milk on blood fat profiles, and some studies even show that the full-fat whole milk performs better in improving beneficial blood lipids. Contrary to USDA advice to choose reduced-fat dairy, low-fat milk has no advantages over whole milk for weight control. In children, the evidence actually suggests greater long-term weight gain with reduced-fat milk than with full-fat milk.

We have vastly over-simplified milk as merely fats and calcium and ignored most of the hundreds of other components that could interact with our immune and metabolic system, the small proteins (branched chain amino acids or short peptides) that could switch ageing or cancer pathways off or on (like mTOR), and even the chemicals lining the fat globules that could be anti-inflammatory, that all play a part in our health, especially as infants. We stupidly believed we could just process the milk industrially to remove the fatty layer, and this would leave all the healthy stuff behind. The fat-soluble vitamins and nutrients get eliminated when you remove the saturated fat content, including vitamins A, D, E and K as well as healthy fatty acids like omega-3 which grass-fed cows will have high levels of. This is another good reason children should not have low-fat milk.

Replacing human mother's milk

Our reductionist view of milk deluded us into thinking we can easily replicate human breast milk with formula feeds for babies. Companies add at least twenty substances to powdered cow's milk to get a close match, but they are nowhere near this goal of achieving a processed complete replacement. New technology shows there are several thousand interacting chemicals in breast milk that have evolved over millennia to be healthy, that will never be replicated by formula milk. These include hundreds or possibly thousands of large sugars called HMOs that are more common than proteins, whose sole role is to feed an infant's gut microbes. They are highly tailored and individualised, changing at every feed according to baby's needs, and although we understand very little about them, they do contain many key immune-regulating proteins (like immunoglobulin and lactoferrin) to help keep babies healthy in the first months of life as their immune systems develop. If you can't breastfeed, don't despair as milk formulas are all tightly regulated and standardised and do a good job whatever the price, as long as you stick to cow's milk. Many companies are working on routinely adding microbes from human breast milk to the new formulas to help the immune system. Wider sharing of breast milk between mothers is another healthy trend in countries like Denmark that we should be copying.

How now brown cow?

The intense breeding of animals for milk production in the last sixty years has narrowed down the gene pool for dairy animals considerably. Cow's milk now comes mainly from Holstein/Friesians who have become milk factories on long legs. They are artificially impregnated to get their milk glands going and then mechanical pumps keep the milk-making feedback loop active, whilst their calves are removed and bottle-fed to maximise yield. They can live off artificial grain diets that other breeds don't tolerate and can produce ten times as much milk per day as more traditional varieties eating varied organic diets. Holsteins produce on average a massive 36 litres of milk per day with less fat, whereas the British Jersey cow manages only about 26 litres with 50 per cent higher fat, but more flavoursome milk. Most of our milk does not come from grass-fed organic dairies, and as milk production per cow has doubled over the last fifty years, our milk is getting cheaper and blander with less nutrients, which as we will see, also affects dairy products.

Other animal milks

Up to the seventeenth century, European health books commonly included tips for drinking human milk. The authors encouraged you to find a willing maiden who was young, happy and healthy, and preferably good-looking to be your own personal milkmaid.[6] This is mostly frowned upon nowadays, despite a brief reprisal in the early Covid days when the miracle powers of human breast milk resurfaced. But the milk you choose should be based on taste rather than some misreported science or myth. Comparing different animal milks at the very primitive macro level, human milk is one of the sweetest, has relatively less protein, but the biggest fat globules. Dairy cows produce three times more protein and 30 per cent less sugar, with about the same fat content on average as humans. Sheep, buffalo and yak milk all have more fat than most cows, while goat is slightly lower in fat content. As a low-fat alternative, try camel milk which has a cheesy savoury taste, or horse milk which has only 1 per cent fat.

Butter and cream

Most cow's milk naturally produces cream of about 20 per cent fat concentration, and it is the close grouping of the fat globules that gives the creamy texture on our tongues that we find so pleasant. Light or single cream is around this 20 per cent mark and double cream around 50 per cent fat. Low-fat creams are difficult to use in cooking, as they tend to curdle and clump into particles, and more than 25 per cent fat is usually needed to retain the fat globules and smooth consistency, allowing it to be whipped and introduce air. Because cream has become synonymous with saturated fat, it had a terrible press in many countries, especially the US where it is still impossible to purchase full-fat non-UHT varieties in many states. The French in contrast, with a more pragmatic view of nutritional advice, have many different types of cream on sale including crème fraîche, which is about 35 per cent fat and is usually produced with microbial fermentation making it a weak probiotic.

Despite its bad reputation, there is no good data to show that eating cream regularly causes heart problems or shortens your life. The artificial alternatives may turn out to be worse. Cream alternatives are now everywhere in countries that followed the low-fat philosophy, with deceptive 'dairy-like' labels making it hard to know what you are buying. In the UK you can buy what you think is a low-fat 'cream' but is actually a mix of butterfat, palm oil, rapeseed and seven other chemicals to give it a similar 'mouthfeel'. None of them taste as good as real cream, but soy creams and coconut cream work well when heated and are considered as good dairy alternatives for cooking in terms of flavour and texture too.

Most butter is made from pasteurised cream with at least 80 per cent fat and a maximum of 16 per cent water, often with 1–2 per cent salt. The colour and aroma of the fat in the butter reflects what the cows were eating; if there are no dyes or carotene added, a good yellow colour is a sign of pasture-fed rather than grain-fed cows. As butter is mainly saturated fat, most countries have reduced intakes. The American Heart Association still suggests a limit of 5 per cent daily calories as saturated fat, which essentially means you can never spread butter on bread, and so can only have processed substitutes. Public Health England (now HSAUK) still advises people to use low-fat spreads instead of butter, without providing any direct evidence to back this up – because there is none. As real butter always tastes better, and it can be rich in vitamins A and omega-3 if from grass-fed cows, I personally use butter over any emulsified artificial spread any day, but we should try not to overdo it, both for our planet and our waistlines.

Five facts about milk and cream

1. Drinking cow's milk does not improve bone health or vitamin D status and likely increases weight.
2. Drinking cow's milk boosts growth but is not necessary for children with adequately diverse diets.
3. Choose organic, grass-fed and whole milk, but be aware the environmental cost.
4. Cream alternatives are increasingly common but beware of excessive chemicals and palm oil.
5. Butter has no health benefits, but is tasty and most alternative spreads are likely worse for us.

25. Fermented dairy (yogurt, kefir and fermented milk)

Yogurt magically appears if you forget where you left your milk, or if you cool it down after heating, allowing lactose-loving microbes to acidify the milk and curdle the milk protein. Yogurt can be made from most animal milk with a high fat content, such as cow, goat and sheep. As I am writing, I am enjoying an unusual organic strained goat-milk yogurt made on a unique Costa Rican farm by ex-vet Carlos Carranza. It is deliciously smooth and flavoursome thanks to the many fat globules, which are smaller than those from cows, and the happy well-fed goats that produce it. As well as the milk, most yogurt makers add microbe cultures after pasteurisation, and commonly these include *Bifidobacterium lactis*, *Strep thermophilus*, *lactobacillus acidophilus* and two types of *lactobacillus delbrueckii*. These all break down the lactose and produce lactic acid, making the yogurt acidic and keeping other (potentially harmful) microbes away.

The fermenting process and presence of live microbes means it is different to milk in many subtle ways, such as a failure to trigger mTOR pathways involved in growth and cancer, discussed in the last chapter. It is likely to have been first eaten regularly in Turkey or possibly Poland thousands of years ago and was just another convenient way to store and drink milk before refrigerators, until in the early 1900s an eccentric Russian scientist (and later Nobel Prize winner), Ilya Mechnikoff noticed that Bulgarian peasants had extremely good health and longevity. He believed like many at the time, that putrefaction in our guts was causing common disease and ill health and could be reversed by the microbes in yogurt. His work in the Pasteur Institute attracted publicity on the possible health benefits and stimulated entrepreneurs such as Catalan Isaac Carasso who founded Danone in 1919, and Dr Shiroto who founded Yakult in Japan in 1930. They transformed yogurt from a peasant food to a specialised pharmacy business, then a multi-billion-dollar food market.

There is a catch. Most yogurt is high in saturated fat and due to low-fat indoctrination it can be difficult to find healthy, natural full-fat versions containing the original nutrients and viable microbes of the milk. Instead, most yogurt found in supermarkets is heavily pro-cessed, using full or partial dairy substitutes and extra protein and starch. Many also now have much added sugar, vanilla or sweeteners to disguise the deficiencies, with children's yogurt topping the charts for added sugar – at least 45 per cent of energy per serving – and mis-leading labelling.[1] In short, children's yogurts should be avoided. Real yogurt is much more expensive and is often now sold as set yog-urt, concentrated or strained yogurt, and takes several litres of quality milk to produce, which unfortunately poses environmental and eth-ical issues. Turkish and Greek natural yogurts are natural full-fat strained versions, while labneh in the Middle East has a pinch of salt added and is then strained to a thick creamy consistency. Through clever marketing, all 'Greek' yogurt has become synonymous with this good thick full-fat strained yogurt but as is often the case, names are deceptive. Most supermarket strained yogurt doesn't now come from Greece or even Greek milk and in the UK is called 'Greek-style' full-fat yogurt; it doesn't even have to be strained to be labelled legally and can officially contain some artificial powdered milk, as well as pectins and thickening starches. It's important to read the label carefully, as market research has found huge variability between different types. Overall, Greek/natural yogurts seem to have a higher percentage of protein, more live cultures and lower amounts of sugar than their fruit- or vanilla-flavoured counterparts.

Fromage frais is another popular yogurt style, often combined with sugary fruit in small pots, aimed at children. It is technically not a yogurt, but a young unripened fermented cheese that has less fat, and by French law also has to contain some live microbes (unlike *fromage blanc*). Although theoretically containing some microbes, most fromage frais contain far too much sugar for the microbes to thrive (averaging around 13 per cent or 3tsp per small pot) with the low-fat versions. Some brands even add sweets to versions for kids containing 19 per cent sugar. As yogurt eating is becoming the norm, companies are seeing opportunities to replace the flagging cereal market with a 'healthy' highly processed alternative.[2]

But good yogurt doesn't need a team of chemists to make it. Making your own yogurt is easy, all you need is a live starter culture. I managed to produce a tasty batch, but need to work on the texture before winning any awards.

Skinny yogurts

Low-fat yogurt is made using skimmed or nearly skimmed (2 per cent fat) milk, and sometimes has some whey protein, sugar or pectin added for texture and flavour. It also has added cultures and can be very thick and creamy, though as we've discovered, the removed fat also means a reduction in micronutrients. Sugars are often added to replace the fat. Skyr is a slightly different low-fat brand (originally from Iceland) as the whey is separated using a traditional straining process creating a mild, creamy cultured product with high 15 per cent protein content. Though marketed as a healthy, superior and wholesome option, there is no evidence that it is any better for our health than regular full-fat milk yogurt. Low-fat natural yogurts have not been shown to be healthier, but the cultures used to make them do still hold some potential health benefits. 'Light' options with added flavourings such as fruit or vanilla and sugars or sweeteners are definitely inferior to natural unsweetened yogurts and should really be avoided, especially for children. As low-fat yogurt uses skimmed milk, fat-loving vitamins are removed and have to be artificially replaced, begging the question, why bother? As long as your yogurt is natural and alive, it's OK. Avoid low fat, unless you prefer the bland taste, extra chemicals and carbohydrates.

Is yogurt healthy?

Whether yogurt is a health food or a clever con, has been debated since the days of Metchnikoff. A decade ago yogurt manufacturers were reprimanded for the exaggerated health claims on their products which they couldn't substantiate and media and public doubted if any healthy microbes made it past the stomach acid, so health benefits seemed unlikely. A 2018 study of mice and a few humans showed that the microbes in yogurt didn't hang around and multiply in the gut as the adverts had suggested.[3] The media proclaimed, 'probiotics don't work'. A 2017 meta-analysis of over nine observational studies from around the world and nearly 300,000 people have shown that for *episodic* yogurt eaters this may be true – it made no difference to heart disease. But for *regular* yogurt eaters of more than 200g per day (two small pots), there were benefits, showing they had less heart disease.[4] As this was based on observational data, this could easily be biased by better lifestyle and other habits, but the conclusion is supported by seven small clinical trials. The yogurt group had beneficial reductions on glucose and fat markers in blood, despite the high saturated fat and calories.[5] Recent research highlights the benefits of yogurt and fermented milks over drinking plain cow juice including reducing the risk of cancers, type 2 diabetes and even heart disease, although the review was sponsored by Danone.

But what about your weight? After all, apart from the microbes, it is a concentrated form of milk, with more protein, fat, minerals and vitamins, and more calories per gram. There are only two randomised clinical trials, both small, short-term and inconclusive. However, there have been ten large population cohort studies following the yogurt habits of over 219,000 people over time. Nine of the ten showed the reverse of what dogma would predict; a positive finding on weight loss or waist size in yogurt eaters, and a clearer benefit than for milk.[6]

How do we put this all together? Yogurt has a mild beneficial effect on heart disease and weight loss, despite the fat and calories, yet the microbes it contains don't multiply in our guts. My team found that it is not the microbes themselves that are beneficial, but the chemicals they produce. In 2022, we looked at the yogurt-eating habits of over 4,000 UK twins and their gut microbes.[7] The microbiome diversity of the regular yogurt users was significantly greater (i.e. healthier) than non-users and they had reduced visceral fat. We had previously found different microbe families (*streptococci*, *lactobacillus* and *bifidobacteria*) that were not in original yogurt were significantly increased. But more importantly, we found many chemical metabolites in the blood and stools of regular yogurt users produced by microbes. These same metabolites appeared to be protective against developing internal belly fat.[8] So, we think that eating the probiotic microbes in yogurt regularly encourages greater diversity of our gut microbes, and these microbes then produce a wider range of healthy metabolites that in turn help regulate our weight and metabolism. We know about prebiotics and probiotics, but this is perhaps a new era of the 'postbiotic' as we learn to harness the healthy chemicals that our microbes produce. We showed this may also be the way that microbes via omega-3 fats can help heart health in our twins.[9]

Yogurt could also help the immune system, and certainly seems to help pigs and mice fight a range of respiratory and gut viruses. Our own unpublished twin studies show clear differences in many immune markers in blood between yogurt eaters and non-eaters, although we don't know their clinical significance yet. Our Covid studies showed that probiotic use reduced risk of severe infections by around 14 per cent, so we might expect yogurt to have a similar effect.[10] We are just learning exactly what these amazing microbe chemicals, such as short chain fatty acids, can do. We do know microbes in probiotics can manufacture other complex sugars (called exo-polysaccharides or EPS) which both protect the microbes themselves, and have beneficial effects on the immune system, increasing our chances of surviving cancer.

Yogurt alternatives?

There is one alternative on the market which could potentially compete with the original. Coconut yogurt is made with coconut fruit flesh which has less fat content than coconut oil and importantly plenty of fibre, and by avoiding dairy is much more environmentally friendly. It tastes good and doesn't have too many additives, but does it confer the health benefits of traditional 'live' yogurt? It seems that it could do, at least in terms of probiotic content, but doesn't compete with milk yogurt's protein content, though fortification can boost calcium. A company creating coconut milk kefir claims to have created the most powerful probiotic currently on the market, with over four-trillion colony-forming units (CFU) and more than forty different types of probiotic strains in just one daily tablespoon.[11]

Fermented milks and kefir

At a national meeting I spoke at in 2017, only one in ten British GPs had ever heard of kefir, but it is changing fast. Soured milks like kefir are a more liquid drink than yogurt and include many national variants, including Scandinavian sour or *ropy* milks, *koumiss* from Central Asia, which is slightly fizzy and alcoholic, and *ayran* from Turkey which is salty and frothy. Kefir is very common in Central Asia, the Balkans and Eastern Europe, and now is commonplace in the UK. Kefir means 'good feeling' in Turkish and may have originated in the Caucasus mountains. Legend has it that the Prophet Mohamed taught the shepherds how to drop special mysterious grains into goat's milk and transform it into something magical. Kefir differs from yogurt in more than just consistency.

Kefir grains contain a whole microbial community in suspended animation, with over ten times more microbe varieties than yogurt. All these contribute different complex chemicals that influence the flavours. What is also special is that they form a community structure around a complex sugar that the microbes produce themselves. This is another EPS called kefiran which has possible immune properties of its own (although studies are small and not convincing) and adds structure to the milk. It is this special mix of bacteria, fungi and the unique EPS sugar backbone in kefir that produces a durable commune of microbes that work together.

Kefir couldn't be easier to make. You can order kefir grains online, which you add to a litre of whole milk in a jar and leave in a warm room for thirty-six hours or until it smells mildly acidic. Put kefir in the fridge and sieve it before drinking. Keep some aside, as the first batch now holds the starter microbes for a new batch. Like sourdough starters, if well fed, you can keep them alive indefinitely. It takes some trial and error by changing temperatures and milks (I prefer whole milk) and grains to get the flavour that suits you. With that many microbes and different conditions there is a large element of luck as well. Alternatively, you can now buy kefir nearly everywhere. Commercial kefirs vary widely in taste, acidity and texture, and some are slightly fizzy, or if from goats stronger in flavour. If you find the sourness difficult at first, one trick is to mix it with yogurt until you get used to having a daily hit.

Mild commercial brands probably have less diverse microbes than homemade kefir. One study compared the microbes in traditional versus commercial kefir and reassuringly found a similar number of microbe species, although the traditional brews had a stronger potential action against other infectious microbes.[12] While there are positive kefir studies, they are all small, usually in a test tube or in animals and of variable quality. Nevertheless, despite the lack of hard data and variability of each product, we should treat it as a super yogurt, for which the evidence is now pretty good and growing.[13]

Both yogurt and kefir can be added to the end of dishes like curry to enrich a sauce and if not overheated will still have live microbes. Though fermented milk products are much better for our health than milk and taste delicious, they do still require litres of milk with its environmental costs. Grass-fed, organic yogurt and fermented milks consumed as a healthy regular dietary boost (but not in excess) may strike the right balance between health and environment. Alternatively, we may have to seriously consider non-dairy as the only truly viable options for the future.

Fermented dairy products in five

1. Flavoured yogurts, fromage frais and fruit or sweetened yogurts are not healthy and should not form part of children's daily diet.
2. Low-fat yogurts are a less healthy choice.
3. Live yogurt and fermented products like kefir support our immune system via our microbes.
4. Natural live yogurt and kefir are generally good for health but we need to be mindful of their environmental impact via milk production.
5. Kefir and cultured milk products are rich sources of healthy probiotics and easy and cheap to make at home.

26. Cheese

Our ancestors worked out that by allowing curdled milk to dry out and leaving it to cool in a cave, tasty cheese could be made. Cheese contains protein, fats, minerals and calories, as well as live microbes, and would have sustained a travelling human for days, if not weeks. I tested the concept of the cheese-only diet during research for my last book, coming off the rebound of my failed vegan experience. I thought that with the help of red wine, it would be quite easy. I had wanted to test the effect of cheese on my microbes using three different raw milk French cheeses (Brie de Meaux, epoisses and roquefort). Day one was a breeze, and I found myself full very easily, and was thinking of writing a new bestseller: *The 28-Day Cheese Diet Revolution*. Day two was fine, but by day three I was feeling bloated, constipated and really struggling. I started craving green things. The cheese diet book deal was definitely on hold, though evidence shows cheese consumption could be associated with a longer, healthier life, although probably *not* as the only source of nutrition.

Traditionally matured in caves, cellars, stables and mills there is no one right way of making cheese, which is why it has an infinite amount of flavour possibilities. To understand cheese better, let's look at the most popular variety in the world – cheddar. At a macro level cheddar is 33 per cent fat (of which 23 per cent is saturated, 9 per cent monounsaturated and 1 per cent polyunsaturated), 25 per cent protein and 1 per cent carbohydrate, plus calcium and other nutrients. Cheddar comes from the tiny village of Cheddar in the west of England in the middle of a gorge with small caves, surrounded by rich pastures. Only one cheesemaker still exists in Cheddar village now, where once there were hundreds. Outside a few artisan producers, cheddar has become a global supermarket cheese. No one quite remembered what traditional mature cheddar tasted like, until a 1917 book by a cheesemaker called Dora Saker was unearthed ten years ago detailing precisely how to make cheddar and describing its distinctive savoury, nutty taste. It should also be made very slowly to help the cheese develop all the flavours, and the curds should always be stacked.

Cheese like cheddar is generally made by mixing milk with a starter culture of a few species of lactose-loving bacteria plus rennet, an enzyme found in the stomach of young calves that cuts up the protein curds, which curdles the milk separating it into curds and whey. The whey is drained off and the semi-solid curds are cut into strips, salt is added, and the mix put into round moulds for pressing. They are then left out in a cool cellar (or cave) for a few months, and the surface rinds allowed to grow a mould to help the maturing process and flavour. Depending on the microbes in the starter culture and atmosphere, levels of acidity and moisture reached at the point of moulding and the speed at which this happens you will have a very different cheese type. British cheeses like cheddar or stilton are typically acidic and low in moisture; soft French camembert is low in acidity and high in moisture; alpine cheeses like comté are dry but have low acidity; and smelly runny epoisses is both acidic and moist.

Cheese microbes keep evolving and changing dynamically over time. Within each cheese type and even within each cheese region the flavours will vary because of multiple factors, including the plants that the animals eat (grain or grass), the genes of the animal being milked, and the various microbes in the starter culture, milk, and in the farm and caves. One traditional cheese maker, Sister Noella Marcellino, used to make cheese according to a French peasant recipe, letting the milk sour in wooden barrels rather than the modern stainless steel. After an outbreak of *listeria*, health inspectors told her she had to stop using wooden barrels. The levels of E.coli in her finished cheeses spiked immediately; it was the bacteria in the wood itself that had kept her original cheese E.coli-free.

The vast majority of cheeses are now made under strictly controlled conditions in factories using commercial rennet and microbe cultures provided by a few global companies to ensure consistency, ideal for high-volume supermarket sales.

Many people claim cheese gives them nightmares or a range of other odd headache symptoms grouped together as a 'cheese reaction'. In 1996 this 'cheese reaction' was linked to high levels of a protein in cheese, called tyramine, a chemical linked to histamine produced by acid-loving microbes present in most fermented foods.[1] Although a few people are genuinely affected, for the majority it is likely to be a placebo reaction, such as the MSG headaches of the 1980s supposedly caused by Chinese food (it wasn't).[2] The longer the cheese matures, the higher the levels of tyramine and histamine, increasing risk, although the balance of microbes used in the starter can now be manipulated to produce less. Rarely, other fermented products, such as chocolate, salamis, pickles, wine and beer can cause similar problems in particularly sensitive people, for reasons we don't yet properly understand but which may be linked to their microbiome.

Industrial cheese

The Canadian Joseph Kraft changed our concept of the farmhouse cheese forever. He invented novel ways of superheating and sterilising cheese, so although it killed any healthy microbes, it could be moulded into different shapes without the fat separating. More importantly it could also be stored long term. The first of these was the Kraft dairy slice that became one of the biggest-selling convenience foods in history. Every packet tasted the same, regardless of the milk, pasture or microbes, and became the backbone of every cheeseburger, grilled sandwich and prepared lunch box. Another of Kraft's popular industrial cheeses is the spreadable Dairy Lea triangle, which probably increased cheese eating among children. Kraft also acquired Philadelphia cream cheese, which originated back in the 1880s in the US. It was made by mixing cream with young cheese and became the iconic New York breakfast with a bagel. It looks highly processed in its plastic tub, but on genetic testing, it did actually contain all the common lactose-loving bacteria – a good sign is that it does develop mould after a week or two. The long-lasting cream cheese Boursin was invented in 1963 by Francois Boursin by adding garlic and herbs to a bland cheese from Normandy.

The 1960s and 70s were the era of butter and cheese mountains across Europe and the US. People were buying less milk because of anti-fat fears and governments wanted to protect the dairy industry as prices dropped. The politically easy solution was to subsidise and encourage other uses of milk, and specifically the leftover fat from skimmed milk production, for cheap ultra-processed cheese, but at the expense of quality, flavour and any uniqueness. Most of this extra cheese was superheated way above a temperature that microbes can survive in, so no longer a living probiotic, and eaten on pizzas, in ready meals and other UPFs lacking in nutrients.

Using hundreds of different chemicals, flavourists can bypass much of the work of the microbes and can recreate the essence of cheddar, camembert or blue cheese. These flavours can either be added to liven up cheap bland cheese or replace natural cheese entirely on ready meal macaroni cheese, crackers and crisps, or as fake cheese for vegetarians. These extra flavours are especially needed in low-fat cheeses that are bolstered with cellulose, egg protein, whey and plant carbohydrates to try and replace the natural flavour and texture of cheese fats. Despite their best attempts they are often bitter and rubbery. You can now buy enzyme modified cheese (EMC) paste which has ten to twenty times the flavour of natural cheese, made from blending curds with secret enzymes and microbe cultures. These concentrated pastes are added to many cheese fillings like cheap ravioli and lasagne to add taste at little extra cost, other than to our health or waistlines.

Pizza cheese

Making pizza cheese has become an industry of its own. Mozzarella cheese is the most popular pizza topping. Traditional artisan mozzarella is made with high-quality milk from herds of local buffalo that is transformed into delicate milky cheesy ovals with relatively low fat levels (17 per cent), and is best eaten fresh with an acid like balsamic vinegar or fresh tomatoes. Although buffalo mozzarella is now made around the world and all over Italy, the top product is called Mozzarella di Bufala Campana which is made in a (DOP) protected area of southern Italy. But where there is money, there is organised crime, the Camorra to be precise, who in 2008 got into the environmental waste business. Rather than processing the waste, it was cheaper to dump large amounts of toxic dioxin waste in grazing areas of the famous buffalo. Not surprisingly, no one wanted dioxin-flavoured cheese and sales plummeted, and six years later many cheeses still had high dioxin levels. In 2021, the area was still suffering with an unusual number of leukaemia cases, so the damage done is long-lasting. The Camorra remained interested in cheese as a money-laundering vehicle and Giuseppe Mandara (who called himself the Armani of Mozzarella) was arrested for substituting cheap provolone cheese and selling defective contaminated products.[3] In 2016 genetic tests still showed that one in four 'local' mozzarellas contained foreign cow's milk from Ireland and Germany. Many Neapolitans now ask to see certificates of purchase from restaurants, but they too can be faked, and with criminals still investing billions of euros in local agriculture and prices high, as the Romans said, 'caveat emptor'.[4]

Pizza was probably invented in the same region of Italy in 1889, though sadly, in a world where one in seven Americans is eating a pizza slice as you read this, the mozzarella used for most pizzas today is rather different. It is often sterilised, frozen and mixed with other cheaper cheeses like cheddar and provolone. Frozen pizza is designed to last for years in a $150 billion world market propped up by analogue cheese, a term for any pseudo cheese that contains ingredients that mimic or blend with the original at lower cost. This is generally made from partly hydrogenated vegetable oil, casein, vegetable protein, binder, stabiliser, emulsifier, emulsifying salt, acidulant, salt, colourings, flavourings, preservatives and water without using starter culture or rennet. Good-quality cheese can be melted without major changes to nutrients, whereas boiled and frozen cheese analogues have less calcium and produce strange fat combinations. Countries vary on how analogue cheese is labelled, but a 2016 survey of British pizza takeaways found one in four were selling analogue cheese as real mozzarella on pizzas.[5]

The French and smelly cheese

In France, culture and national pride favour small cheesemakers in their fight against big food. Lactalis is the world's largest dairy company owning Italian Galbani (mozzarella) and many other global brands such as Seriously (cheddar), Société (roquefort), and Président (brie and camembert). Its massive factories produce a cheese called Camembert Fabriqué en Normandie, a consistent pasteurised product with a cosmetic white fungus rind of *penicillium camemberti* and a good shelf-life. A few kilometres away, another type of camembert with a similar though protected name, Camembert de Normandie, couldn't be more different. It is made locally by a few dedicated cheesemakers from raw milk cheese from local Normandy cows and uses ancient methods of ripening (*affinage*) and real fungus. It tastes much richer and more complex as you would expect. The artisans are so far resisting huge pressure to rebrand all Normandy cheese under the same lower standard AOP label. As a home experiment, put a mass-produced Président Brie on a plate at room temperature next to a Brie de Meaux and watch them over a few days. You will soon know which has more microbes and fewer chemical preservatives.

The British public took a while to warm to eating blue mouldy cheeses such as gorgonzola and roquefort. But Stilton is a village in Cambridgeshire that started making cheese with a blue streak of mould in it sometime before 1724. This first mention came when a passing traveller noted the local cheese was eaten with a spoon and, as well as the mouldy blue bits, he was encouraged to eat the moving mites and maggots. Stilton is now maggot-free and is made by stirring in dry fungus spores – usually *penicillium roqueforti* – along with the starter culture, and after the moulding, the cheese is punctured with needles to produce air holes which allow the fungus to breath and multiply. In order to be called stilton and be protected, the cheese has to adhere to strict rules and be pasteurised, so that ironically the only raw-milk artisan cheesemaker based in Stilton, has to call his excellent cheese 'Stichelton'.

Some of my favourite cheeses, including epoisses, munster and

Pont l'Évêque, have a bacteria called *brevibacterium linens* on the surface that gives the rind an orange tinge, and produces a chemical methanethiol and a powerful odour. The same microbes that like to eat cheese also live on our skin and especially in the same moist conditions on our feet, producing the same 'cheesy feet' chemical.

Mimolette, made in the French city of Lille, depends on tiny little cheese mites that look like dust, but are in fact alive, to really bring out the flavours. The mites can usually be seen crawling over the bright orange cheese, even with a naked eye. The ever-squeamish US authorities of course banned it, leading to great publicity and a thriving black market. The Sardinians make another famous but rare cheese called Casu Marzu, which cannot be legally sold and which uses maggots to get that distinctive taste by stimulating a second fermentation in the pecorino-type cheese. Eating wriggly maggots isn't everyone's cup of tea and they didn't bother asking the USA for an import license.

Other European cheeses

Ricotta, made since the bronze age in Italy, is arguably not a cheese, as it is not fermented in the normal sense. It is made from the leftover whey from other cheesemaking (traditionally pecorino), using acid in the form of vinegar and boiled to high temperature, killing any microbes, making it a tasty, low-fat but useless probiotic. It is a very versatile cheese and commonly smoked, baked, salted or sweetened as a dessert or filling (as in Sicilian cannoli). It is surprisingly easy to make at home by heating whole milk, salt and vinegar (or lemon) together and straining the resulting curds. Cottage cheese is similarly not really a cheese and is made from acidifying the curds into chunks and with a high protein-to-fat ratio, is popular with weightlifters and in weight-loss recipes.

Feta is an ancient salted Greek cheese, mentioned in Homer's *Odyssey*, made from sheep's milk (or up to 30 per cent goat's milk). It is made in the normal way then mixed with salt in several stages, usually lying in a tub of brine with 7 per cent salt for several weeks. Salt encourages the right microbes to grow and up to twelve varieties of healthy bacteria have been detected that protect the cheese. Hard varieties are considered better quality than soft, and it has plenty of equivalents around the world. To be called feta it needs to come from Greece, and most others are called white cheese.

The squeaky textured semi-hard cheese from Cyprus called halloumi contains live microbes, and is made from cow's or sheep's milk. The industrial forms are best fried before eating. A new tasty British version made in Hampshire is called Buffalomi – made from buffalo and cow's milk – that has a softer texture.

'Risky' raw-milk cheese

In 2016 in Lanarkshire, Scotland, Errington Farm Dairy, a raw-milk dairy famous for its blue cheese, hit the headlines for the wrong reasons. A three-year-old child had tragically died of *E.coli* infection and kidney failure; over a ten-week period twenty-five others in the same area had become unwell and seventeen needed hospital treatment. Health protection Scotland traced the outbreak to a particularly nasty strain of the microbe called *E.coli* O157. The officials instantly suspected the dairy and carried out tests showing that the same microbe was present in some cheeses. They were shut down overnight. Errington sought independent advice from microbe experts who found no evidence any of their cheeses had levels of the microbe sufficient to cause the outbreak, and started a public and legal campaign to get compensation. The cheese ban was finally overturned, and criminal proceedings were dropped a year later, but not without near fatal stress for the dairy. The true cause was never found.

All raw milk dairies fear contamination with pathogens like *E.coli* or *listeria*, which from time to time will get into the cheese. Usually the other acid-loving microbes kill them off or suppress them to very low levels. But while raw-milk cheese can sometimes cause problems, pasteurised milk cheese is not completely safe from contamination either, if not well supervised, transported and stored, which can happen because of greater complacency.

Listeria was only linked to food poisoning in 1983, because infections were rare. In the US the most reported outbreaks of *listeria* food poisoning (listeriosis) are related to a young soft Mexican home-made cheese called queso fresco, which is very moist and lacks acidity, which without good hygiene is very susceptible to infection. According to the US media and health agencies the risks are horrifying. Eat raw-milk cheese and you have over 800 times the risk of infection and forty-five times the risk of being hospitalised.[6] When someone dies it makes national news; in spring 2017 two people died and four others were ill after buying raw-milk cheese from a Whole Foods store in Connecticut.

As always, risk statistics can be misleading. Raw-milk poisoning in the US accounts for roughly one death every three years and an estimated 720 illnesses per five million regular consumers. Thus, while the relative risk is high, the absolute risk to an individual is tiny, yet importing soft cheese is illegal in the US, although there is a growing internal local industry in some states. What is also clear is that many people can be 'infected', but are protected by their own gut microbes, and never develop symptoms. Many of us permanently carry inside us small numbers of *Listeria* and *E.coli* bugs without any harm. Individual cases are tragic, but this risk needs to be put into context.

Even if the risks are tiny and raw-milk cheese has a wider variety of healthy microbes, does it taste any better than pasteurised cheese? The BBC Radio 4 *Food Programme* organised some blind tastings, and while experts agreed that raw milk often added a depth and complexity of unusual flavours, well-made pasteurised cheeses can be excellent. We should support our artisan dairies to maintain this wide diversity of flavours, textures and microbes and remind us what real cheese really is. If we don't, we could all soon be eating long-life analogue cheese sprayed with flavour molecules.

The environmental cost of cheese

Unfortunately for me and cheese-lovers everywhere, cheese, even in the artisanal form, is terribly inefficient in terms of energy needed to make it. The production of raw milk is a major contributor, but there are many other reasons why cheese is so energy-demanding. Traditional cheesemaking consumes a large volume of fresh water to ensure a sanitary processing environment and generates large volumes of whey by-products that still contain highly valuable proteins. The long ripening times of hard cheeses may also require cooling facilities. Cheddar cheese normally has a carbon footprint of 14kg CO_2 equivalent for every 1kg of cheese, but by changing milk production and introducing anaerobic fermentation of whey to produce biofuels, cheddar cheese production could possibly become carbon negative.[7]

*

Until microbes help solve the cheese-whey problem, to help the environment eating cheese should be a rare, occasional treat focusing on artisanal, organic and grass-fed options from small producers.

Top five cheese facts

1. There are thousands of different types of cheeses, containing varying amounts of fats.
2. Traditional cheeses are a rich source of live microbes, protein, calcium and vitamin D.
3. Cheese contained in ready meals, burgers, frozen pizzas and some cheese snacks is ultra-processed analogue cheese and confers none of the health benefits of the real thing.
4. Raw-milk cheese can be enjoyed safely if properly stored, and supports artisanal, probiotic cheesemaking in its traditional form.
5. All cheese has a big environmental footprint related to the large quantities of milk and water used.

27. Dairy alternatives

Many of us are turning to plant-based 'milks' such as soy, rice, oat, hemp and almond for ourselves and our children. As well as health and allergy concerns, many people cite the effect on the environment. Many of the alternative milk producers claim that more than 80 per cent less land is used and 30 per cent less emissions result from the production of a pint of soy or oat milk than cow's milk.[1]

Plant milks are all processed in factories and involve squeezing the fat from the grain or nut to form an emulsion of the fat globules in the protein and water, which is the essence of milk. Various additives, proteins and chemicals can be added to provide the right texture and taste. I never personally found soy milk easy to drink, although many Asians are brought up on it. Almond milk is just about OK, but Swedish oat milk exceeded my low expectations and was quite pleasant with tea. I was surprised to hear that potato milk is gaining momentum, and who knows where this market will go.

As the plant milk market grows around the world (at around 7 per cent a year), so are specific allergies to these new plant milks, showing there is nothing special about animal milk protein. People already on poor diets, who now avoid animal milk, run into other nutritional problems in many western countries. These include rickets (low vitamin D), iodine deficiency, and a change in acidity in blood causing muscle weakness.[2] A worrying recurrence of an old epidemic in the UK after 100 years is iodine deficiency. This used to be called cretinism, due to iodine-poor soils leading to deficient pregnant mothers, producing mildly developmentally retarded babies.

Iodine is key to normal brain development and most teenage girls in the UK who avoid milk are now iodine deficient, potentially impacting the reading age and IQ of their future children.[3] Poor quality, non-diverse diets, lacking natural iodine from dairy or other sources such as seafood, are at risk in countries that do not routinely add it to salt (unlike the USA who iodise salt). Though there are exceptions, some milk-replacement drinks lack any iodine so it is important to read the label if purchasing these milk alternatives for regular use. Generally, plant milks do not convey the same complete nutritional benefits as cow's milk; they have less protein and readily available calcium, and have more sugars and potential anti-nutritional factors that inhibit micronutrient absorption. Dutch girls who still drink cow's milk don't have the same levels of iodine deficiency as British girls. Alternative iodine sources to milk include seafood, seaweed, eggs and prunes. But the plant-based milk industry is catching up and adding micronutrients to their products, which do make these more environmentally friendly alternatives a good option to include in varied diets in countries where other calcium-, iodine- and protein-rich foods are easily consumed. However, readily available sugars in these plant milks produce a very different response on our bodies to cow's milk so we should be wary of treating any of them like a health drink.

Butter alternatives (fake butter)

Because of the scaremongering fat warnings, many people replaced butter with a pale synthetic oily mix we call margarine. This started life in 1869 in France as a poor man's butter, consisting of beef fat, milk and a hint of butter flavour. It became a vegetable-based product thirty years later when the chemical process of making liquid vegetable oils solid (hydrogenation) was invented, but it still needed a yellow dye to make it palatable. Its popularity came not from its taste, but from the publicity of the 'healthy' fat content, being mainly unsaturated fat. In one of the biggest health scandals ever, we were told to use 'heart-friendly' margarine and vegetable oils and give up high-fat butter and cream. This positive public health message came without any proper tests of the safety of margarine, because experts were blinded by the simple fact that it contained less of public enemy number one – saturated fat. They ignored the fact that it contained many other chemical substances and often extra sugars to reduce the fat content. The clever chemists that had managed to make liquid vegetable oil solid via hydrogenation had also created a novel chemical bond linking the fat molecules that our body couldn't deal with, called trans fats, which are so harmful to our health they are now completely illegal in some countries.

Between 1990 and 2005 margarine outsold butter in most countries. To the horror of my butter-loving Belgian wife, I insisted for about ten years on buying spreadable (healthy fat) margarines, and then olive oil spreads with pictures of Italian olive groves on the tub. They all carried positive health messages on how they reduced cholesterol (which they did very slightly, but without improving our health). As well as containing many unwanted chemical additives, emulsifiers, flavourings and dyes, my olive margarine spread only contained a tiny amount of low-quality olive oil residue, as well as about eighteen ingredients including palm oil, sunflower and rapeseed oil with negligible amounts of any beneficial polyphenols. To reduce trans fats, margarine and other vegetable oils are now either made by partially hydrogenated methods or increasingly by a trick called 'inter-esterification' which bombards the more solid fats in a liquid mixture with heat, chemicals and enzymes until they harden. It is then blended with salty water using emulsifiers, starch and often milk powder. The question remains whether this kind of tinkering with fats will turn out to be harmful in the way that trans fats are.

While *probably* safer than hydrogenation, the original esterified fats were shown to have a 'safe' blood profile, but we know nothing yet of the long-term effect of these ingredients on our bodies. Studies have shown that the latest complex mixtures of esterified fats used in UPFs, although not as bad as trans fats, worryingly can have negative effects on lipids and metabolism that require much more data.[4] We appear to be repeating the mistakes of the past. I have since thrown my processed spreads away, and returned to adding butter or extra virgin olive oil to my bread. I am not alone in this. The world's largest manufacturer Unilever, maker of Flora, Stork, Becel and the 'I can't believe it's not butter' range decided to sell its non-dairy spread business as worldwide sales continue to fall. Butter, unlike margarine, is a unique and versatile emulsion in many cuisines, that holds its structure naturally between zero and 32°C without chemical help, and luckily shows no signs of going extinct or causing a devastating numbers of deaths.

Organic nut butters (like Vegan Block) are a new addition to the 'fake butter' vegan market, made with shea butter plus other vegetable oils such as coconut and rapeseed and slightly more natural ingredients with no hydrogenation, and the taste is slowly getting closer to butter.

Fake cheese

Vegan food manufacturers and vegans who used to be cheese aficionados have tried many different ways to create the perfect vegan cheese. It is still a work in progress, but in 2022 it is already valued at $1.1 billion with a 12.8 per cent projected annual growth rate. Around six years ago, I tasted a few vegan cheeses and found them universally unpleasant and an important reason why I could never be vegan, but I have since changed my mind. There are broadly two main types – those made of starch and vegetable oils, and those made with nuts.

The market-leader is Violife, a bland, inexpensive but salty starch-based cheese. It has too smooth a surface to be natural, but some of my dinner guests were fooled and enjoyed it when I served it blind. But being based on refined carbs and oils and low in protein, it has little to offer nutritionally: the same as highly processed cheese – but without the animals. To replace parmesan, a sprinkle of nutritional yeast makes the most sense in terms of delivering on the umami flavours and still holding some nutritional value at a very low cost to the environment.

Nut-based cheeses, especially the artisan variety, made by Andrea Orlandini of The Greencheese Experience, and others, cost as much as artisan cheese and use the whole nut, often adding other seeds and herbs like basil. Most of them have live microbial cultures via coconut milks or plant-based kefir to add flavour and longevity and are best eaten after storing and drying for weeks or months. Getting the right balance involves endless, sometimes costly, experiments. My favourite is a Greencheese Experience nettle cheese made with brazil nuts and fermented koji miso paste, then dried for six months. This had many of the qualities of an aged parmesan without the aromas. Others have mixes of other nuts, like cashew, almonds, walnuts with balsamic vinegar, and figs, and are probably healthily high in poly-phenols and protein.

According to several google searches, Violife also makes a good parmesan and Miyoko's makes good vegan mozzarella but I have yet to find a convincing alternative. In the US, Treeline cheese is one of the most popular for its environmentally friendly tree nut and cashew probiotic spreadable paste with garlic herb flavour. In the UK, blind taste tests reveal that packaging and fancy marketing don't top the charts, however, as some supermarkets' own brands made with the predominantly less heart-healthy coconut oil win the votes.[5]

When choosing vegan cheese, it seems the best option for taste and probiotic benefits rests firmly with small-scale artisanal 'dairies'. The best option for the environment would be to replace analogue cheese in frozen and ready meals with fast-improving vegan cheeses, such as vegan probiotic cheeses as in this recipe which uses whole cashews and is surprisingly simple to make: 'The Minimalist Baker, 'Easy Probiotic-Cultured Vegan Cheese': minimalistbaker.com/easy-probiotic-cultured-vegan-cheese/. Whether we call it cheese or fermented nut paste is another matter.

Dairy alternatives in five

1. Plant-based 'milks' generally don't contain as many calories, proteins and vitamins as cow's milk, and are often highly processed.
2. Vegan cheeses are a mixed bag, and while nut-based products have some health benefits, starch-based ones do not.
3. The dairy industry has adverse environmental impact, so finding more sustainable alternatives is important, and fortified plant milks and vegan cheese, although not perfect, seem to be an evolving solution.

4. Fake butters, although variable and improving, are not beneficial to health.
5. Eating high-quality extra virgin olive oil, or smaller quantities of butter or homemade buttermilk, is a better option.

28. Eggs

Eggs are a perfectly contained source of nutrition for baby birds, equivalent to the seed of a plant. They can hugely impact children's growth and are usually stored in the dairy section in shops and in our fridges as a staple food in most countries in the world. Considered a whole food group by themselves, one egg contains a superb range of nutrients with 13 per cent protein (over 100 different proteins), 11 per cent fat and vitamins A, D, B12, B6, calcium and magnesium. It also contains the carotenoid eye pigment lutein and zeaxanthin (though much less than berries), and many still unexplored bioactive compounds. The vast majority we eat come from chickens, though eggs from other birds taste surprisingly similar. For many children it is the first food they ever cook, but we appear to have lost our love of eggs as well as our technical skills.

A 2016 survey found that a third of British twenty-five to thirty-four-year-olds couldn't boil an egg, and one in ten students tried cooking them in a microwave (Tip: don't try it – they explode). This could be due to excessive parental pampering or a sign of the times; breakfast cereals with positive health messages and additives have replaced eggs, with their unhealthy connotations of salmonella and cholesterol. Before saturated fats, cholesterol was public enemy number one and in the 1970s was to be avoided at all costs. But like most nutrition advice, it was based on faulty data and assumptions, as cholesterol is an essential part of every cell in our body and found in many healthy foods, including fish. The smear campaign was so good that fifty years later many people still associate eggs with heart attacks, despite large, well-conducted systematic reviews and meta-analyses clearly outlining that this is not the case.

A randomised trial in 2018 compared fifty people breakfasting on two eggs or porridge, and after four weeks showed the egg group had better blood fat levels and higher eye pigments and lower hunger hormones than the oat group.[1] Similar results are seen in other longer-duration egg studies.[2] Back in the 1980s and 90s, doctors, backed by (biased and unreliable) observational epidemiology studies, suggested that eating eggs increased risk of heart attacks. Now with much more data, over sixteen studies have shown no relationship whatsoever between eggs and any type of heart disease, with a large study in China showing that up to one egg a day might actually be protective for our hearts.[3,4] So, an egg a day may not make you live longer, but now appears perfectly healthy, even if you have heart disease or diabetes.[5] (In the future we will likely be personalising advice on egg intakes, depending on how well you process fats.)

There are roughly the same number of laying hens as humans on the planet. This intensive breeding and farming has made their eggs susceptible to infections like *salmonella* and *campylobacter*, so that a small percentage of battery-farmed eggs are always infected. *Salmonella* infection is the traditional problem in commercial farms and mainly comes from contamination of the shells. In America, eggs are treated rapidly after laying with powerful disinfectants (including chlorine sprays) and only one in 30,000 is infected. In Europe this doesn't happen. In Britain in the 1980s a major outbreak occurred, followed by the health minister declaring that most UK eggs were contaminated. This led to panic and the collapse in confidence in eggs, the culling of millions of chickens and demand dropping 60 per cent. Although the UK has improved its procedures and infection rates dramatically, it is a global market and egg infections continue to be problematic. In 2017, 700,000 Dutch eggs imported into the UK were contaminated with high levels of Fipronil – a pesticide illegally used to treat lice in chickens, and millions more infected eggs in Europe were destroyed.

Which eggs are best?

For the past thirty years, many governments, including the UK, advised against at-risk groups (infants, the elderly and pregnant women) eating raw or runny eggs. This advice was rescinded in 2017 after vaccinations against *salmonella* in over 85 per cent of British hens (as indicated by the red lion stamp on the egg). Raw-egg-only regimes are occasionally popularised, by Rocky Balboa to gain muscle to become a Hollywood boxing champ, or by art collector Charles Saatchi who ate nine raw eggs a day to lose weight (to the annoyance of his then wife Nigella Lawson). Raw egg lovers claim they are better for you. While they may contain marginally more vitamin D, and choline (which increasingly looks as though it may be important for neurological development and brain function in the first two years of life), the downside is that, compared to cooked eggs, only around half of the protein is absorbed.[6]

Brown-shelled eggs seem more natural, organic and wholesome, but shell colour is just related to the species of hen and the region they come from. I don't think anyone has formally tested if blondes taste different to brunettes, but shell colour, like hair colour, makes no difference to taste or nutrition. What about big eggs compared to small? Bucking the usual trend, European eggs are on average larger than American varieties, but there is no evidence their size makes them taste any different.

What about organic versus battery-farmed eggs? The EU and the state of California have now banned battery-farmed hens in tiny cages. In Europe this was only a pyrrhic victory for the chickens, as the cages became so-called 'enriched cages' – just slightly roomier prisons increasing personal space from 600cm^2 (the size of A4 paper) to 750cm^2. In the UK in 2020, about 40 per cent of eggs sold were from these enriched cages that contain forty to eighty birds and include a 'luxury' pecking area. The other 60 per cent are now free-range or cage-free. Countries outside the EU, including the US, still raise chickens in smaller cages. These birds have a short lifespan of only twelve to eighteen months before being killed for processed foods. Free-range hens can lay eggs for over ten years and the world-record layer managed thirteen years. For other farms, a whole range of different options exist for keeping and advertising 'cage-free animals'. These can include being allowed just an hour a day to stretch their legs, or a more relaxed regime roaming and pecking free outdoors most of the time. Most hens are fed a cheap mix of grains and soy proteins and lay up to 300 eggs per year. In the last eighty years, hens have tripled the number of eggs they lay, which are also larger and cheaper, now sometimes costing the consumer as little as 10p each. Consequently, the ratio of white to yolk has increased, but luckily the total nutrients have not declined since the 1980s. There has been a slight decrease in total fats, and slight increases in vitamin D and mineral selenium, which is found in different amounts in soil and increasingly being linked to deficiency problems that may accelerate ageing.[7,8]

Studies have shown some differences between organic eggs and cage or barn eggs, with larger yolks in less albumen for caged eggs, and a brighter-coloured yolk from barn eggs. More importantly, organic eggs are more nutritious with a higher amount of polyunsaturated fatty acids (PUFAs) and comparatively less saturated and monounsaturated fats. What's more, feeding organic hens different types of herbs is a well-researched topic, with combinations of basil, chicory, nettle, aromatic herbs and fresh-foraged grass all bringing eggs a unique combination of polyphenols and PUFAs that we know are good for us.[9]

Can the discerning palate tell organic free-range eggs with bright yellow yolks from happy hens? A couple of food writers have performed blind tastings comparing identically prepared organic, free-range, caged and omega-3 boosted eggs.[10] The consensus was that the omega-3 eggs tasted a bit fishy, and most preferred a darker orange yolk regardless of the source. The colour of the egg yolk depends on the right nutrients in the hen's diet, but the feed is continuously manipulated to reduce costs, change the balance of fats and make the yolk look appealing. The clarity and amount of albumen is more difficult to manipulate, though, and it seems that happy foraging hens have more transparent egg whites, and more of it too. When the eggs were stained blue, the tasting panels couldn't distinguish the eggs, though if anything, had a slight preference for the factory-farmed variety. Again, our visual senses are easily fooled and can override our taste buds.[11] The lesson here is that organic eggs will taste better as long as you clearly tell your guests they are expensive and organic. Most hens are given cheap soybean feed as protein, but adding flaxseeds, for example, increases omega-3 levels. Having a reddish yolk may come at a price. New methods are being used, such as replacing the traditional soy protein feed for pulverised soldier ants, which increases the carotenoid levels and as a bonus the redness of the yolk.[12]

On a brighter note, trends are changing: the organic egg market in the UK is enjoying double-digit growth according to government statistics, accounting for 10 per cent of egg sales, with many EU countries showing similar numbers. The trend is also clear for caged vs free-range eggs with the latter on a steady increase and intensively farmed eggs on a downward trajectory. Globally, while few eggs now have detectable *salmonella* on the shells, this may be because of clandestine use of antibiotics. One in five Vietnamese eggs tested had high levels of antibiotics in 2017, contributing to drug resistance.[13] Even so, it's best to know where your eggs come from.

How to make the best scrambled eggs is one of the most controversial subjects for any food writer or chef, but most large kitchens, hotels and caterers use pre-cooked packets that can be microwaved, or egg and milk powder mixtures, making it impossible to tell its origins. If shell colour, redness of yolk, animal feed or humane conditions of the hen make little difference to taste or cooking properties – what does? One consistent factor is freshness.

An egg eaten within a few days has a better structure for frying or poaching, and holds up better in emulsions and sauces than one a month old. Older eggs, depending on storage, don't always need to be discarded. They can still be used for baking when over seventy days old or several weeks past the expiry dates. Most supermarket eggs can sit around for one to two months in the system and even longer in your fridge. The Chinese found different ways to keep their eggs longer without refrigeration by soaking them for several months in an alkaline solution of tea, lime, ash and salt until they smell of sulphur and the yolks turn dark green. These 'century eggs' are delicious if you can stomach the smell. As a normal egg ages, the air will increase in pockets at the wider end and the egg becomes more alkaline. If in doubt, don't use the expiry date on the pack: put your egg in a pan of water and, like the old medieval test for witches, if it sinks, keep it – and if it floats, throw it away.

Eggs are a great source of protein, nutrients and good fats and in the UK we each consume around 192 eggs per year. For most people up to one a day appears healthy, and many can handle more. If you believe all Netflix documentaries, you'd think that eating any form of animal protein, especially eggs, is deadly for us and the planet. Current estimates place eggs as the least damaging form of animal protein, producing 2.1kg of CO_2 per 50g protein, or per egg. Per 50g, tofu weighs in at about 1kg and beef a whopping 17.7kg of CO_2. So, while eggs definitely have a smaller climate footprint than other animal proteins, plant-based foods, especially pulses, are still better for the planet. The EAT-Lancet commission on healthy sustainable diets recommends that we consume one egg every other day.[14] This would help to support our own and the planet's health by reducing the number of intensively farmed hens necessary to supply our demand. The tastiest eggs, which are probably best for us and the environment, are fresh ones, so buy local eggs, from healthy hens that are free to roam outdoors.

'Ethical' eggs

Since 2005 there have been reports from China of completely fake eggs being sold, and more recently exported to India. It is hard to prove the veracity of these stories, and could be 'fake news'.[15] But eggs made by labs instead of chickens are now available to buy, with several companies vying to rule the roost. VeganEgg uses ten ingredients including algal flour, whereas Neat Egg uses only chickpeas and chia seeds. JUST eggs are another with a big PR budget and though they can replace eggs for certain uses such as baking, none of these offers a true versatile replacement. Vegan-friendly egg replacements are great for egg allergies and could form part of a more planet-friendly diet, but you can't yet recreate nutrient-dense dippy eggs with toast soldiers with any of the existing products.

Eggs in Five

1. Eggs are a great source of nutrients, containing over 100 types of protein and all of the essential amino acids and multivitamins.
2. Choose organic eggs from chickens who have plenty of access to the outdoors – they should have a clear transparent egg white when cracked.
3. An egg a day is not harmful for your heart or general health, and many people can handle more.
4. To identify a rotten egg, simply float it in a pan of water. If it sinks, it's fresh, if it floats to the top, it's a bad egg.
5. Eggs are the most environmentally friendly form of animal protein if you eat three to four eggs per week, but they still require billions of caged chickens and the systematic culling of male chicks.

29. Sweet treats

At the heart of most of our sweet treats lies one important ingredient: sugar. This simple carbohydrate comes in many slightly different forms and under many obscure names. At least 250 names have been invented for food labels to dupe consumers into thinking they are buying healthier products free from added sugar – from dextrose and maltose to corn syrup, grape sugar, trehalose, fruit concentrate, malt syrup, invert sugar, granular sucrose, corn sweetener, fructose, fruit juice concentrates, glucose, raw sugar, sucrose, sugar syrup, cane crystals, cane sugar, crystalline fructose, evaporated cane juice, coconut blossom extract, and corn syrup solids, to the mysterious silan syrup, popular with health foodies on Instagram. But don't be fooled – they are all sugar, and any differences are trivial. Maple syrup and honey are often promoted as healthy options without any evidence other than our willingness to believe. But they contain similar chemicals, are sweet and in excess our studies show they cause rapid blood sugar spikes and subsequent dips and hunger.

Table sugar is sucrose – a combination of two other sugars (fructose and glucose) and is contained to some extent in all plants. It is predominantly made from sugar beet in Europe, from corn in the US, and from sugar cane in tropical zones like the Caribbean and Brazil. We like it because it is our brain cells' preferred energy substrate, allowing rapid and easy metabolism for thinking, speaking, memory-forming, pleasure and all the other wonderful things our brains can do. So where did it all go wrong? To understand why we all crave sweetness, and why we adjust to increasing amounts, it's important to understand the biological advantage of sugar in evolutionary terms. Sugar is high in calories per gram, so it delivers instant energy for our brains and muscles. For our active ancestors, finding sugary sweet berries and honey was a huge advantage, providing quick access to a boost of energy to hunt or escape being hunted. We are programmed to prefer sweet tastes from tasting our mother's relatively sweet milk at birth, to choosing sweet tea over a bitter green tea. The food industry knows the power of sugar, so it's no surprise that the sweet stuff is added to everything from breakfast cereals to readymade Bolognese sauce; it's a cheap way of ensuring our primitive brain feels rewarded and ready for action, even if it's just pushing the remote control.

Sugar never used to be a rare treat when I was a kid, mainly added to food or drink at the table and easy to control. The average American teenager now consumes 30tsp sugar per day (in all its forms), while the WHO only recommends a maximum of 6tsp for women and children. The UK NHS recommends a maximum of 30g for an adult (around 7.5tsp) per day and less for children, but the average consumption is way higher; around 80g for adults and 110g for teenagers.[1] The majority of the sugar intake is embedded in the food itself with cereals, soft drinks, ready meals, biscuits and snacks accounting for 13 per cent of total calorie intakes. As discussed (see page 27), sugar in our food can cause large blood sugar spikes that cause short-term hunger and inflammation and longer term a higher risk of weight gain and heart disease. So, how did a product that started out as a rare and pricy food medicine end up being so cheap that it's added to virtually every UPF?

For early Europeans, used to honey, the first time most people heard of 'sweet salt' was during the Crusades in the early Middle Ages. The closest they may have come to it was perhaps dried dates which can reach 70 per cent sugar and have been eaten for millennia. Pure sugar had been around in India and then China for thousands of years, and as for most rare food items, it was first used sparingly as a medicine, then as a luxury confection for the rich. Now it is so cheap it is used in most processed foods to actually *save* money. These days, as taxes begin to bite and public opinion starts to change, manufacturers of sugary drinks and confectionery are changing their future products. However, the average adult can detect a mere 7 per cent drop in sugar content, so to maintain brand taste and loyalty, just dropping it can be tricky. The small company Doux Matok in Israel uses mechanical tricks to halve the sugar content of its version of hazelnut chocolate spread without affecting the perception of sweetness. This secretive process involves getting sugar molecules to interact more than usual with your saliva to fool your brain into thinking it is sweeter than it really is – and doesn't contain palm oil or any added chemicals.

Sugar hypocrisy and health

The pendulum has recently swung again from blaming all our ills on fat consumption to blaming the 'white poison' called sugar, which has been simplistically blamed for the obesity epidemic, as well as heart disease, cancer and dementia. Yet while governments tell us to eat less sugar and pretend to be acting tough by imposing punitive sugar taxes, they continue to subsidise the sugar beet industry to keep prices cheap. Thanks mainly to the EU agricultural policy, manufacturers will continue to pay less for sugar, as the subsidised prices plummet and the global price is nearly half per pound than in 2011. They pay so little for sugar – around 12p per 1lb – you can buy a two-litre bottle of fizzy supermarket lemonade in the UK for less than 25p per litre. Even a 100 per cent tax on sugar will have limited impact.

Most observational studies support disease associations based on high intake of sugary drinks, but meta-analyses generally are less conclusive as it is hard to separate them from other aspects of diet without a large clinical trial. Large sugar and soda companies have largely given up promoting these 'empty calories' as a 'natural source of energy'. While experts concur on the need to limit calories from added sugar, because of the lack of data and the different food contexts it is used in, tooth decay is the only clear side-effect where there is consistent data.[2] The WHO and most developed countries now suggest an upper limit of 10 per cent calories to be taken as sugar, and many now suggest lowering this to 5 per cent, or less than a can of soda. There is disagreement on which component of sugar is the main culprit. Several prominent writers and scientists have blamed the fructose component of sugar in particular for metabolic problems and diabetes, as it is metabolised differently to glucose. The topic of fructose and obesity has been controversial for the past ten years, but evidence is accumulating that fructose does impact sugar metabolism, possibly inducing metabolic dysfunction. While fructose may be theoretically worse for us than sucrose, in practice it may make little difference. Too much sugar of any kind clearly isn't healthy, especially when that sugar is consumed artificially, as opposed to in a whole piece of fruit. Increasing pressure on manufacturers and sugar levies have led to drops in sugar intakes in several countries and regions, replaced by a massive increase in the use of artificial sweeteners (see page 39) which are not much better for us.

Real sugar comes in many different guises. Many people use brown sugar in the hope that it may be healthier, but it is usually just white sugar mixed with molasses from the boiled sugar syrup. This makes brown sugar absorb moisture more easily and become clumped after a few months. Molasses is exactly the same as treacle and is the cheap waste product of extracting sugar from cane (not from beet, which is inedible). Molasses has little nutritional value, and in many countries it is used as a temporary, inexpensive, but smelly tarmac for covering dusty roads. Variations in white sugar mainly depend on the size of the crystals. Finer caster sugar is used because it allows air pockets to be trapped in the fat in the dough for baking, making it lighter. Very fine crystals are used for smooth icing sugar.

Sugar is unusual in that it has no nutrients or complex flavour in its pure form. But when heated or caramelised it releases all kinds of flavour molecules giving it a sweet and nutty taste. This caramelisation is a chemical browning reaction that occurs above 160°C and is helped by a drop of water to set it off. When sucrose is caramelised it separates into its original sugars (fructose and glucose) and fructose will convert earlier at a lower heat, explaining why high fructose fruits like apples and pears caramelise easily. Sugar can turn bitter if cooked for long enough. Burnt sugar is used widely in sweets, toppings and as a food colourant in many products like Coke and Pepsi, and some of the pigments produced in the process have preservative or antioxidant properties. The complex flavours of caramel, often when a bit of salt is added, have strong 'addictive' properties that are part of many bestselling sweet snacks. But however strongly we are programmed to prefer sweetness, the evidence that sugar is truly addictive has been overhyped.

Canadian and Mexican sugar

Canadians, who produce 70 per cent of the world's supply, will proudly tell you that maple syrup is an amazing natural product. It was originally produced by the indigenous North Americans by boiling up the sap of the maple tree. It is about 30 per cent water and the rest is sugar, mainly sucrose. It does have a few trace mineral elements and a number of polyphenols and, according to mapleologists, over eighty different flavours. While it appears to have more non-sugar chemicals than sucrose, there is no hard data on its health benefits.

Agave syrup is made from cactus before it is distilled into tequila. It is similar to maple syrup with slightly less polyphenols and nutrients. It is often flagged as a healthy alternative, but is made of fructose plus a small amount of glucose, making it *very* sweet. It is highly refined and has little else to commend it, unless you are a tequila fan.

Sugar or syrup made from coconut, date or oil palms may sound exotic, but have nothing to recommend them either nutritionally or especially environmentally. Brown rice syrup is hailed by some health bloggers as 'nature's sweetener'. Unlike honey and agave, it is fructose free. Unfortunately, it is 100 per cent glucose – 40 per cent higher than table sugar, so consumption leads to a massive blood sugar spike. Additionally, it's highly processed and made from fermented cooked brown rice that is boiled into syrup, completely removing any other nutrients. Not only is this empty calories (75 per tbsp), but it's also the highest-scoring sweetener on the GI index, causing impressive peaks in almost everyone's blood sugar.

Is all sugar the same?

In terms of sweetness, fructose ranks top, followed by sugar (a mix of fructose and glucose), and then glucose. Honey varies in sweetness depending on the composition, but is usually slightly higher than table sugar because of the higher levels of fructose. This all comes back to the GI index, the scale of how much a certain food increases blood sugar relative to drinking glucose. The index is only a rough guide as it is based on average, not personal responses. Our studies are showing that individuality in a number of factors including the gut microbiome determines how quickly we absorb glucose and how fast our insulin response is.[3] How the microbes precisely control the release of sugar isn't yet clear; this could happen in the small intestine, an area which is as yet very hard to study microbially, or by signalling molecules from other parts of the gut.

It is hard to reconcile the general consensus that high-sugar fruits and berries are healthy, and honey may have some benefits, while refined sugar with virtually the same principle ingredients is considered deadly. This is another example of our muddled reductionist view of nutrition. Clearly, as we have seen before, the other less-studied parts of the food such as fibre and polyphenols may be more important in offsetting the pure sugar. We may even find chewing on a piece of sugarcane or a dried date is good for us, but honey has always had star status for us humans.

Honey

The Hadza tribesmen and women who have been resident in Tanzania for at least 50,000 years would forgo even meat for a chance to get a handful of fresh honey. One afternoon during my visit, they decided the time was right to revisit a tall baobab tree that the previous year had held a nest. There was a three-man honey team: a young adult hunter in charge, assisted by an adolescent and an eight-year-old boy. Sometimes they were led to a new tree by the distinctive call of the local honeyguide bird in a rare human-avian pact. This bird works together with the bee hunters to find a new nest and pick up the leftovers and grubs after the humans have taken their share. But this was a well-known tree and a smoky fire was lit underneath. Using a knife, branches were cut into pointed stakes, then hammered into the trunk at intervals as footholds to scale the massive tree. The hunter finally made his way to the top about 30 feet above ground. It was a long way to fall, and a common cause of broken limbs and, occasionally, death.

Bees were buzzing around him angrily and although stung many times he was grinning and oblivious as the small boy passed a burning clump of twigs up to the top. He wafted the smoke over the nest to stun and confuse them so they couldn't communicate with each other. Amid the chaos of the smoke and angry bees fleeing the nest, with his hands, he scooped the honey from the nest and filled a bucket. After taking a few mouthfuls for himself and smiling even more, he passed it down the makeshift ladder. As the tree was near the camp, a crowd had gathered below. They descended on the bucket, and twenty hands dived in, not waiting for the guests. When I managed to wriggle through the crowd and finally got a soft nugget, it was the brightest colour orange, and with a mix of honeycomb, larvae and honey, it was an unbeatable treat. I finally understood why they risked life and limb for this delicacy.

Honey is probably the earliest guilty pleasure our ancestors encountered after breast milk. It is part of our inheritance, well documented since 2000 BCE, and awarded mythical or religious status in many cultures. Yet, honey is really bee vomit. It is produced by hundreds of species of bee from the sugary nectar found in flowers. The bees swallow the nectar, which mixes with their gut microbes, and regurgitate it several times.

There is a plausible evolutionary theory that the ability to hunt honey and rapidly get calories enabled our brains to grow in size much faster than other apes. Whether this use of fire to make smoke was more important than learning how to use fire to cook is unclear, and both skills will have probably contributed to human success. The Hadza tribesmen can gorge themselves on honey for days at a time, occasionally eating an estimated 7,000 calories a day. They like it so much, it makes up to 15 per cent of their calories over the course of a year (far higher than Western recommendations). Despite this sweet tooth, they are pretty healthy, with no obesity, allergies, heart disease or diabetes. The fact that they eat 70–100g

fibre per day and have twice as many microbial species as Western-
ers may also help . . .

Honey as medicine

Reviews published in the medical and web world extol the virtues of
honey for everything from bronchitis, asthma, diabetes and wound
healing, to cancer. Honey is mainly made up of simple sugars, the
majority is fructose and then glucose, plus about ten other simple
sugars (oligosaccharides). What else could there be in it that potentially might explain its special reputation? Or is it hype? One thing is
its complexity. It has over 200 major constituents, plus over 500 volatile compounds that give it its special flavour and perfume. Many of
these are potentially important for health like polyphenols, organic
acids, carotenoid-derived compounds, nitric oxide (NO) metabolites, ascorbic acid, aromatic compounds, enzymes, trace elements,
vitamins, amino acids and proteins. The composition of honey can
vary markedly with the diet of the bees, as essentially its nutrients
and distinctive flavours come from the plants they feed from. Some
varieties of honey even contain a tryptophan metabolite (responsible
for many brain chemicals) allowing speculation of possible brain
effects and even anti-inflammatory nanoparticles.

Of the hundreds of studies performed on animals and humans, the
vast majority show a beneficial effect of honey. The important caveat
is that the numbers of good human trials are tiny, most are in test
tubes, paid for by the honey industry, and the overall quality of the
trials is poor. Claims of benefit in cancer are baseless with no good
human data. There are some notable exceptions; one is for a tickly
cough. A review of fourteen studies showed that honey improved
cough frequency and severity in adults with upper respiratory infections (the common cold).[4] One consistent finding is that honey also
seems safe to eat, or to put on your eyelids, or to help wounds heal.
Feeding honey to infants under one year old may be risky; because of
their weak intestinal immune system, they are very susceptible to
microbial spores of botulism which don't harm older kids or adults.
Many cultures and countries ignore this advice and regularly give

honey to babies, believing it helps prevent other illnesses, as botulism, though life-threatening, is very rare indeed. Anyone strolling in
the mountains near the Black Sea in Turkey should avoid eating
rhododendron honey (aka 'Mad Honey'), however, which does
exactly what it says on the tin, because of a chemical in these plants.

Some human studies have shown that ingesting locally sourced
honey can significantly improve hay fever symptoms.[5] It seems that
honey might well have anti-allergy benefits. The best theory is that it
has an anti-inflammatory effect, and that it may also be presenting
the local pollen allergen in a way that allows our gut microbes to
recognise it as a harmless protein, thus avoiding an itchy nose.

How do we explain honey's possible benefits for our skin and
reducing lung irritation? It is likely to be the hundreds of other non-
sugar ingredients that are important. Many of these are antioxidants
or polyphenols that can have direct effects or help our microbes.
Studies have shown that five polyphenols – galangin, kaempferol,
quercetin, isorhamnetin and luteolin – are found in all honeys, plus a
whole range and concentration depending on the type of nectar the
bees are feeding on. Honey also contains microbes, but most are in an
inactive spore state as they can't survive the sugar and acidity for very
long, so we don't know how useful they may be. Studies of the bees
themselves show that their own microbes benefit from the quality of
the honey, which in turn depends on the environment, pesticides and
antibiotics.

Manuka honey from New Zealand is supposed to be full of even
greater magical properties in cosmetics and health, and is one of the
most expensive honeys in the world with some jars costing $500. It is
named after the plant the bees feed off, in this case *Leptospermum sco-
parium* or the manuka plant. The term manuka is currently protected
but Australians are now claiming that Tasmania grew the manuka
plant first (they called it the tea tree) and first used it for honey in
1864. It is best known for its antimicrobial properties on wounds and
dressings, as it slows growth of skin bacteria. Most honey varieties
are useful in skin wounds as they contain hydrogen peroxide which
works as an antiseptic but this can be inactivated by the body's fluids.
But specialist honeys like Manuka or Malaysian Tualang may be even

better theoretically as potions, because of extra chemicals such as methylglyoxal, which act as a mild antiseptic but without affecting your gut microbes.[6]

The honey industry is big business and has led to intensive over-farming. Farmed bees now produce more honey using fewer flowers and travelling and pollinating less than in nature, leading vegans to argue that eating honey is just as cruel as drinking milk. Bees do play a critical role in the survival of so many species, including our own. Without bee pollination, we wouldn't be able to enjoy most of our flowering fruits and vegetables. Whether you are using your honey for hay fever or for flavour, remember that it takes twelve worker bees their entire lifetime to produce just one teaspoon of honey. Choose good honey from your local beekeeper and enjoy it in small doses as one of nature's finest treats, which our ancestors risked life and limb for.

Royal jelly

Royal jelly, the special food the queen bee is fed, is a honey by-product which since ancient Greece has been given special status due to its reputed healing powers. It is an earthy and acidic liquid that contains even more components than regular honey, including extra B vitamins, amino acids and added polyphenols. This nutrient-rich jelly keeps the queen bee alive for years when her workers age faster and live just a few weeks, so it is of great interest (and profit) to the cosmetics industry as a luxury ingredient in face creams and shampoos (though it sounds less classy when you know it is produced by the saliva of nursing bees and smells of phenol). It has been shown to extend the life of worms and is widely advertised as a miracle anti-ageing compound, but sadly there is no evidence that it extends life in humans. However, it does have some proven antimicrobial properties. Propolis is a resin-like substance that bees use as glue that contains large amounts of polyphenols and has been touted as another health remedy, sold for a large markup without any good clinical studies. You can also find propolis as a tincture for sore throats and in honey lozenges, which may work for tickly coughs as we have seen, thanks to the honey as well as the 'magical' propolis itself.

Fake honey

The amount of honey consumed (much of it in the US) far exceeds
the number of hives capable of producing it. There are, for example,
over three times more sales of New Zealand Manuka honey than is
physically possible based on the number of hives, and so much of the
honey we buy in stores is effectively counterfeit – usually a mixture
of real honey, sugar and cheap corn syrup and unlikely to have many
healthy polyphenols or benefits.

Ten years ago Europe banned all Chinese honey imports following
discoveries of cheap, often fake honey contaminated with lead, antibiotics and other chemicals. The US had already effectively banned it in
2001 by imposing an anti-dumping duty, as the Chinese were allegedly
selling huge amounts of it on the US market, causing the local honey
industry to collapse. Chinese producers still needed a home for their
product and in 2008 a German import company in the US was found
to be relabelling the banned Chinese honey, and selling it as organic
Polish honey at a massive profit. This is a global scam involving many
countries, and many arrests each year, with illegal shipments of 60
tons confiscated annually, but many more landing undetected.[7]

Since the 'honeygate' scandal of 2013, honey launderers have
become smarter and, after milk and olive oil, honey is the third most
faked food in the world.[8] A recent EU survey showed that up to one
in three European labelled samples were likely fake.[9] This counterfeit
honey may not be particularly bad for us, but this huge illicit business
drives down real honey prices, putting genuine beekeepers' live-
lihoods at risk. So, buy honey from a supplier you trust. And if it's
cheap, it's probably not made by hard-working bees.

Bees in danger

Bee populations are dying off at a rapid rate in many countries because
of pesticides and a loss of their healthy microbes and habitats, which
even if you are not a bee-lover, should be a wake-up call. Common
pesticides (such as neo nicotinamide) damage bees directly and are
decimating populations. Herbicides (such as the world's favourite,

glyphosate) are also a problem, both by destroying their food sources and directly perturbing their gut microbes. These changes to the bee microbiome are now linked to changes in their behaviour and altered feeding habits. From an estimated 20,000 globally, the US has 4,000 native bee species, but recently 20 per cent of the most common Massachusetts species have just disappeared. Most wild bees do not make honey, and are crucial in pollinating plants and fruits that we eat, including pears and strawberries. In the US almond-growing business, farmed bees are flown in every year to pollinate the trees as there are no longer enough local bees to do the job, further disturbing the delicate ecosystems. Bees are a good barometer of the health of our planet, and the signs are not good.

Chocolate and cacao

How this bitter Amazonian fruit pod of the *Theobroma cacao* tree became, first, one of the most popular drinks, then the most pleasurable confectionery on the planet is a mystery. Cacao trees grew in Equatorial South America as far back as 10–15,000 BCE, and Ecuadorians were fermenting and enjoying cocoa in 3500 BCE. The cacao bean then spread across South America and up into Mexico where it was cultivated by indigenous tribes that then migrated to Central America. These guys passed it on to the Mayans and then the Aztecs. Cacao (also called cocoa) pods were treasured items and also used as currency. According to Spanish records in the 1540s, three pods bought you a rabbit and ten a quickie with a local sex worker. Cacao pods contained around twenty to thirty large bitter seeds that needed a lot of effort to convert them into a luxury chocolate drink that included herbs, flowers and spices and sometimes blood. The story goes that Montezuma drank the froth of over fifty cups of chocolate to invigorate himself before having a romantic night in with his many wives. By the end of the 1580s, chocolate had reached Spain and then Europe where it was drunk, warmed up and even had papal approval. After a while, milk was added to the mix by a chocolate-loving Brit called Hans Sloane, founder of the British Museum and Chelsea Physic Garden.

It took another two centuries to work out how the liquid could be dried out in a solid form. The chocolate bar was invented in 1847 by the English firm Fry and Sons. Richard Cadbury from Birmingham in 1868 used novel pressing techniques to extract the cocoa butter and found a marketing niche when he produced eating chocolate in a heart shaped box. Thirty years later, this dark chocolate was first combined with powdered milk to soften and sweeten it by the Swiss Nestlé company, and Hershey's in America later blended it with milk fat that is partly broken down by enzymes, adding a mildly rancid cheesy flavour that blends with the cocoa. Hershey's only contains about 13 per cent cocoa and doesn't export well to those not raised on it, and many Europeans, like myself, think it smells unpleasantly of vomit.

Fermented chocolate

Many people don't realise that chocolate is a fermented food. The cacao seeds lie within the sugary pulp of the pod and are mostly protein and fat to feed the newborn plant, plus a range of chemical defences to keep predators away, including polyphenols and the bitter alkaloids theobromine and caffeine. They then become beans, which can't germinate after fermentation. Farmers break up the pods and pile the pulps and beans together in vats and wait for the sun and moisture to work. Microbes quickly feed off the acidic pulp, and the natural yeasts are key to kick-starting the complex process and making the mixture brown. These yeasts first produce alcohol, then die off and are replaced by lactic-acid-loving microbes who are in turn replaced by vinegar-producing (acetic acid) microbes. These acids eat into the beans, altering their structure and, after a few days, allow a mixing of many other chemicals that produce rich aromas. The farmers then dry the beans by spreading them out in the sun for a further few days. Once dry, the microbes can't feed and die off, and the beans can be transported for the roasting stage.

This manual harvesting and fermenting process has to be done immediately on the farms, leading to variable quality. But rather like with cheese (see page 314), starter cultures are just beginning to be used effectively, instead of natural fermentation. These will improve the overall standard and reduce failures, but we risk losing some of the unique chocolate flavours because of the diverse mix of local microbes.

The fermented vinegary beans are roasted gently either as the whole bean or broken up into the kernels of the seeds, called nibs. A major difference of mass-produced chocolate is that they roast only the nibs, which is more efficient but reduces flavour, whereas craft varieties always roast the whole bean, providing more complex flavours. After roasting, the nibs are then ground into smaller grains to release the oily cocoa butter and give it a smooth consistency. The granularity varies by country, and US chocolate is usually rougher in larger granules than European and can be felt on the tongue. The next stage for most chocolate is a vigorous mixing stage called grinding and 'conching' (so called because of the original shell-like mixing machines), where either sugar, milk, vanilla or other extras are blended together with both friction and heat, which liberates even more flavours and mellows acidity. Finally, before repeated heating and cooling to stabilise the fats (a process known as tempering), and moulding it in blocks, more cocoa butter (or vegetable fats and palm oil) and lecithin, a natural emulsifier, are usually added.

The finished product is so far removed from the original bitter cacao seeds, it is hard to imagine how our ancestors came up with the crazy idea. Chocolate has over 600 flavour chemicals and a huge variation in tastes and aromas thanks to the fermenting microbes and is one of the most complex foods we get to taste regularly. There are hundreds of polyphenols released primarily in the raw and fermented states, but the polyphenols that survive the drying and roasting stages can vary enormously, depending on the exact methods used.

In making cocoa powder, some large factories employ short-cut processes like 'Dutching', which reduces the acid content to make the product milder, but probably destroys many healthy polyphenols.

How healthy is chocolate?

For most of the last hundred years, chocolate was assumed to be a sugary treat, just designed to make you fat, give you acne and rot your teeth. Our own twin research disproved any strong link between acne and chocolate, as susceptibility is strongly genetic.[10] But what is the evidence that chocolate is good or bad for you? And do the polyphenols and fermentation process offset the sugar content? The observational data suggests it may. Based on fourteen studies and over half-a-million people, eating three to six portions of chocolate a week had a 10-15 per cent risk reduction in heart disease, stroke and diabetes.[11] But the data is flawed as the types of chocolate eaten varied widely in each study, and were not well documented. Clearly there will be big differences between eating a mass-produced milk chocolate with only 13 per cent cocoa (such as Hershey bars), the rest being sugar and fats and many chemicals, and artisan 90 per cent dark chocolate with no additives. And as it's made from a bean, there is actually a reasonable amount of fibre in chocolate – per 100mg 70 per cent cocoa bar, 7–12g in dark; 3g in milk. These are significant levels when you remember that the average European eats a total of 15g or less a day, and one portion of chocolate is double that of a slice of wholegrain bread.

The evidence from clinical trials is much weaker, because the ten studies using actual chocolate products are small and all very different from each other. Milk or dark chocolate was used in different doses to explore effects on the heart and on blood markers. It was hard to see any patterns, apart from a suggestion it worked best in patients with existing diseases rather than in healthy volunteers. An independent summary of thirty-five studies showed a probable but very small benefit in reducing blood pressure by about 2mmHg.[12] More promisingly, a 2017 randomised study sponsored by Hershey's found that a combination of almonds and dark chocolate reduced some blood markers of heart risk in overweight patients.[13] Most of the evidence suggests consuming chocolate may be protective for heart health, though this may only be true for high-quality dark chocolate.[14,15]

The purest form of dark chocolate is made simply by mixing cocoa solids and cocoa butter with sugar. Adding other ingredients generally reduces the quality and potentially health benefits. The cocoa percentage should be on the label, and the higher it is the purer and more bitter the chocolate. The consensus is that above 70 per cent seems to be the right health balance when the fermented products and polyphenols outweigh the fat and sugar content, although this is arbitrary, and I would only advocate small daily amounts. Added hazelnuts and other nuts, although healthy, lower the cocoa percentage. The caffeine content in a high-percentage cocoa bar is similar to having a cup of tea. Unlike milk versions, dark chocolate is more filling and you will be unlikely to ever finish even half a bar in a sitting. Don't throw strong dark chocolate under the table for your dog though; dogs lack the enzyme that breaks down theobromine which, along with the caffeine content, makes it very toxic.

Chocolate genes?

Many Anglo-Saxons find dark chocolate above about 50 per cent hard to eat. This is not genetic, as we showed in our twin study, but cultural. One reason the UK (and the old empire) still prefers milk chocolate is that their early experience of dark chocolate was limited to products such as Cadbury's Bournville plain. This mimicked continental varieties, except for a few key points. Most of the expensive cocoa butter had been removed and sold for cosmetics, and it has only 36 per cent cocoa (just making the minimum EU standard of 35 per cent). I tried it again recently after a gap of about thirty years and found it unpleasantly sweet, with no smooth texture or complexity. It is still the UK market leader in dark chocolate and costs just over £1 for a 100g bar. If chocolate is eaten sweet and milky as a child it can be difficult to appreciate more bitter flavours later in life. Most Europeans in contrast have more early exposure to bitter dark chocolate and conversely often find milk chocolate too sweet. Tastes can luckily change over time. I was brought up on Cadbury's milk chocolate (23 per cent cocoa), but now love the dark variety, and have slowly with practice moved up the cacao percentage scale with less sugar. White chocolate is a misnomer – with only rare artisan exceptions, all the cocoa and helpful chemicals have been removed and any smells eliminated, so it contains just sugar, milk solids and emulsifiers, and is not technically chocolate. The Milkybar kid of the UK TV ads in the sixties and seventies would have been unlikely to have any teeth left, as white chocolate bars are usually over 50 per cent sugar.

Commercial chocolate milks made with low-quality chocolate powder contain little real cocoa, fibre or polyphenols. The most common brand contains around 20 per cent cocoa powder, which is then treated with alkalis, stripped of its natural fat content, and the expensive cocoa butter is replaced with palm oils, making it an ultra-processed food with 20g (4tsp) sugar per glass. Most manufacturers fortify the sickly mix with vitamins so they can claim this is a 'healthy' drink.

The world's best-loved chocolate spread, Nutella, has around fifty roasted hazelnuts per jar (its production uses a quarter of the world's hazelnut supply), 58 per cent sugar, 10 per cent saturated fat and very little cocoa. But you can make your own healthier version fairly easily: blend together toasted hazelnuts, good-quality dark chocolate, a pinch of salt, a dash of flaxseed oil and some vanilla extract, et voilà.

Chocolate and brain chemicals

Along with polyphenols, most chocolate contains other chemicals that could alter our mood and melt our hearts, even if not served in a pink heart box. Some people report warm feelings of wellbeing on eating chocolate and Phenylethylamine (PEA), nicknamed the 'love drug', and tryptophan (which helps serotonin production) have both been suggested as the cause. Whether these are present in sufficient quantities to have a real influence is dubious. Of eight small studies exploring mood, three showed clear evidence of a positive effect, although whether it was the physical or chemical properties of the chocolate is uncertain.[16] Since 2005, giant companies like Hershey or Mars have financed hundreds of research articles on the benefits of chocolate, and not surprisingly virtually all have some positive feel-good findings. Some scepticism is needed, however, as usual.

One German research article made the headlines in 2015 when it reported that eating chocolate helped weight loss. The world press lapped it up and the public followed. However, the paper was a sham, written deliberately badly from a non-existent research institute and submitted to several online journals who accepted it without proper peer review in return for a lucrative 'open access payment' of £3,000.[17]

Artisan chocolate tasting

An estimated thirty volatiles from over 600 chemicals are key to the aroma of chocolate. Individually, they may mimic cabbage, peaches, soil, sweat and lard, but together can be delicious. At my first chocolate tasting recently, I was told not to just bite and swallow the chocolate, but to break it into small pieces first, which if of good quality, should produce a crisp snap; the surface should be shiny, and the texture smooth. Before chewing, let it sit on your tongue to warm for at least thirty seconds. As the cocoa butter in chocolate changes from solid to liquid at 36°C (around the same temperature as our bodies), it melts slowly and gives a cooling effect, then move it round your mouth to liberate all the aromas, before swallowing.

The difference between artisan-made and industrially made bars can be guessed from the label and is instantly noticeable on tasting. As with other mass-produced foods, the latter's long list of ingredients might include emulsifiers, soy lecithins, E-numbers, flavourings and vegetable fats with no specifics of origin. In contrast, craft bars will just have three or four ingredients: cocoa solids, cocoa milk, sugar, maybe milk. The best producers, such as Tony's Chocolonely, will also work to ensure safe and fair working conditions for their cacao farmers. A good guide to quality and healthy potential is cost, as less than £3 suggests an inferior chocolate; the next is number of ingredients, preferably no more than three or four; thirdly, you need to know the precise area where the beans are from (farm estate or cooperative) and who made it. Note that EU law does not require this so it is only the good producers that bother to put it on their packaging. Finally, as a practical test, find out how much dark chocolate you can eat in one sitting. If you can eat the whole bar, you need to switch to a darker, healthier variety. I've tried valiantly but it is really difficult to demolish a high-quality bar with 70–80 per cent cocoa, and two small squares for dessert is now my preferred medicine.

Good chocolate should always be eaten slowly. Knowing how it is made should make you appreciate it in a different way. Happily, it is now moving back to its seventeenth-century roots and becoming a medicinal product again. You can buy cacao tablets in pharmacies and bars with added fibre (prebiotics) and there are even probiotic chocolate bars for sale with (apparently) a million live microbes.

Using chocolate as a base for other chemicals is becoming mainstream. There is a new trend emerging for edible semi-legal psychedelics (see page 238) in 'shroom' chocolate. There are also companies that have added live probiotic cultures to chocolate. The healthy way to eat chocolate is to avoid added emulsifiers, colourings, artificial sweeteners or ultra-processed fats.

The dark side of chocolate

Mass-market sales of chocolate are slowing down, partly because of global sugar health fears. There is also a growing desire for an individual artisan product that has a distinctive taste related to the origin and qualities of the bean. The global companies that own most of both the cheap and the exclusive brands have tried to go upmarket with clever advertising to reverse trends. But none of these major brands actually describe where the beans come from, or where it is made. Very little Belgian chocolate is now actually made in Belgium and is more likely to be made in places like Poland or Romania.

Then there are ethical concerns. Eighty per cent of the world's cocoa comes from Ivory Coast and Ghana, where prices are low and farmers struggle to make a living, earning as little as 40p a day (78 US cents). There are also significant concerns about child slave labour in cocoa production, involving over a million children working in appalling conditions, especially in Ivory Coast, which the big manufacturers ignore.

Chewing gum and 'no added sugar'

Sugar has been sold in many imaginative ways, including chewing gum, the famous US invention which came about in 1869 by mixing chicle – a form of latex from the sapodilla tree chewed by Mayans for thousands of years – with sugar. Bubble gum was invented shortly after using an even stretchier version of the latex. Most gum is now made synthetically with a polymer – similar to one used in bicycle tyres – sugar and sugar alcohols (polyols, a hybrid of sugar and alcohol, like dextrose, xylitol) and the more surprising erythritol which pops up in mushrooms and soy sauce as well as being an unusual sweetener that passes through the gut unchanged.

'No added sugar' chewing gums taste so sweet thanks to sugar alcohols. Xylitol is mainly produced from corn cobs or beech trees, or hardwood in China, while erythritol is made in vats by genetically tweaking yeasts in industrial quantities. The results are sweet-tasting chemicals with almost half the calories of regular sugar and the beauty of it, of course, is that manufacturers can add this to food and put 'no added sugar' on the packaging.

Low-sugar gums include more artificial sweeteners like aspartame or sucralose or natural sugar alcohols like xylitol and less sugar, often as a cocktail. Whether chewing gum itself is good or bad for your health is disputed. My primary school teacher made it very exciting as she told us it caused acid which could bore holes in your stomach, and if you swallowed it – you could die. Science hasn't backed up her claims, but it is possible to overdose. The consequences for heavy users can be diarrhoea and flatulence, as well as jaw ache.

Xylitol, if you don't mind the gastro side-effects, is absorbed more slowly than sugar and so may help in reducing sugar peaks and insulin response, and possibly slowing gastric emptying in people trying to lose weight. Studies in mice have shown a major shift in gut microbes, with a suggestion these changes are unhealthy for fat metabolism, although others have suggested digestion could release short chain fatty acids and have beneficial effects. As usual most studies are in mice and no good safety studies exist in humans.[18,19] Erythritol is even more complicated as only 10 per cent reaches the lower gut and appears hard for microbes to ferment, and although it is associated with internal body fat, it can also be produced inside the body, so we don't yet know if this is cause or consequence.

The evidence for artificial sweeteners such as aspartame is even more confusing. A recent review of the patchy evidence suggests that we cannot assume that their chemicals are metabolically inert.

Some studies suggest they may actually contribute to metabolic disease, though better-quality studies need to be conducted before we can draw conclusions.[20] In the meantime, I would steer clear of artificial sweeteners and mixtures of pseudo sugars.

The big manufacturers claim chewing gum, whether low-sugar or not, reduces tooth decay which is related to microbes in the mouth feeding off the sugar. Gum certainly does stimulate the cleansing effect of saliva and improves our feeble mastication muscles that have wasted away due to soft, processed food. But the data shows that sugar-containing gums actually increase dental caries, as the sugar feeds unhelpful microbes. A number of randomised studies using xylitol gums for a month or more do show a protective effect against tooth decay via modest reductions in *strep mutans*, the bug that causes tooth decay, and a possible advantage in reducing plaque, but only if you are fastidious in also brushing your teeth.[21,22]

Chewing gum is banned in Singapore not for health reasons, but because of the polluting effect of the sticky gum on the pavements; it never degrades and costs fifty times more to clean up than to buy. People spit or drop 86,000 square meters of chewed gum each year on Oxford Street in London alone. It costs the UK over £60 million a year to clean up, and then it washes into our water supply, ending up inside some fish and birds. A biodegradable solution has been found with gums like the organic Mexican brand Chicza that degrade, but they are currently much more expensive.

Minty fresh

Mints are very popular to reduce or mask bad breath, and surveys show one in five people use them for this reason. Bad breath (halitosis) has many causes, but poor dental hygiene, gum disease (periodontitis) and a dry mouth are common reasons. Microbes are jointly responsible for most of these odours as they produce the smelly volatile chemicals. They are even responsible for the doggy morning breath when we wake up. During our sleep, the normal daytime microbes residing in our mouth lose their oxygen supply, stop reproducing and get replaced by species that like dark spaces without oxygen. These so-called anaerobic microbes produce the early morning bad-breath chemicals, before oxygen and coffee drive them away. Though mints may provide short relief from some odours, they are mainly sugar with little room for peppermint. Tic Tacs were born in 1970 and are one of the most popular global brands that are 95 per cent sugar, but in some countries claim cheekily to be calorie free, as each serving (i.e. one tiny Tic Tac) has less than 1g of carbohydrate. Other traditional mints like Polo mints with a hole or the even older US Lifesavers have added peppermint, which is a natural oil-producing plant. This produces aroma polyphenols such as menthol, which has a unique cooling property on the tongue, and stimulates temperature receptors, fooling them into sending brain signals that they are 5–6°C cooler. Spearmint has less menthol and doesn't have the same effect. But there is some evidence that long-term mint use may actually make your breath worse as the sugar will encourage the wrong microbes to grow.

Mint-flavoured mouthwashes and toothpastes are a big market and one that is set to change soon. Studies have shown that using mouthwashes containing antiseptic agents such as Chlorhexidine causes a major shift in salivary microbiome. The microbes in our mouth work hard to maintain pH levels and prevent gum disease, as well as fight off the nasty microbes which cause cavities, so artificially shifting microbe populations is not a good idea. A new generation of microbe-friendly toothpastes, lozenges and mouthwashes are entering the market supporting our helpful bugs, and shown to be effective in treating gum disease in some early clinical studies.[23]

There are some studies suggesting that regularly eating yogurt and apples is a better substitute for breath problems, while other studies show that garlic and lime mouthwash outperforms most of the chemical mouthwashes available.[24] The family of mint plants do have some genuine medicinal properties and have been historically used to soothe the intestines in minor infections and in longstanding conditions like IBS (see page 449). However, any benefits are dwarfed by the sugar or artificial sweetener content, so fresh mint tea is a better option.

Liquorice

I inherited my love of soft Australian liquorice from my mother and I don't consider it to be in the same category as most other sweets. But am I right? Liquorice is made with the roots the *Glycyrrhiza glabra* plant, and its distinct flavour is known for its thirst-quenching and refreshing properties. Chewing on liquorice roots is actually quite pleasant and could be good for us in calming acid reflux, but when we extract glycyrrhizic acid from the root to make liquorice sweets in their processed glory, beneficial effects decrease and the resulting processed product could be lethal. Chronic liquorice ingestion is associated with increased blood pressure and a drop in plasma potassium levels, with reports of daily liquorice addicts dying from sudden cardiac arrest.[25,26] But for the record, this hasn't completely put me off.

Faking the sugar

The world's most common sweeteners are now sucralose and aspartame, added to over a third of all soft drinks sold. Both Diet Coke and Diet Pepsi have steadily grown in sales since their launch in the 1980s. The idea was that the synthetic molecules, which are hundreds of times sweeter than natural sugar, tickle our taste receptors pretending to be just like sugar but, as they have no calories, don't alter our metabolism and pass through the body unnoticed like stealthy ninjas. Food health campaigners have tried to prove for years that these chemicals cause cancer in humans and have convincingly failed.

So these harmless compounds should be excellent substitutes for sugary drinks which many of us have become addicted to. When we switch we should lose weight. Early scientific studies supported this, but increasingly the evidence doesn't stack up. A 2017 review by independent epidemiologists from the UK, USA and Brazil looked at all the studies and found no clear evidence that artificially sweetened beverages (ASBs) help weight loss.[27] They found many biased studies, which could go in either direction; positively if funded by the diet drink industry, and negatively if sponsored by the sugar industry. Their conclusion was that no country should recommend these drinks as part of a healthy diet. Other studies and reviews by independent researchers have reached similar conclusions of no evidence of benefit and a strong suggestion of long-term harm in regular users.

So why don't ASBs work as they should? Two studies shed light on this. The first was a small but clever 2017 study using fifteen normal-weight volunteers who were fed five different drinks over a few days while lying in functional brain scanners.[28] The brain scanners were used like lie detectors to avoid possible bias. Although the drinks had a different mix of maltodextrin as calories and sucralose as sweetness, they couldn't be told apart. The researchers found the reward centres of the brain lit up more when given a sweet drink with no calories than one with calories. They speculated that the mismatch between the perception of sweetness and lack of energy perturbed the normal responses of the brain, which sent out signals to the body to try and regain energy.

The second study explored the effects of a range of ASBs on the gut microbes of mice and humans. This had evolved from previous findings that people who drank ASBs were more likely to have an abnormal microbe profile, with a recent study linking ASB consumption in human pregnancy to altered microbiome and obesity in the offspring.[29] These studies showed that all the common sweeteners (sucralose, aspartame and saccharin) altered the microbes of the mice leading to abnormal blood sugar levels despite having no 'actual' sugar in them. When transplanted from sweetener-fed mice to germ-free animals, these altered microbes increased the blood sugar levels of the new hosts. They then added antibiotics to kill many of the gut microbes and showed that these abolished the blood sugar response.

To confirm this finding, they then gave seven human volunteers saccharine and found in four this caused high glucose peaks, and their microbes when transplanted into sterile mice had similar metabolic effects in the animals. There have now been multiple studies with similar conclusions, although most are in mice with some doubts about appropriate dosing and quality. The rate of absorption of the chemical, and consequently how much reaches the microbes, may be important. A newer sweetener, AceK, which is more rapidly absorbed than older sweeteners, is increasingly used, often mixed with others, but studies show it too is likely to have similar negative effects on our microbes and our glucose response as a consequence, which we have seen is crucial for our metabolism and inflammation.[30]

The evidence shows ASBs are far from inert and are not a healthy substitute for sugar in drinks or other processed food products. Worryingly, many are being combined with other types of sugars known as sugar alcohols like xylitol, erythritol, mannitol or isomalt, which are less sweet than sucrose but have fewer calories (see page 39). This increasing complexity of chemical mixtures, which we have not encountered naturally before, risks confusing our body and microbes even more, potentially altering our normal metabolism and behaviours. Sugar originally comes from plants, so could we find a natural substitute?

Stevia – the new miracle saccharine?

Stevia has the potential benefit of coming from an actual plant, *Stevia rebaudiana*, a shrub native to Paraguay and Brazil. Its main leaf component, stevioside, tastes about 300 times sweeter than sugar. In 2008, the FDA awarded its first 'Generally Recognized as Safe' (GRAS) status to the refined extracts; the EU granted it novel food status in 2011, and in 2017 permitted it for most sweets, chewing gum and other sugary confectionery to reduce the calorie content. Coca-Cola created a 'natural' version of their 'chemical' beverage with the more natural stevia calling it Coke Life. Unfortunately, despite running it past taste-panels it had to be discontinued, as too many consumers complained of the liquorice-like aromas and a bitter aftertaste. This comes from the main stevia chemical, glycoside Reb A, which stimulates both sweet and bitter receptors at the same time, which many people are sensitive to. Entrepreneurial companies are now fermenting stevia leaves in industrial quantities with alcohol and yeast to let the microbes produce the rarer glycoside chemical (Reb M) in large amounts, that produces the sweetness without the bitter liquorice aftertaste. This fermented stevia could be the holy grail of sweeteners.

Stevia has some antimicrobial effects, which may be useful in preventing pathogens like *listeria* and *salmonella* growing on food, but could have adverse effects on beneficial microbes in our guts. No proper human gut studies have been performed, although worryingly it reduces gut bacterial growth in mouse models in the same way as saccharine.[31] With anti-sugar pressure growing, versions of stevia are now added to nearly every type of processed food containing sugar and it's no surprise that investment is booming in this area. But we should be wary of calling such an industrialised product 'natural' and are still not sure if our microbes will react badly to it. Until stevia is proven to be safer on human gut microbes we shouldn't use it to replace the 'poison' sugar with yet another 'miracle sweetener'.

*

Although many people got healthier during the Covid-19 pandemic lockdowns, according to a 2021 study, the average Brit consumed significantly more sugar, mostly through snacking in the form of biscuits, cakes, patisseries and muffins.[32] The report highlighted the hidden sources of our additional sugar intake: a single KFC milkshake can contain up to 19g sugar (nearly 5tsp); kitchen staples like ketchup, salad cream and popular pickles like Branston or mango chutney contain a surprisingly high 30 per cent sugar. We also have to beware of the marketing of 'sugar-free' products. Remember: 'light' cigarettes in the 1980s were no better for you than regular ones, and many sugar-free or low-sugar confectioneries are just a way of rebranding the same unhealthy UPF product. Sugar in itself is not the problem, but the way it is packaged, renamed, hidden, processed and then replaced with other chemicals. As far as sweet treats go, nature has provided us with myriad fresh fruits to savour and the cocoa bean to make chocolate with. Save sweeties, cakes and biscuits for rare treats.

Key facts on sweet treats

1. Honey produces a similar effect on the body as table sugar, but it may help tickly coughs and hay fever thanks to its active ingredients.
2. Dark chocolate has large amounts of polyphenols and fibre and is good for your gut. Look for the high-quality dark chocolate bars with only three or four ingredients.
3. Most commercial chocolate bars are highly processed with dubious ethical credentials – pick high-cocoa varieties where possible.
4. Beware of the many sugar aliases on food labels.
5. 'No added sugar' products can contain sugar alcohols or sugars by other names, which are not necessarily good for us or our gut microbes, or artificial sweeteners, which may have a negative impact on our metabolism.

30. Nuts and seeds

Nuts are single-seed fruits with a hard shell; seeds are basically just mini nuts and nutritionally similar. Until recently nuts were regarded by many as an unhealthy snack food with a high fat and calorie content and best avoided. After all, they are one of the most calorie-dense foods you can eat, most being over 50–60 per cent fat, more than a fat steak and double that of rice or pasta. So, a high-fat, high-calorie snack food often with added salt shouldn't, according to conventional nutritional wisdom, be any good for you. No wonder a small randomised trial of walnuts raised a few eyebrows when it reduced blood cholesterol levels in the 1990s, but given the institutional dogma that fat was bad, this didn't change common perceptions or our nut habits for a long time.[1]

The high fat content of nuts is, as usual, a mix, consisting mainly of unsaturated fats like healthy oleic acid, found in olive oil, and can be either in poly- or mono-unsaturated forms, usually with omega-3 fats, plus about 10 per cent saturated fats. Everything, in a nutshell, is there for a reason; namely to nourish and protect the future plant. As well as the central portion containing fat as an energy source, nuts also have decent amounts of fibre (5 per cent), and very high levels of protein (10–30 per cent). As the seed's energy source, most nuts store fats, but some, like chestnuts, are an exception, and also have variable amounts of carbs and free sugars. Cashews also have high levels of starches, allowing them to be used to thicken sauces and soups. In the outside layers, all nuts have high levels of B vitamins, folate and antioxidants like vitamin E and polyphenols, mostly concentrated in the skin under the hard shell. This can be bitter but keeps away predators and stops them rotting. Many nuts with high oil contents are made into cooking oils (see page 409). Nuts can usually be eaten raw once the shell has been cracked, but most benefit from being lightly roasted for a few minutes: this helps to dry them out and extract some extra flavour chemicals.

From pine nuts to coconuts, nuts come in all shapes and sizes and mostly grow on trees, though we commonly include in the category the bean known as peanut (see page 175). Most observational studies of nuts have focused on heart disease and, unexpectedly, have shown beneficial results. An influential 2017 Harvard study combined three large population studies of over 200,000 people with over five million years of observations. People who ate one portion (28g) five days a week had a roughly 20 per cent reduced risk of heart disease compared to non or occasional eaters.[2] They also looked at types of nuts, with some evidence that walnuts were very slightly more beneficial than nuts in general, though introducing nuts and seeds to our diet overall seems to have beneficial effects.[3]

Other meta-analyses from around the world of large observational studies combined with multiple small short-term randomised trials found that many heart health markers improved. By far the largest long-term clinical trial performed comes from the PREDIMED study of around 7,000 men and women in their sixties followed for up to seven years. One group was given 30g nuts per week and compared to those on a low-fat diet. The nut group had around 30 per cent less heart disease, stroke and death over the next five years. They also appeared to be protected against developing new breast cancer. The results of the randomised clinical trial were similar to using the observational data on the same people, which showed a 39 per cent reduction in mortality in regular nut eaters.[4] The study has been under intense scrutiny and was re-analysed because of concerns over the methods used to allocate treatments in some people and towns. The re-analysis produced broadly the same findings, namely a 30 per cent reduction in mortality in the nut-taking arm of the trial.

Similar findings that nuts reduce mortality by around 25 per cent came from eighteen prospective observational studies, with all cancer deaths reduced by a more modest 13 per cent.[5] The main benefits for mortality were seen when people ate around 12g per day, equivalent to half a portion (a small handful). Other studies with less convincing data have suggested benefits for mental function, macular degeneration, and other ageing problems that merit more studies.

So even if nuts helped your heart, all those extra fatty calories should make you fatter, right? A US study gave one group of volunteers specially prepared fruit and nut bars with about 350 calories on top of their normal diets and found no weight increase after three months. Another gave nutty snack bars to one group while the control group ate regular snacks for three months, and found the nut-bar group actually lost 1–2 per cent of total body fat and central visceral fat.[6] Another review found consuming dried fruits and tree nuts in their pure form was beneficial for health as opposed to the equivalent highly processed snack bars.[7] A recent meta-analysis looked at over 400,000 people and over seventy short-term feeding studies and concluded that nuts definitely *do not* make you fat. In fact, they can reduce your risk of obesity by about 4 per cent per portion per week, meaning for me a 20 per cent overall risk reduction for my five portions a week regimen.[8] The PREDIMED trial also showed that daily nuts slightly reduced weight gain and waist size by about a centimetre, over five years. In theory, as well as making us all slimmer, over four million lives per year could be saved if everyone ate a handful of nuts which could, if we want it, expand our lifespan by two years. This is likely wildly optimistic, as the same result would come from curing all cancer, but it makes the point that nuts are healthy and since they are easy to transport they are your best portable snack option.

Diet nuts

So how might nuts keep you slim? It could simply be the lack of sugar and unhealthy fat peaks that lead to extra hunger and inflammation; the high protein and viscous fibre content could make you feel fuller faster as it slows digestion; or it could be direct effects of the fats and chemicals in the nuts themselves, altering and speeding up resting metabolism and energy expenditure. Others have suggested that, as we don't fully chew nuts, many of the fats don't get released so they trigger fullness but aren't absorbed in our small intestine as calories. Perhaps therefore we have overestimated by a quarter the calorie content of many nuts, like almonds, cashews and walnuts, giving them a bad name, as well as making us sceptical of any official calorie estimates, with some countries recalculating their estimates for labelling.[9] Finally it could be due to a general anti-inflammatory effect of the polyphenols and prebiotic fibre thanks to our gut microbes. A trial conducted by my colleague Sarah Berry showed that a simple swap to eating almonds instead of typical snack foods reduces 'bad' LDL cholesterol levels, so snacking on nuts has benefits.[10]

Do microbes like nuts?

There have been a few nut microbe studies. One three-week ran-domised crossover trial of a large daily portion of walnuts (42g) in eighteen healthy people found that it improved the composition of gut microbes. It increased some beneficial anti-inflammatory species like *F.Prau* or *Roseburia* that produce the short chain fatty acid butyrate and decreased fat digestion bugs.[11] Another trial of fifty-four patients showed specific healthy changes in microbes related to walnuts.[12] Some of these beneficial microbial species modify the nut's fats to healthier forms that could explain the heart benefits.[13] Other small clinical studies with almonds found similar results, showing these microbial benefits are probably general to most nuts.[14]

Walnuts have come out in many studies as being particularly healthy, and the Harvard group estimated that taking occasional handfuls of walnuts conferred the same benefits as regular mixed nuts. Why would walnuts be any better? Compared to other nuts, they are pretty average in terms of composition with 15–20 per cent protein, around 60 per cent fat and 15–20 per cent carbs, and in many countries, the name 'walnut' is also the generic name for 'nut'. One possible reason could be that they are usually eaten raw with zero processing and still with their dark-brown skin, which critically con-tains many of the antioxidant polyphenols that are lost on peeling or roasting other nuts. Walnuts have high levels of omega-3 linoleic fats which, though healthy, means they can go rancid if not stored in cool places (keep them in an airtight jar in the fridge). The macadamia, originally from Australia but now growing well in Hawaii, has over 70 per cent oil content (mainly healthy oleic acid) and also should be stored carefully.

Almonds are now the world's biggest nut crop. Before modern breeding, their ancestors were bitter almonds that produced the ultimate deterrent, cyanide, but also produced the pleasant almond flavour, benzaldehyde. The nutrition content of modern almonds is similarly impressive to walnuts, though they last longer as they have far fewer polyunsaturated fats (and more monounsaturated), and often have the skin removed and are blanched or roasted. Some countries sell almonds with their skins covered in paprika, an excellent combined source of polyphenols.

Brazil nuts and the cashew, both of which hail from the Amazon, are eaten without the outer shell, which in the case of the cashew is a good thing as it is poisonous.

Pine nuts can have up to 75 per cent fat in some varieties and have amazing aromas and taste on light dry roasting. They are a vital ingredient in Genovese pesto and Middle Eastern cuisine, but are becoming very pricy.

Healthy seeds

A number of high-fat seeds (think of them as baby nuts) are worth mentioning for health and cooking. Flaxseed (or linseed) is one of the best sources of omega-3 alpha linoleic fat, but they are not a complete replacement for the DHA omega-3s found in fish. About 30 per cent of linseed's weight is made up of fibre and it is now often used in microbiome experiments. Several short-term human experiments have shown brief improvements in glucose and lipids after eating, which prompted a larger study using a gelatinous flaxseed extract called a 'mucilage'. Fifty-eight obese women were given 10g mucilage, a *lactobacillus* probiotic or placebo for six weeks. Only the mucilage had a significant effect on the gut microbiome and also significantly improved insulin and glucose profiles. The main benefits appeared to be from the prebiotic fibre in the seeds.[15]

Summaries of fifteen flaxseed trials have also shown modest benefits in reducing blood pressure by about 2 per cent if eaten daily for three months. Flaxseeds have a tough outer coating, and much of the oil and nutrients may not be absorbed unless they are chewed very thoroughly or ground up. Grinding slightly reduces the amount of available fibre, but releases a lot more omega-3. An alternative is to soak them in warm water for twenty to thirty minutes (cold water takes longer). Over forty-five small studies have now looked at weight loss and overall show a small benefit (about 1kg) after about three months, but suggest you may need to eat at least 30g daily to see bigger effects. One tablespoon of flaxseeds is equivalent to 7g, so to get the full benefits you need about 4–5tbsp daily, which is quite a mouthful.

There is also some weak evidence flaxseeds help protect against breast cancer or improve conventional cancer treatment. The data comes from a number of observational studies, plus studies of breast tumours in mice. In humans, a single study looked at existing breast cancer and gave flaxseeds or a placebo to women six weeks before surgery. The results showed improved tumour markers in the flaxseed group, possibly because they contain lignans which have anti-oestrogen effects, although it could be other chemicals like omega-3 or the many polyphenols. There is also a suggestion they may enhance hormonal therapy-type drugs (like tamoxifen) via promoting specific groups of the gut microbiome known as the 'estrabolome', producing key enzymes for steroid hormone regulation. But without bigger studies, conclusive proof of benefit in cancer is currently elusive.[16]

Chia seeds, from a flowering plant in the mint family, were a staple crop of the Aztecs, used in a wide variety of foods, as well as religious offerings. They are billed as having amazing 'superfood' properties. They contain around 34 per cent fibre, 20 per cent protein, 30 per cent fats, mainly unsaturated linoleic acid, and a high concentration and variety of polyphenols. These are impressive stats, suggesting at least some of the media hype could be true. They have higher amounts of protein than oats, and compared to flaxseed, slightly higher fibre, with similarly high levels of omega-3, and slightly more linoleic acid. They are a lot more expensive than flaxseed and other oily seeds. Like flaxseeds, they absorb water and swell up to nine times their dry weight at an amazing rate, making them popular in chia puddings and to thicken smoothies and porridge whilst also providing plenty of fibre.

Also, like flaxseeds, chia can be used as an egg substitute to bind cakes together, which is particularly helpful for vegans. Sadly, there are no good human studies for chia, and a 2018 review agreed, saying that the existing twelve small studies were all of 'low or very low quality', meaning you couldn't draw any conclusions.[17] Until we get some decent studies in humans, I would cautiously expect them to be similar health-wise to flaxseeds. They are now increasingly being added to other snacks and foods like butter and margarine to boost the ingredients' labels and justify health claims. Europe currently imports 20,000 tonnes of chia from Central and South America with large environmental impacts, but demand produces opportunities, and production is now stepping up in countries like France – a much better use of land than growing ever more EU-subsidised sugar beet.

Poppy seeds are tiny and are mainly made up of oil, altering their colour in different lights. They are famous for producing opium when the plant is very immature and their latex juices are drained. If you do eat a large poppy-seed cake, be aware that you can still fail a drug test for opiates, although the levels are minute, and you are unlikely to feel any effects.

Sunflower, pumpkin and sesame seeds are also full of fibre, fats and protein, as well as a rich source of micronutrients, and likely to all be healthy for us and our microbes. In Japan, I discovered great restaurants where customers are given their own mini wok to gently dry roast sesame seeds before adding the rich smoky aromas to a succession of dishes.

Hemp seeds are now legal in most countries, as long as they have a low (<0.5) per cent of the THC chemical (cannabis). Hemp has a high protein and fibre content, with mainly omega-6 fatty acids. They are increasingly being added to superfood smoothies for novelty.

Nigella seeds are not in fact named after the British celebrity cook, but are a tiny black ancient seed, sometimes called black onion seeds, because of taste, not genetic similarities. Lightly toasted, they add a useful kick when sprinkled on foods or in Asian breads like naan, with a complex 'pepper-like' taste with spicy, smoky and sweet notes. They are lower in fat content, but have over 40 per cent fibre. There are many wild health claims, including for weight loss, headaches and acne, but you would need to eat kilos of them and none are substantiated, so it's best to add them for variety and taste in normal doses.

Nut and seed butters

With seeds, milling them makes their nutrients easier to absorb, but studies show that nut butters do not confer the same benefits as eating whole nuts, and minimal processing is crucial, allowing the nutrients to stay intact. This may mean that a handful of whole almonds is better than almond butter on an apple, for example. However, with seed pastes like tahini or pumpkin seed butter, you can get more beneficial nutrients and minerals when the seed has been broken down into a paste. The key is to choose brands that use high-quality nuts that don't need any palm oil or artificial flavourings, and always look out for added sugar and salt.

*

Far from being bad for us, there is now strong evidence that high-fat nuts and seeds are good for our hearts, and for avoiding cancer and living longer. There are also potential unproven benefits on mood, brain function and ageing. Like many complex high-fibre foods they probably act via our microbes. Eating a handful every day or a larger portion three or four times a week looks ideal. Walnuts tend to come out as especially good because of the omega-3 fat content and the fact that they are usually eaten with the skin, unprocessed. Other nuts may equally be as good (including peanuts), but ideally, eat your nuts with the skin intact, and try a mix of different nuts and seeds to cover your bets. Flaxseeds have the best health data currently, though the more expensive chia seeds may turn out to be as good.

Key facts about nuts and seeds

1. It's hard to have too many nuts and seeds, ideally in their unprocessed form.
2. There is reasonable evidence that both seeds and nuts have health benefits against heart disease and cancer.
3. They are increasingly being used as vegan dairy alternatives and are a great source of protein and healthy oleic acid fats.
4. There is better health evidence for some (such as flaxseeds) than others.
5. Eat a mixed variety of nuts and seeds to boost your weekly plant intake. Keep a jar of mixed seeds and ground-up nuts to hand and add to yogurts and smoothies, sprinkle onto salads or into baking dough.

31. Seasoning, herbs and spices

Our world order, history and civilisation owe much to salt and spices and the human quest for them. Our craving for salt was designed to keep us alive, as the sodium it contains is essential to keep our trillions of cells intact. Salt was probably the first major spice commodity and the forerunner of the stock market.

Spices are also used to preserve ingredients and enhance the flavour of basic foods. Most important spices came from India, China or southern Arabia and they soon gained popularity with the rich, as the Greek and Roman empires gathered them from their eastern provinces and transported them back to Europe, where their powerful aromas were seen as mystical symbols of a land of paradise few could ever imagine. After the collapse of the Roman Empire, Europe was cut off from its spice routes, and the Dark Ages were a pretty bland time for its cuisine. In the Middle Ages, sixteenth-century Venetians found themselves at the heart of the lengthy, newly opened spice routes – from India through Afghanistan, Iran, Syria, Turkey and the Balkans, then to Venice – from where they were distributed to the rest of Europe by sea and land at great prices, making it by far the richest city in the world.

Today the popularity of spices has not waned, and we are consuming more novel spices from around the globe. Twenty years ago two American neurobiologists looked at 4,000 recipes in ninety-three cookbooks from thirty-six countries around the world. The spiciness of the dishes correlated with the average temperature of that country. That was not surprising, but they also correlated the spiciness of the foods with the predicted number of disease-causing microbes killed by cooking with the spice. This suggests that we have evolved a love of spices because we survived infections by eating spicy food.

All spices are vegetables or fruits in some form that can be stored for years when dried. They are so full of antioxidants and protective polyphenols that they are usually toxic to humans. But when eaten in tiny doses they have so much chemical complexity that their aromas can transform the blandest of foods, with accompanying health benefits or sometimes hazards.

Salt

Salt has been around for a long, long time. It makes up around 3 per cent of our oceans and was a treasured additive in food and a source of wealth from ancient times. The first European city, Solnitsata in Bulgaria which flourished in 4500 BCE, was believed to have been founded on a salt mine, as were others like Salzburg and Droitwich, which had a brine spring. Roman legionaries were paid with bags of salt, thus the word soldier (*sal*dare) and salary in English, and cash in modern Italian (soldi).

After I became unwell at the top of the Italian mountain with sudden raised blood pressure, I immediately cut back on salt. My lecturers had drilled into me at medical school that salt was the key to reducing blood pressure, strokes and heart disease. There were a few isolated critics, but the evidence from around the world seemed rock solid. Observational data showed salt levels in diet mirrored blood pressure, and when people with low levels and no hypertension migrated to new locations with high intakes, their risks of high blood pressure also increased. The evidence was so compelling that it was not just a question of cutting down, but more a question of how drastic the reduction needed to be. By 2010 in American nutrition guidelines, the recommended sodium intake for everyone aged over fifty or with heart problems or diabetes was less than 2g salt per day, which is just under ½tsp. While 6g is suggested as a maximum for everyone (around 1tsp), actual average intakes are much higher at around 10–12g. This implied a need for some serious reduction. Estimates in the US suggest eating over-salted food was costing about 1.6 million lives annually and an optimistic UK model estimated a net saving of £1.3 billion if we reduce salt intakes to 5g per day by 2050.[1]

Hidden salt

Anti-salt advocacy groups correctly point out that many highly pro-cessed foods have high levels of hidden salt, including breakfast cereals and biscuits, ketchup and canned soups. In 2018, a survey of Chinese takeaway restaurants in London found that 97 per cent had over 2g sodium per portion; two hoisin pancake rolls with soy sauce had 3.8g.[2] Fast-food customers regularly under-estimate their salt intakes sixfold, often ignorant that their favourite muffin, doughnut or bagel is laden with salt to enhance sweetness and prolong shelf-life.[3] In fact, eating out in restaurants or eating any processed food is virtually impossible if you want to keep below 2.4g per day, let alone 1.5g for over fifties.

Recently we have arrived at a new concept of salt sensitivity. Studying thousands of participants, we observe a huge variation in how we respond to high or low salt. If you have African ancestry, you are likely to respond more than Europeans or Asians on average, but within every group there are big differences on a continuous scale. So, even if the average is a 1–3 per cent drop in blood pressure, many people, maybe the majority, will have an undetectable change, and 10 per cent may have a large (say 8 per cent) benefit.[4] We know from twin and family studies that genes are important in salt response and again, Black populations tend to be more sensitive. Sadly, with-out being tested intensively in a clinic for three days, we can't easily tell from genes or blood tests what category you are in.

In the UK, average salt intakes have fallen by 11 per cent since 2005, which although remaining much higher than advised, is hope-fully saving lives. In fact, in 2013 when writing *The Diet Myth*, I didn't even think it worth mentioning salt restriction. It turned out I was wrong. The turning point came recently when randomised clinical trials of patients with diabetes on low-sodium diets showed that rather than improving, they were consistently dying earlier of heart disease than those on average intakes.[5] As diabetic or pre-diabetic individuals now make up a large proportion of our population, tell-ing these people to reduce salt to low levels could be paradoxically killing them. Salt is crucial for many of our life functions, and restriction has other adverse effects on the body. A few people woke up and scrutinised some of the old discrepant results. A 2017 independent meta-analysis of 185 randomised studies and 12,000 people confirmed the good news that salt restriction did definitely reduce blood pressure.[6] But, and it's a *big* but, for most healthy people, this reduction as a result of lower salt consumption is surprisingly small and clinically trivial. Despite many trials, there is no consistent evidence that low-salt diets reduce the risk of actually suffering an event such as heart disease, heart failure, stroke or earlier death.[7] Within this same 2017 meta-analysis of salt reduction they also looked at blood tests indicating increased stress to the body. Kidney hormones increased 55–127 per cent; adrenaline and noradrenaline 14 and 27 per cent; cholesterol 3 per cent and triglyceride fats 6 per cent. So while high blood pressure is related to high salt intakes, reducing it doesn't make much difference for most individuals, and can in certain groups make you more likely to die due to a disruption in other vital systems such as our heart, for which sodium is a key electrolyte.[8]

This is starting to sound worryingly like the cholesterol/saturated fat story of the 1980s, but, while there is still evidence that low salt reduces high blood pressure, again we see a failure to see the bigger picture and the complexity of our food interactions. A 2016 *Lancet* study of forty-six countries shows that the health problems of salt are at the two extremes, a bit like alcohol, a so-called U- or J-shaped curve. Eating massive amounts of salt on a regular basis, especially when hidden in processed foods, such as breakfast muesli, is evidently a bad idea, and we should focus primarily on reducing UPFs. I think it is a mistake, however, to bow to puritanical reductions in salt content and replace it with other chemicals, as that could be harmful at the other extreme.[9] The pressure on manufacturers to reduce excessive salt is good, but adding ten more chemicals as preservatives to the mix – to maintain shelf-life or improve flavour – creates other problems, especially in meat products.

'Low-salt' substitutes, like potassium chloride mixed with sodium chloride, taste salty but with a faint metallic taste. A 2022 meta-analysis of 26 trials surprisingly found that using salt substitutes reduced blood pressure by 4.7mmHg and reduced strokes and heart disease more than lowering salt intake.[10] Plants like bananas, beans or leafy greens are good sources of potassium and useful in preventing cramps in muscles, but potassium overdoses can be deadly, and one of the best ways to have abnormal rhythms and stop the heart. Potassium also interacts with about half the tablets people take to fight blood pressure, like diuretics and ACE inhibitors.

If you are eating too much salt, it is either because you are eating too many UPFs, or you work in a Michelin-starred restaurant, where salt goes into everything. Salt is added to food in every country in the world and in every restaurant simply because it tastes better. It accentuates nearly every flavour, and every good chef will tell you the first skill to learn is how to salt your food, and the biggest crime is under-salting. Some experts advise not salting during cooking but adding it at the table to your taste. By all means experiment, but you will probably find you need to add more salt on your plate to enjoy the flavour as the sprinkled salt doesn't enhance flavours nearly as much as it does when added during cooking. There are exceptions, as in salads where you might want flaky sea salt crystals to have an effect on the palate. Salt can also alter the structure of foods, as in salting cucumbers to soften them in salads; salting (or quickly boiling in salt water and draining) aubergines before cooking to collapse the number of cells so they don't become swamped in oil with cooking; or salting fish to dry out the moisture.

All salt is not equal

Salt is not just sodium chloride, identical in all its forms. Chefs are very fussy about their salt, which should be sprinkled carefully with hands and fingers, not spoons, and swear to different crystalline structures having different taste properties. Table salt is refined salt with small even grains that usually contains 2 per cent of other anti-caking chemicals such as magnesium carbonate or sodium alumina-silicate to stop it clumping. It is often 'iodised' to help prevent thyroid deficiencies and mental retardation. Different countries vary widely in their salt additives, and nearly half of French table salt also contains fluoride to help reduce tooth decay, as they don't generally add it to water; Germany and Hungary also offer fluoride varieties. Other countries add some dangerous sounding (but approved) chemicals like sodium ferro-cyanide or folic acid and iron. Kosher or kitchen salt, preferred by chefs, is a purer form of table salt without additives and with larger irregular granules, so a pinch is a third less concentrated (and salty) than table salt. Salt is best added from a height (and a flourish) to the pot or food so it disperses evenly. Sea salt, if unrefined, has a much wider surface area and irregular crystal structure. It contains several minerals like calcium and magnesium and can contain algae and sometimes a fishy smell. It is good for adding to plated food where these subtle differences can be picked up by the tongue, but is much more expensive and wasted when added to the pot.

Gourmet salts

Some variants of sea salt are already a billion-dollar global business. You can now find Himalayan pink salt in local supermarkets around the world or even grate your own from a pure crystal. Some of these products have a 5,000 per cent markup compared to table salt. Bay or sea salts are well known and the market leader is Fleur de Sel (salt flower), collected for centuries from the coasts of Brittany and the marshes of the Camargue, with similar versions from Spain, Portugal and Catalonia. British sea salts from the coasts of Essex (Maldon), Wales and Cornwall, are also popular and less moist with a distinctive flavour. Black salt is found in India in black lumps or brownish-red powder and comes with a smoky sulphurous kick.

The most expensive natural salt is probably Korean bamboo salt, a delicacy at around £50 for a tiny 2oz jar, made by progressively heating up grey sea salt in a sealed bamboo stick coated with clay until it becomes molten and recrystallises. It is apparently very strong, salty and mineral in flavour with medicinal claims, so you can't eat a lot of it, which at that price is just as well.

Salt in food and guts

As well as being a key nutrient, salt is essential to numerous dishes and food preservation methods. Most fermented foods, including sauerkraut and kimchi, involve soaking in brine to help certain friendly microbes survive and kill off others. Other salt-loving microbes (like *lactobacilli*) reproduce and start producing lactic acid which makes the salty solution more acidic, eventually leading to a stable state for storage with little microbial activity. This basic method is also used to ferment soybeans to make soy sauce, which many Asian countries use at the table rather than refined salt. Fermenting food in this manner is a delicate business: too little salt and *lactobacilli* can't flourish, too much and they stop reproducing and can die.

Our human guts may be similar. In 2018 our group was the first to link diversity of gut microbes with differences in the stiffness of blood vessels, which are key to heart failure and blood pressure. We looked at 617 women in detail and saw that particular fibre-eating bugs (like *ruminococci*) were protective and kept blood vessels flexible, probably by producing chemicals like butyrate.[11] These effects were four times larger than seen for traditional risk-factors like obesity or blood sugar alone. In the ZOE PREDICT study of 1,003 people, we found several species of microbe associated with increased salt intakes, most of which were beneficial probiotics, including some found in yogurts.[12] In mice overfed with big doses of salt, *lactobacilli* species die out, disrupting immune cells that could be preventing raised blood pressure. The effect was reversed with probiotics containing *lactobacillus*. Similar results were seen in twelve human volunteers given an extra teaspoonful of salt per day for a fortnight, which although modest was effectively doubling their normal (healthy) intakes.[13] The volunteers that had the friendly *lactobacillus* species at the beginning ended up losing them, showing that our gut health and metabolism, just like sauerkraut, depends on getting the balance of salt to microbe right.

If you are not keen on all the psychological and physical side-effects of salt restriction, probiotics or fibre-rich fermented foods could help. Meta-analysis of multiple small randomised controlled trials of fermented milk containing *lactobacilli* in healthy people and those with high blood pressure has shown them to be effective.[14,15] What we don't yet know is exactly which preparation is most effective and at what dose.

The majority of healthy people probably have the right level of salt intakes to suit their gut microbes to ensure they are happy and produce chemicals to keep the immune system healthy and blood vessels relaxed. In general, while you should avoid eating heavily salted foods regularly, most people can take current strict guidelines with a big pinch of salt.

Black pepper

Most of the world also has another shaker on the table, black pepper, as the other crucial spice, but it was mainly chance and history that made it dominate. Black pepper was the reason the Americas were discovered, as fourteenth- and fifteenth-century European adventurers set out in flimsy vessels to discover the source of the peppercorn, and a new quick way to get to the original source in India. Columbus optimistically thought he had arrived in West India, when he had only reached the Bahamas, where he proceeded to plunder many other treasures, subjugating and murdering the indigenous inhabitants in the process. In Roman times, pepper was used as ransoms and some Egyptians were buried with peppercorns as well as gold. Nearly every medieval European city had a spice street, and pepper was the predominant aroma, and street name. In the Middle Ages pepper was ten times the price of any other spice, and largely controlled by the Venetians who made a fortune. Once Britain controlled India by the eighteenth century, the price of pepper fell dramatically and became synonymous with token payments, like a peppercorn rent.

The peppercorn is the fruit of a vine that grows wild in India. Red, white, green and black peppercorns all come from the same vine and are just at different ripening and processing stages. Black peppercorns are unripe berries left in the sun to ferment (thanks again to microbes) and then dried out and left to wrinkle. Green peppercorns are unripe berries that are not allowed to dry, and white peppercorns are just the peeled inner fruit of the soaked black whole peppercorn which slowly turns red when the husk is removed. They, like other spices, are rich in protective antioxidants and, in ground powder form, retain chemicals and aroma for about three months, but the whole peppercorn keeps for years and is best ground into food just before eating. The key to pepper is the aromatic chemical piperine, that has both complexity and pungency and can increase the flow of saliva and gastric juices. Black pepper has quite a few relatives that, under different historical circumstances, we would have been grinding on our dinner tables every day, such as its spicier cousin long pepper, which was used by the Greeks and in medieval times. They all contain piperine as the main active alkaloid compound and give dishes a pleasant kick, but are not all that different in composition, making the price tag on some of the colourful varieties questionable. Confusingly, pink peppercorn isn't pepper at all, but dried berries from the baies rose plant, imparting a pricy, aromatic, but not hot flavour. If you are allergic to pistachio or cashew nuts, beware the cross reactivity with pink peppercorn, but not with real black pepper.

When Christianity lost control of Constantinople in 1453, and the trade routes were cut, the pepper price soared and the search for a cheaper alternative began in the New World. Spanish sailors reported a fiery spice used by the Aztecs, and they called it *pimiento*, the Spanish name for pepper, forever confusing these very different species. The Spanish and Portuguese subsequently exported these around the world, including to India and the Far East, changing their cuisines and palates for ever.

Aromatic plants

Popular on our windowsills are the humble basil and coriander plants that we can buy at our local supermarket. With their vibrant green leaves, it's no surprise that they are polyphenol-rich powerhouses of flavour and nutrients. Basil is popular in Mediterranean cooking and in Ayurvedic medicine, as well as crucially to make pesto sauce. A study looking at polyphenol content of tomato sauce cooked with different herbs, showed that adding basil, marjoram and oregano to finish a traditional soffritto-based tomato sauce increased the overall nutrient and polyphenol count well beyond shop-bought tomato sauces.[16]

Parsley and coriander (cilantro) have similarly rich nutrient profiles with vitamins A, C and K as well as anti-inflammatory polyphenols. Mint grows well nearly everywhere and tastes sweet as well as fresh. It's rich in polyphenols and is traditionally used to soothe indigestion as well as lull us to sleep, especially in a mojito.

Rosemary is enjoying a revival due to its supposed antibacterial and liver-protecting effects, without much science to back it up. Any benefits of rosemary are likely due to it being a hardy plant with lots of polyphenols to help it survive in the hot and dry climates it loves growing in.

Rosemary and thyme, being quite dry leaves, are easier to package and transport without losing too much of their essential oils and chemicals. Basil, parsley and coriander probably retain more of their benefits eaten fresh. To keep dried herbs fragrant for longer, store them in a cool area in airtight containers as exposed most will lose their magic within six months.

Spices

Cumin, mostly produced in India, is a fragrant seed spice with great depth of flavour and over 100 chemicals and volatiles. Many claim it helps people lose weight, though the research isn't that strong. A systematic review of twelve small trials, half of them performed in Iran, suggests cumin at doses of as little as 75–225 mg/day is helpful for weight loss.[17] A trial using 1 small teaspoon of 3g per day gave similar results.[18] We can all add it easily to our cooking, and who knows, we might all be slimmer. Many people use cumin for its possible antibacterial and anti-inflammatory properties too, making it a popular spice for upset stomachs.

Turmeric is both a spice and a medicine in India and China and it is also used in cooking in Iran, Malaysia, Indonesia, Thailand, Vietnam and many more. It is used as an antiseptic, in cosmetics, as a dye, a food ingredient, and to treat and prevent a vast range of diseases including depression, heart disease and cancer. It is the root of the flowering turmeric plant of the ginger family, originally domesticated because of its colour as a cheaper saffron substitute. Fresh turmeric is now available in places such as the UK and is present in most curry dishes and increasingly as an ingredient in many dishes.

It is not a strong spice, but it is used as a balancing agent, usually rounding or completing a dish and staining every surface and bit of the body it comes into contact with. Turmeric is a complex substance; a mix of carbohydrate (69 per cent), plus protein, fat, minerals and water. Curcumin is the main active ingredient making up about 5 per cent, which if you want to impress your friends is actually called 1,7-bis-(4-hydroxy-3-methoxyphenyl)-hepta-1,6-diene-3,5-dione, or its snappy nickname: diferuloylmethane. There are many other ingredients, and curcumin itself forms many other metabolites, each with their own actions. Eating only curcumin has little effect on the blood, something we call low bioavailability. Black pepper helps the absorption of curcumin into the blood according to several studies. This tendency of turmeric to stay in the gut worries more honest supplement companies, but could be important if microbes are involved, which has yet to be properly explored. As curcumin and capsaicin have some common effects on pain receptors, they could affect the gut in similar ways, slightly altering the acidity and improving the health of the gut community.

Test-tube studies consistently suggest it has effects on key immune and cancer pathways (which we can largely ignore) but there are now over a hundred clinical trials, though most are small, using different doses, and the results and meta-analyses often published in low-ranking journals lacking rigour. Nevertheless, a recent systematic review of its effect in twenty-two small clinical studies with cancer patients in addition to chemotherapy was encouraging and showed even high doses of 10g per day appear safe.[19] One study showed shrinkage of intestinal polyps that can be a precursor of cancer when curcumin was combined with pepper, while others of curcumin alone showed no effects.[20] When you combine the small number of available studies you can see some consistent benefit of pain reduction in osteoarthritis patients (ten studies), where it seems as effective as ibuprofen, and based on six tiny studies, possibly severe depression.[21,22] In twenty studies there is also some encouraging data that it may be helpful in blood sugar control in type 2 diabetes.[23]

The exact quantities needed are uncertain, but as a guess, taking 2tsp turmeric per day is worth doing if you suffer with arthritic pain, and probably as an addition to chemotherapy. There is no good data to support claims in autoimmunity, or dementia. While we wait for more definitive proof with larger independent studies, turmeric appears quite safe, so ingesting it ideally with chillies, a pinch of pepper and some yogurt or kefir seems a good bet.

Saffron is one of the most expensive substances by weight on Earth. The word comes from the Arabic for thread, and its intense colour comes from polyphenol carotenoids like the carrot. It is currently about half the price of gold and ten times more expensive than the next pricy spice, vanilla. For many centuries this colourful crocus was used by rulers and nobles to show off their wealth. As well as its extravagant use on food to add colour and flavour, it was used to dye hair and fabrics and even used on skin as a quick but expensive tanning agent, producing a golden glow. Henry VIII is supposed to have had his golden tights dyed with saffron and crazy amounts of the spice were used in making one of his favourite court dishes, Golden Swan. In the sixteenth and seventeenth centuries, a small arid area replaced Iran as the world centre of saffron crocus production: a small corner of Essex around the town of 'Saffron' Walden, known as the driest place in the British Isles. Production continued for 200 years, using intensive manual labour to extract the three red-orange stigmas from the purple petals. It takes around 150,000 flowers to produce just 1kg dried saffron. The industrial revolution spelt the end of this colourful spice farming, as the cheap workforce moved to the cities. A brave and dedicated saffron farmer has recently started up production again near the original site where the ground is still ideal. The plants are too fragile for any modern machinery, and manual labour is still needed. Saffron is now also being grown again in Cornwall, for the first time in many years.

High-quality saffron has plenty of the bitter carotenoid chemical crocin. In tiny amounts this will stain even more than turmeric.

When fresh it has a warm honey or straw aroma that is used in many curry and rice dishes. Brought to Europe by the Phoenicians, the Spanish adopted it for their paella, the Italians in risottos and the French in bouillabaisse fish stew. It quickly degrades and should ideally be stored in an airtight box in the freezer. To maximise its qualities, take a few threads of fresh spice and let it soak overnight in water and alcohol. While, like all spice, it is purported to have health benefits, no one has yet invested the millions needed to do the clinical studies to prove it. It is also the most lucrative spice to doctor and substitute other cheaper products like turmeric and dyed grass. In the Middle Ages, the penalties for this deception were often death (or worse), but now the risks are small, the profits large and sadly fraud is common. A 2016 investigation using the new tools of chemical fingerprinting (metabolomics) showed that around 50 per cent of high-quality Spanish saffron now actually comes from lower-quality plants in Iran and Morocco, although reassuringly the PDO-certified super-expensive varieties from La Mancha were usually genuine.[24]

Ginger is reported to have a range of different antioxidant, anti-inflammatory and anti-cancer properties. Gingerol is the main component responsible for its biological properties. A recent meta-analysis found it works well for weight loss but sadly only in lab animals, not in humans.[25] Ginger extracts have been shown in a few clinical trials to slightly help osteoarthritis pain, and can also help nausea after anaesthetics, but again the effects are small.[26,27]

Cloves have been well known since ancient times to help tooth-ache, and oil of cloves is still sometimes prescribed, as human trials have shown it to be as effective as anaesthetic gels.[28] Cloves are a safe and effective ways of soothing teething babies too. Eugenol, the active principle from clove extract, is well known for its anti-inflammatory and antimicrobial properties, and is also found in nutmeg and cinnamon which also have some potential benefits, but so far lack human evidence. Outside dentistry there is no good human data to support other uses of cloves, apart from being a great addition to baked apples or mulled wine. Various health properties have also been suggested for cinnamon and the Middle Eastern spice sumac.

Chilli peppers

The new pimiento found in the New World was the chilli pepper of the Capsicum family and the active chemical producing the burning sensation is capsaicin, which is concentrated in and around the seeds. The Capsicum family includes bell peppers, cayenne, paprika, jalapeno and thousands of others which contain this protective chemical to stop them being eaten by animals or damaged by sunshine. Larger sweet bell peppers are the black sheep of this family – they contain a recessive gene which means they produce no capsaicin. Paprika is the powder of the dried fruit of the milder and sweeter capsicum varieties, and was first cultivated in Hungary from the seventeenth century, where it was known as Turkish pepper, and used in goulash. Other sweet varieties are Spanish *pimenton* and Italian *pepperoncini*. Cayenne pepper is made from the seeds of the spicier chillies. The word chilli is a general name for the Capsicum family, but the capsaicin content can vary widely, both within the fruit (most being in the core and seeds) and between and within species, some now being intensively bred for their spiciness. This means that every chilli is unpredictable in its kick. In Spain, a traditional dish called *pimientos de padrón* serves a dozen grilled peppers, most of which are mild but usually one will be much spicier, making it a bit like Russian roulette.

Hot sauces and spices are increasingly popular, but why do we enjoy burning our tongue? The trigeminal nerves of the face and tongue are responsible for a dual role of detecting burning as well as cool sensations. The capsaicin in chilli affects these nerves by releasing a chemical called substance P, which is picked up by a pain receptor, first irritating then numbing the nerve. Psychologists describe deliberately eating hot chillies as benign masochism that releases endorphins. Humans are the only animals apart from birds who can tolerate and enjoy these hot chillies and so spread their seeds. Love of hot chillies clearly has a cultural component, but within distinct populations, there are marked differences between people. In Europeans using our twin study we found a strong genetic influence

(58 per cent), which may be related to genetic differences in personality or in pain thresholds.[29]

Capsaicin, as well as causing pain in your mouth, is also a painkiller that I have prescribed regularly as a cream for rubbing on painful joints or muscles, shown in trials to be effective. After rubbing on, it is initially painless then stings for a few minutes, before relieving symptoms. I always warn my patients to wash their hands and be careful about touching their eyes and other sensitive body parts. Most people don't repeat the mistake. You can build up tolerance to eating chillies or strong curries with practice. Vindaloo is believed to be the hottest classical curry, but phall curries are believed by other 'experts' to be even hotter. The phall is not Indian and was apparently invented in Birmingham in the 1970s by Bangladeshis who boasted it was the hottest curry sold in the UK.

The worst thing you can do with a fiery curry or chilli is reach for a fizzy drink. The carbonated liquid just tickles the trigeminal nerve even more and prolongs the agony; plain water doesn't help either. Mexicans swear by sucking on a lime wedge, but I find the best remedy is full-fat milk or yogurt to coat the tongue, hence the popular fermented milk-based lassi drinks in traditional restaurants.

Every country has its own hot sauce contribution. Korean *gochujang* is made with chilli, fermented soy and sticky rice. The Indonesians have spicy sambals and the Thais sriracha. In the Caribbean, superhot scotch bonnet pepper sauce is on every dining table, while Portuguese peri-peri sauce is almost ubiquitous now in the UK. Tangy Cajun pepper brand Tabasco ages its sauce for three years to achieve its flavour. Harissa paste is North Africa's most loved condiment, with a thick and smooth but slightly grainy consistency, made with ground red chillies, cumin and coriander and a bit of olive oil, making it less processed and possibly the best hot sauce around in terms of polyphenol content.

Are chillies a health food?

To compare the strength of chillies' burning power, the Scoville heat unit (SHU) was invented. At the maximum, the 100 per cent pure capsaicin chemical has a score of 15 million, while at the other end, an average pimento in an olive is only 100 SHU; Tabasco 2500; and a good vindaloo curry scores only a feeble 100,000 SHU, but that's quite enough for me. For hardened chilli fans, specially bred fiery chillies compete to be the world's strongest. These include ghost peppers, moruga and reaper varieties which can reach 2 million SHU, ideal for macho eating competitions and the basis of police pepper sprays. Eating them normally causes no more harm than severe sweating and a wish to cut your tongue off, but people do suffer worse trouble. A Turkish man had a heart attack after eating concentrated cayenne powder, and another thirty-four-year-old man was admitted to hospital with severe thunderclap headaches, two days after eating a whole Carolina Reaper chilli, billed as the strongest in the world. The capsaicin had caused spasms in his brain arteries leading to the headaches, but luckily he recovered. But don't let me put you off: regular eating of chilli peppers in moderation could be beneficial.

A 2017 observational study of 16,000 Americans followed for nineteen years found the regular chilli eaters had a 13 per cent reduction in mortality and vascular problems compared to non-eaters.[30] Other studies have shown similar results; a massive study that followed 488,000 Chinese from ten regions for seven years found that those eating more chillies reduced their risk of early death by about 14 per cent.[31] For cancer, there are probably an equal number of studies saying chilli eating prevents cancer as those that show the opposite. Most of these studies are poor-quality and dubious test-tube studies dropping chilli on cancer cells, or case-control studies, which are often biased. A meta-analysis of thirty-nine of these studies in 2017 concluded that no clear protective or adverse effects were seen for cancer.[32] The only exception that needs clarification might be a large 70 per cent increased risk for stomach cancer seen in men (but not women), which is now rare in the West, but still quite common in Asia. There is reasonable human evidence from trials that long-term chilli eating paradoxically reduces symptoms of heartburn and discomfort, perhaps raising your pain thresholds.

Good studies on the effects of chillies on gut microbes were absent until 2017 when mice given capsicum along with a high-fat diet had reduced normal weight gain. This is likely because of effects on the microbe community. Chilli reduced the generally unwanted *proteobacteria* (that include *E.coli*) and increased the levels of *Akkermansia*, associated in mice and humans (in our studies) with weight reduction. Another well-conducted mouse study demonstrated that chillies reduced low-grade inflammation, which is likely to be another causal factor in obesity.[33] This anti-inflammatory effect was due to gut microbes, predominantly the *ruminococcus* family which seem to like chillies and produce more butyrate, thereby maintaining gut diversity and a healthy gut lining, reducing inflammation and weight gain.

In humans, there have been four randomised placebo-controlled trials of capsaicin treatment for weight loss in 288 subjects.[34] None were very convincing on their own and they used a variable range of doses from 6–600mg per day. But overall they did show slight weight loss, metabolic improvements and reduction in appetite, suggesting they could be effective. Much of the data is based on one ingredient, capsaicin, ignoring the 200 or so other chemicals in a chilli pepper that may have a wider effect. Producing the whole chilli as a medicine would also be tough, as even seasoned chilli eaters can't tolerate the same levels of capsaicin when given out of context as a drink or medicine, rather than as real traditional food. So, my advice for the moment is cautiously positive; if you like spicy food, carry on eating chillies and curries, but avoid highly processed ready meals.

Mustards

Mustard seeds are derived from a plant of the cabbage family, and have a pungent odour only when crushed or added to liquid. Chemicals in the mustard are released into the air and go up your nose at room temperature, but when the seeds are roasted or added to the pot, the enzymes are deactivated and the effect is much milder. Mustard seeds were used by the Romans who crushed and mixed them with unfermented wine grapes (must), so mustard was invented and the practice continued in medieval Europe. Black mustard seed is the strongest and contains most of the chemical *sinigrin*, but is harder to grow than the brown seeds now mainly used in Europe. White mustard contains a milder chemical (*sinalbin*) used mainly in American mustards. Dijon mustard has been made in this French town since the thirteenth century and is now made with brown mustard seeds from Canada mixed with wine vinegar, but other versions have whole black or brown seeds added to it. English mustard, such as the most famous brand Colman's (until recently when the company was acquired), has been made since 1814 in Norwich using Indian brown seeds and is the strongest, most concentrated mustard. American mustard, such as its most famous brand French's, is bright yellow due to added turmeric and mild due to dilution and the use of white seeds. German mustards come in many varieties and can often be darker and sweetened.

Wasabi is the Asian equivalent and comes from the root of an Asian cabbage that also uses *sinigrin* as a defence against insects. Fresh wasabi should be grated directly from the root onto the dish, releasing many different chemical aromas. The strength is greatest five minutes after grating, but after twenty minutes the overpowering aroma dissipates and it has a milder rich complexity. Most shops and restaurants outside Japan cheat and use dyed horseradish with mustard which is much cheaper. As the demand for sushi and wasabi surges, there is not enough farmland in Japan to grow it, despite the rewards for one of the world's most expensive vegetables. In 2015 a farmer in Hampshire, southern England, started growing it successfully alongside his watercress for the first time in Europe. He keeps his address secret, but he is still growing his own wasabi and is now selling grow-your-own wasabi rhizomes, showing increasing popularity for this slow-growing and delicate vegetable.

Vanilla

The vanilla bean is the seed pod of a climbing tropical orchid native to Mexico, now mainly grown in Madagascar. It is the next most expensive spice after saffron because it is so delicate, and requires a lot of heating, drying and storing. Its price also goes up and down twenty-fold depending on growing conditions and yield, and in 2017 the bean briefly reached over $500 per kg. Although it has potential anti-oxidant and antimicrobial effects, the vanilla bean is best known for its unique aroma from the release of the chemical vanillin. Most of us find vanilla aroma relaxing and it has been found to calm new-born babies nearly as well as breast milk and is used in some milk formulas.

After the European colonisation period, when Madagascar became the vanilla capital of the world, the local government formed a cartel and wanted to keep the price high and so destroyed many other potential vanilla farms, pushing the price up further. More recently, prices rose dramatically after a series of tropical cyclones destroyed yet more crops. In the face of this uncertainty, US chemists working for big food companies started synthetically producing vanillin from lignin in tree bark. This was chemically identical, but was produced in a lab by burning pine tree bark at only a fraction of the price. This also explains why smoking other meats and fish and drinks like whisky can produce vanilla aromas. Most vanillin now comes from a by-product of the petrochemical industry, with a minority coming sustainably from trees in paper manufacture, which apparently has a more interesting flavour. This synthetic product is the usual ingredient in most cheap and pre-prepared foods and cake mixes, and is routinely added to yogurt in many countries. Americans appear addicted to it. In the US, it can be hard to find 'natural' yogurt without added vanillin, even in high-end health food stores. Vanillin is used widely as it has the advantage of enhancing the depth of many dishes and flavours, such as chocolate, caramel and coffee and can make them appear sweeter than they really are. It is now being combined with artificial sweeteners such as aspartame to disguise the unpleasant tastes.

One in fifty people lack the taste receptor for vanilla and there is wide variation within this group, some of whom will find most ice cream or vanilla drinks unpleasant.[35] In cakes and biscuits, blind tasters cannot usually tell the difference between natural and synthetic vanilla, but in ice cream the effect is most noticeable. Around 99 per cent of the world market is now made from vanillin, and accounts for over 95 per cent of the market in the US and UK, but less than 50 per cent in France or Italy, where the extra flavours of the 171 other chemicals in the bean are more appreciated; even if it adds to the cost of the crème brûlée or ice cream. While many food companies announced they wanted to return to natural vanilla, with tiny and unpredictable crop production, this will be impossible. Sneaky alternatives now involve making 'natural' vanillin from fermenting rice bran with yeast or, now the vanillin gene has been discovered, from genetically modifying microbes to make it for us.

A word on 'adaptogens'

Adaptogens are the latest craze sweeping the nutrition blogs and supplements market, but the term is only a pseudo-scientific way of describing the anti-stress properties that chemicals in plants have on our bodies. With dubious studies reporting hormone-balancing results, improved conception rates and reduced cortisol stress levels, the focus is mainly on a few select herbs and exotic spices, some especially obscure, grown in Tanzania, the Chilean mountains and other far-flung locations. In my time spent in Tanzania, I had the opportunity to try baobab porridge for my breakfast which was surprisingly zesty, filling and delicious. Baobab is supposedly able to help mop up excess cortisol levels, and it certainly made me feel healthy when I ate it, but I'm sceptical as there are no decent studies to confirm this power. The humble maca root is one such so-called super spice. Ground into a powder and added to smoothies from LA to London, maca is supposed to help with regulating reproductive hormones as well as improve sleep and reduce anxiety. Again, there is little hard evidence to support this, but a diverse source of phytonutrients and fibre cannot hurt. Other supposed adaptogens include mushrooms, moringa, nettle, turmeric and ashwagandha. Whether you are trying to improve your progesterone levels for successful pregnancy or reduce cortisol levels due to a stressful lifestyle, a whole-foods dietary approach will undoubtedly be more helpful than focusing on just one 'adaptogen'.

*

Using multiple different spices is a good way of getting a range of potentially healthy chemicals and fibres into your body. An intriguing randomised study in Chinese men has shown that adding 6–12 g daily mixed curry spices to our diets (turmeric, cumin, coriander, amla, cinnamon, clove and cayenne pepper) significantly and rapidly improves our gut microflora composition, encouraging all the good bugs to grow and make us healthier.[36] So it's worth adding those spices from your beautiful but unused spice rack to your dishes. What we can't yet say with any certainty is what the precise effects are, nor can we give recommendations of the best doses to give and how we respond differently to them. It would seem sensible to consume a wide variety of spices in their natural complex form as logically they increase fibre and polyphenol content, as well as plant variety.

Many chefs will encourage you to use fresh herbs wherever possible and to grind whole spices at home with a pestle and mortar to release the delicate flavours right when you need them, and they are probably right. Though phenolic compounds seem to remain intact in dried herbs, vitamin C and carotenoid content greatly suffer from drying, but the consensus seems to be that processed herbs are still a fantastic addition of antioxidant capacity for our diets, so whether fresh, dry or in a paste, add those herbs and spices.

Five spicy facts

1. Adding salt to food improves flavour and is not harmful for most people in normal amounts, but regularly eating hidden salt in UPFs should be avoided.
2. With a few exceptions, salt restriction to low levels is not helpful for most people.

3. Spices are good sources of polyphenols and added fibre, good for your gut microbes and contribute to your optimum thirty plants a week (excluding salt and pepper).
4. Turmeric may have special health properties, though we need better studies to confirm this.
5. Adding mixed spice blends to to your food is likely to increase fibre and polyphenol counts and improve your gut microbes, but make sure you replace them every six months for freshness.

32. Liquids, oils and condiments

Liquids

In a book all about food, it's hard to completely ignore the liquids that we consume every single day. More than 90 per cent of the world's population drink tea or coffee daily and all of us drink water to survive. Countries differ widely on reported alcohol consumption but it's safe to say that a large majority of us also consume some alcoholic drinks throughout our lives. The impacts of these common drinks that we ingest daily for most our lives on our health are surprisingly controversial: from choosing the 'right' bottled water to debates on the benefits of coffee consumption, and even whether drinking red wine can actually be beneficial for our health.

As you will know well by this point in the book, we are all unique and our responses to these liquids vary. With the exception of water, which is essential in some form, choosing which of these liquids to drink every day often boils down to personal preferences and reactions. One of the liquids with the biggest variety of reactions between individuals is coffee.

Coffee

Coffee can indeed be fatal. A lethal dose of caffeine is 10g, which is only 100 cups of coffee. No one to my knowledge has drunk this much in a few hours to test the theory, although a Nottinghamshire twenty-three-year-old died after downing 2tsp of pure caffeine powder bought legally on the internet, equivalent to fifty espressos. Coffee used to be high on doctors' lists of dangerous drinks, mainly because caffeine speeds up the heart rate and could cause heart flutters. However, these were myths based on feeding nervous rats massive doses that gave them heart problems as well as in some cases cancer.[1] But caffeine at normal doses has now been shown to be generally safe and does not cause cancer. The data comes from both large observational studies in many countries and more importantly clinical trials of high-risk heart patients fed large daily doses of 100mg of caffeine.[2]

Coffee is of course much more than just caffeine. The cumulation of seventy-six epidemiological observational studies based on over a million people suggests that coffee drinking reduces risk by about 20 per cent for heart disease and mortality and possibly diabetes, with the best effects at around three cups per day.[3] This heart protection is backed up by other massive studies of over half a million people.[4] Another recent study from UK Biobank found similar lower mortality in coffee drinkers (excluding instant coffee).[5] Other summaries agree that several common cancers (breast, colon and prostate) are also reduced.[6] There are now even studies showing coffee drinking helps survival after heart attacks.[7] So, we can now dismiss the myth that coffee is harmful, with the exception of pregnancy where the evidence shows it would be wise to cut down. Despite the large numbers of studies, researchers cannot yet separate what component of coffee might be beneficial, but the likely benefits of decaffeinated coffee drinking suggest it is to do with the range of plant polyphenols as opposed to just caffeine.

Coffee is also a reasonable source of fibre – a cup provides more fibre than a cup of orange juice; two cups of Americano provides more fibre than a banana. Tea also contains polyphenols though those from black tea are hard to absorb especially if you like adding milk to your brew. Green teas have higher polyphenol counts than black tea, but for higher fibre intakes as well as polyphenols, a ground matcha green tea is the best and tastes delicious when whisked in the traditional way.

Water, water everywhere

We are told to drink eight glasses of water a day by national guidelines, although there is no good data to support this in normal healthy people.[8] This is very helpful to global drinks companies that now sell more bottled water than sodas.[9] There are three main categories of commercial water: spring water, natural mineral water and purified water. Spring water is derived from defined natural sources but has a variable composition. Mineral water, on the other hand, is defined as coming from 'a source', but in addition has to have a minimum mineral or electrolyte content (total dissolvable solids greater than 250 parts per million). Some mineral waters, such as Italian San Pellegrino and French Badoit, contain enough calcium (over 180mg) to help avoid calcium deficiency, whereas many others have virtually none. Purified water has the least minerals and is usually made cheaply from reprocessing and inefficiently repackaging our tap water. Despite water being so important to our health, manufacturers are not required to list the source of the water or any additives on the label. Both Coca Cola and Pepsi had to admit that their bestselling Dasani and Aquafina brands were in fact just re-filtered tap water. Often so little taste remains after purifying that key minerals have to be replaced. Ironically, most still lack the extensive range found in tap water whilst still containing many of the disinfectants and chemicals people are keen to try and avoid.[10]

Surveys tell us that people switch to bottled water because it tastes better and they believe that it is safer than tap water with fewer chemicals and less risk of infection or poisoning. They also believe that as long as they recycle the plastic, it is environmentally safe. However, safety controls on bottled waters are much less stringent than with our mains supply, which is tested several times a day under strict regulation. In the UK and Northern Europe there have been no major scares about tap water safety for years. In larger countries like the US with no central controls, there are the occasional glitches, but for most people in developed countries the chance of getting ill from tap water is much less than your chance of dying from a lightning strike. But fear is a powerful marketing tool, particularly when combined with images of purity, such as a bikini-clad nymph rising from an icy volcano with a stylish bottle in her hand. Also, most people buy bottled water without knowing whether it's spring water or simply bottled 'filtered' tap water. Many health scares and recalls of bottled water are reported – Pepsi had to recall its 'purified tap' water in 2013 when it was found to have excessive levels of bromate, a suspected human carcinogen – and likely many more are kept under the radar. And what of the environmental concerns? Many bottled waters travel thousands of miles to get to cities where there is little typhoid or drought to justify it. The maths just doesn't add up.

Other 'soft' drinks

Many of us also drink juices, tonic waters, sparkling drinks and colas. The main issue with virtually all of these drinks is that they are invariably no better for us than water, and cause health issues. Colas, fizzy drinks and most sports or energy drinks are either sweetened with sugar, which increases obesity and dental caries, or artificial sweeteners which have less well understood but likely unhelpful effects on our metabolism and microbes. Fruit juices (see Orange juice, page 130) are the ones that are most often marketed as 'healthy' and even as one of our 'five a day' which is causing real damage to our health and especially our children's health. Without the beneficial fibre we usually find in whole fruit, juices offer a huge amount of sugar that quickly passes into our bloodstream without the benefits which whole fruit consumption confers. A standard glass of orange juice typically contains the juice of six juicing oranges, which nobody I know could actually eat in one sitting, and even if they could it would take them a lot longer than downing one glass of juice and they would be getting the benefit of the fibre.

Booze

The final group of drinks that so many of us enjoy, and abuse, is alcohol. The science and societal context behind all of these different drinks is vast and warrants an additional book by itself (watch this space!) and I should confess upfront that I thoroughly enjoy a glass of red wine with my dinner. The reason why alcohol consumption is so contentious is that it's deeply engrained in many of our societies and our social interactions, but there is some good science out there.

Of all the alcoholic drinks available to us, we know that red wine is the highest in beneficial polyphenols such as resveratrol, which has gained cult status. Drinking red wine for its polyphenol content alone is of course not a good reason because fresh berries are healthier, but it does help us to understand why some studies show a beneficial effect of drinking red wine. White wine has less polyphenols, so you have to drink more to get any benefit, which rather destroys the point. Other alcoholic drinks don't seem to have any beneficial effects and the detrimental impacts of drinking alcohol are well known – from reduced cognitive function to vomiting and loss of consciousness. There is a well-established increased risk of almost all diseases with increasing alcohol consumption, but the point at which the risk becomes meaningful is unclear.[11] My view is that one unit or small glass three times a week is relatively safe, although we all vary in our responses. If you do fancy a drink, the current data does seem to leave a sweet spot for drinking a glass of red wine daily with friends as beneficial for overall longevity and a healthy heart; perhaps due to the polyphenols or perhaps due to the social context, or maybe a cocktail of both.[12]

Olive, seed and nut oils

We have learned to extract fats from plants as diverse as coconut to palm, avocado to olive, all with their own claims, followers and flavours. As we discussed in Chapter 3, the food matrix is crucial when considering how we digest fats from foods. We know that whole almonds produce a much more favourable blood fat response than almond butter, and even more than almond oil. Once extracted, fatty acids have a measurably bigger impact on our metabolism, and this applies to all fats in this state. The only exception to this rule seems to be extra virgin olive oil (EVOO), as the olives are simply pressed to extract this high polyphenol condiment and cooking fat. In general, the more extraction the oil has had to undergo, the worse it is likely to be for our resulting blood fat response. Our blood fats (like triglycerides) change a few hours after we eat fat in foods. High blood fat that hangs around rather than being cleared efficiently leads to local inflammation and oxidative stress which is bad for our blood vessels. Whilst all fats will cause a blood fat change, those that have high levels of antioxidants (or polyphenols) like EVOO will help to combat the associated inflammation. Unfortunately fatty bacon doesn't have this same calming antioxidant effect, making EVOO healthier than animal fats.

Olive oil

Olive oil is unusual in that it is used as both a seasoning and a cooking oil, and still today as a medicine. There is also a vast gap between the three main classes; the most expensive EVOO and the range below this of the virgin olive oils, moving to the cheapest blended olive oils (just called olive oils), both in flavour and nutritional value. Olives are actually a fruit that nourishes itself by producing fat rather than sugar, and classified officially as a berry as the stone is in fact a seed. So olive oil could be considered a fruit juice, but not one we would normally have by the glass with breakfast. Without marinating, the ripe fruit is virtually inedible due to the tannin polyphenols that protect it, which are also beneficial to us. They are one of the earliest cultivated fruits that ancient civilisations depended on as a multi-purpose ingredient used for cooking, preserving, lighting, massage, medicine and washing. The olea tree is extra hardy – it survives droughts and can live for a thousand years. Although it started life in the Eastern Mediterranean, with recent climate change olives can be cultivated in many countries, although they are labour intensive and need a cheap workforce to make it profitable.

EVOO as a health tonic

This strange fruit juice has since classical times been used for nearly every ailment. The high intakes of EVOO have been suggested as a major contribution to the remarkable longevity of Greek islanders and Sardinians, as well as Italians and Spanish, despite the large amounts of grains and dairy they consume. According to official figures, the average modern Greek consumes nearly 0.5 litres per week closely followed by the Italians and the Spanish. The British now import around 60 million litres annually; a tenfold increase since 1990 when it was only found in pharmacies.

This UK consumption averages out at only around 1 litre per person annually, which is similar to the US, but pales into insignificance compared to the Mediterraneans: the tiny microstate of San Marino consumes a hefty 24 litres per person every year. Early tourists to Spain in the 1970s were horrified by the unexpected sight of food floating in greasy EVOO which, with its high calories and mixed saturated and unsaturated fats, was labelled as dreadfully fattening and even unhealthy. However, health surveys of European populations kept finding that southern Europeans lived longer and had less heart disease than the rest of us, despite these higher fat intakes. It turns out EVOO was the likely reason.

The Mediterranean diet

Ten years ago the unique clinical trial called PREDIMED enrolled 7,500 mildly overweight Spanish men and women in their sixties at risk of heart disease and diabetes.[13] They were randomly allocated two diets for five years – one a low-fat diet recommended by doctors in most western countries, and the other a high-fat Mediterranean diet supplemented with either EVOO or nuts. The Mediterranean diet group had a third less heart disease, diabetes and stroke than the low-fat diet group. They also lost a small amount of weight, had less memory loss and reduced breast cancer. Extra portions of EVOO seemed to particularly protect against heart arrhythmias. Traditional stubborn defenders of low-fat diets say that the Spanish didn't lower their fat intakes sufficiently to properly compare the two diets, but this misses the point. Any long trial also demonstrates the real-life practicalities of sticking to a diet – and the Mediterranean diet wins hands down. Picking through the data they found that the EVOO-supplemented group did slightly better than the extra-nut group but both were undoubtedly superior to mildly low-fat diets.

Our own ZOE PREDICT study data tells us that those who follow the recommended whole-plant and wholegrain-based diet naturally tend to get around 39 per cent of their energy from fat-rich foods such as avocados, whole nuts and full-fat dairy. This is the same percentage as achieved in the Mediterranean diet arm of the PRED-IMED study that had the best outcomes, true even in the free-living data outside of clinical trial conditions, for those who have the healthiest blood profiles. A smaller but more rigorous intervention study looking at epigenetic markers of ageing and cancer risk asked 219 subjects to use EVOO for all their cooking and dressing. They were also told to follow a Mediterranean diet pattern of eating whole grains, fruits and vegetables, more fish and less meat, and only a few portions of dairy per week. The results clearly showed a reduction in ageing biomarkers compared to the exercise-only group.[14]

Benefits often can't be narrowed down to any one single food, though EVOO is possibly the closest thing we have to a real 'super-food', as the evidence points to the EVOO itself being the most powerful factor. The unique chemical composition of EVOO is likely due to the fact that extracting the oil from the olive fruit does not require high temperatures or solvent extraction and bleaching like with many other seed oils, leaving the polyphenols and beneficial fatty acids, such as oleic acid, intact in the final product. Interestingly the cheaper forms of olive oil (those labelled regular or virgin) don't have as dramatic an effect on blood fats – it had to be extra virgin as shown in a recent trial in Australia.[15] Extra virgin is a bit of a joke, a bit like being 'extra dead', made using the best, ripest fruit with the highest polyphenol count (up to 65mg/100g). Nearly all basic olive oil is virgin, i.e. from olives crushed without solvents, but the top-grade oil called 'extra' has the lowest acidity levels, with less than 0.4 per cent in the finest oils, less than 0.8 per cent in EVOOs and 2 per cent in the normal virgins. The time between picking and crushing as well as the extraction temperature (cold is best) is key in making sure the level of peroxides stays low. As the number of peroxides increases, the oil becomes less fruity, more rancid and less 'extra'. Standard virgin olive oil has a less complex flavour and is oilier; and those simply labelled 'olive oil' have the least amount of polyphenols, none of the fresh fruitiness and can often be made of many mixed olive oils from different regions and with less than ideal picking times and extraction temperatures. But even poor-quality olive oils generally have more healthy polyphenols than equivalent seed oils.

Extra virgins

The tenfold difference in price between the best EVOO and the standard supermarket olive oil is a reasonable guide to quality. In the UK and US, olive oil labels, especially from large suppliers to supermarkets, can be very deceptive, looking authentic with words like 'artisan' and 'classico' to describe the cheapest blends of oils with as little as 1 per cent extra virgin. When buying your EVOO, consider buying from a single producer from countries like Turkey, Greece, Italy and Spain that have a non-intensive olive farming approach and traditional extraction methods using pressing and water with no need for additional solvents. Another good tip is to find the EVOOs that have their vintage on the label – the more recently the olives were pressed, the better the polyphenol content and the lower the peroxides. This date is a better indicator than the sell-by date which tells us when the oil was bottled but not necessarily pressed so if you can, look out for the actual date the oil was harvested and pressed, not just bottled.

In countries that grow and harvest olives for EVOO, you will find elderly pensioners and young students shaking the olive trees and manually picking the ripe fruits that fall in large nets with as little bruising as possible, to then carry them straight up to the stone mills for cold extraction. The quality of the olives is influenced by many factors: the time at which they were picked (some varieties want picking early in the season, others towards the end of the summer); knowing which soil your olive trees like (chalky or volcanic, for example); and a wide diurnal range which is how much sunshine and heat there is in the day compared to cooler, humid nights that also create the typical morning mists of the rolling Tuscan hills. Finally, minimising time between picking and pressing is key as is the use of technology to ensure the temperature and humidity of the olives at extraction are ideal to maintain the high polyphenol count in the oil. Some good single-estate cold-pressed EVOOs now reach over 60mg/100g of polyphenols, which is four times the recommended minimum amount to be considered a fine EVOO. These elderly pickers tend to ask for oil instead of cash as payment, making sure that their precious freshly picked, polyphenol-rich EVOO comes home with them.

High-grade extra virgin olive oil is the only one worth buying for dressing and cooking and has at least thirty different antioxidant polyphenols, including tyrosol, lignans and other flavonoids that appear to have beneficial effects on ageing and inflammation, particularly on the heart and brain. Rather than drinking a bottle of oil, some small Italian companies now produce concentrated olive oil polyphenol shots, which are the equivalent in a tiny glass of super bitter polyphenols, but drizzling EVOO on real food is probably better.

As well as the polyphenols helping our microbes and reducing inflammation in our bodies, the many other chemicals involved potentially explain the paradox of why drinking fat in the form of oleic acid may actually reduce total blood fat levels. As a partner of an EU research project we gave forty unhealthy overweight southern Italians an intensive eight-week Mediterranean diet with plenty of fibre and extra virgin olive oil, and saw that all the blood parameters for fats and inflammation improved.[16] Other clinical studies have shown that EVOO performs better than butter in blood fat profiles, but these underestimate the heart benefits conferred by the antioxidants in EVOO which lower inflammation and thus reduce the risk of cardiovascular diseases such as heart attacks and stroke. High oleic sunflower and rapeseed oil can confer similar antioxidant effects when used raw in dressings but are less versatile and become quickly oxidised when heated.

Good EVOO is not like vintage wine and doesn't last very long especially if kept in the light, so is best stored in the cupboard in dark-coloured glass bottles. If not, they can go rancid after only six months, so use it up, and never buy oil in a clear bottle.

Fake EVOO

EVOO is relatively expensive and, as expected, is in the top three most doctored products. Italy produces more bottles of oil than is actually possible, counting the number of olive trees, and much is rebottled from Spain which produces the most oil, or from Greece which produces the most high-quality EVOO. Substituting low-quality tasteless products lacking any polyphenols is a growing crime at all levels. Recent estimates from a 2016 CBS survey suggested 40 per cent of Italian EVOO is adulterated with other substances, and over 75–80 per cent of US imports were not what they seemed, with many tested failing to meet minimum standards.[17] In 2019, a Europol-coordinated operation arrested twenty fraudsters and seized 150,000 litres of low-quality oils that had been adulterated with yellow colourants to make them appear like EVOO. Methods of verifying labels, contents and producers exist, and need to be implemented, but now organised crime is involved on this scale, it is hard to police and reverse it.

The best way of spotting fakery and grading quality is with a combination of technology and good old-fashioned expert tasting panels. To gauge the quality of your EVOO, sniff it or slurp it around your palate with plenty of air like wine. As well as grassy or even smoky aromas, you should detect some peppery, fresh and fruity notes from the polyphenols: if good quality, it sometimes makes you cough. My Italian friends tend to stick to EVOOs from single growers they know and trust and would never think of buying a surprising bargain.

Smoke points and cooking oil

People use olive oil in different ways in different countries. In the North of France and Italy it is used mainly for adding to foods or salads, while in the south and all over Spain and Greece, it is also used as the main cooking oil. Critics of EVOO point out its lower smoke point of 200°C is a health problem when frying and cite this as a reason to avoid it (see page 78). But, in my opinion, the overall stability of olive oil and its high polyphenol content still makes it the best option for cooking, even if you do like to burn your oil.

Highly processed, solvent-treated 'pure or Lite' olive oils only sold in the Americas have higher smoke points of over 240°C and are best avoided. But there is much more to oil than just smoke points;

another key oil characteristic is its stability. The less saturated fat and the more PUFAs (polyunsaturated fatty acids) an oil contains, the less healthy it is (see page 78). As a rule, therefore, avoid regular portions of cheaply fried fish and chips or greasy kebabs every night. EVOO is one of the more stable oils in these tests, as it contains plenty of saturated fats, as well as very low levels of PUFAs, making it a great option for cooking. In addition, EVOO improves polyphenol availability when used to lightly sauté vegetables such as onions, carrots, garlic and celery.

Randomised human trials produce better evidence than small animal studies. The thousands of Spanish participants in the PRED-IMED trial cooked all their food for six years with EVOO, presumably sometimes deep-frying and burning it, reassuringly with less health problems than with other vegetable oils. By investing our money in buying and eating high-quality EVOO early in life, we have a chance to make our gut microbes healthier, although we may never catch up with the Greeks.

Sunflower and other seed oils

Sunflower is an ancient staple oil in many countries. I was surprised when I visited Georgia recently that with its Mediterranean climate there was no EVOO culture, despite being the home of fine wine. They love their sunflower oil and have many grades and varieties, and a bowl of the golden liquid is presented on every table to dip your bread into. It tasted better than anything I'd had before, showing the importance of unrefined and local oil versus the mass-produced, highly refined versions. Sunflower has been billed 'the healthy oil' in the last thirty years, as it is lower in saturated fats than EVOO and high in polyunsaturated fats, oleic acid and omega-6, but like most oils, is a complex mix of many sub-fractions. Most of the world's supply comes from Ukraine and Russia so has become rarer. Semi-refined sunflower oils have less flavour but a high smoke point of 232°C so despite their instability, many chefs prefer them for frying. There are now at least four different types of sunflower oil, with high-, mid-, low-oleic-acid varieties, all with different cooking properties and health effects that are hard to generalise, and with its neutral taste, often hidden from the consumer. Sadly none has any measurable level of useful polyphenols.

Rapeseed oil (also called canola, as Canada produces most of it) is often touted as a healthy alternative, being derived from the brassica or cabbage family, and so contains some polyphenols. It is very popular in North America and is the third most common oil globally; virtually unknown as a crop in the UK before 1985, it then steadily increased, changing landscapes of green fields to bright yellow. It can be used as biofuel or as a lubricant, but most rapeseed in Europe is used for animal feed because of the high-protein content. Some of its chemicals (like erucic acid) are thought to be harmful to animals and so it needs to be heavily processed to reduce these to levels considered safe in humans. An example of the dangers is when a variant of rapeseed was used illegally as a cheap oil substitute in Spain in 1981 and gave hundreds of people toxic oil syndrome with nasty effects on the heart and lungs.

Good-quality rapeseed oil is unlikely to be toxic or cause inflammation, and can be a good source of ALA omega-3 fatty acids when eaten raw, which is why it has been used to feed farmed salmon.[18] There is little detailed human health data other than that the highly processed form (including fully hydrogenated processed forms) has been passed as safe by US and European authorities, and a widely held (traditional but dubious) belief of its benefits due to its low saturated fat levels. On the downside, it can make food taste a bit grassy, has a lowish smoke point of 190°C and is four times less stable to oxidation than EVOO, making re-frying a potential problem. GM versions in North America have changed the fat composition to increase its smoke point, but I have not tried them. As with other oils, there is a wide range in quality and it is possible to buy high-quality cold-pressed rapeseed oil that is a reasonable alternative on salads, though it still won't confer any of the antioxidant benefits of EVOO, as nicely presented by a study that tried replacing EVOO with rapeseed oil in a Mediterranean diet.[19] When buying rapeseed oil, opt for a hi-oleic brand which will remain more stable if you're using it to cook, but it's best only for low-heat cooking. Whichever type you buy it is unlikely to contain much in the way of healthy polyphenols and is beaten even by cheap olive oil.

Sesame and flaxseed oils have low smoke points of under 110°C and low saturated fat levels, making them less stable, so it is best avoided for frying and using on salads instead. As discussed, flaxseed oil is a great plant source of omega-3 fatty acids, so is worth adding to your pantry, especially if you don't eat much fish. Mustard seed oil can liven up a dish and makes roast potatoes taste a bit special.

Coconut oil is not really an oil, as at room temperature it is usually solid and should be called coconut fat. It has a pretty high smoke point (if refined), of 204°C and is very stable to oxidation, so it hardly ever goes off. Because of powerful marketing, it has been touted as a cure for all ills, whitening teeth, and extending healthy lifespan. People around the world now add it to their coffee, in their cooking and in their baking, based purely on celebrity endorsement. It has a natural defect, however: everything tastes of coconut, which is great if you like coconut desserts or Thai green curries, but can be overpowering. It also has a uniquely high 89 per cent saturated-fat content, mostly lauric acid and other unusual medium chain triglycerides (MCTs), which we are right to be wary of. It is also lacks both the fibre to slow down lipid absorption into our blood, and the polyphenols found in coconut flesh that act as antioxidants. Coconut oil is, however, very, very energy-dense and has many unusual fat components, in particular MCTs, which have been shown in some studies to increase feelings of fullness and don't increase common blood fats as readily. This data on pure MCT has been used to hype coconut oil, though of all the fats it only contains 14 per cent MCT and butter also contains them too. I will stick with tastier butter.

Rave reviews on nutrition websites and claims from some influential chefs of wondrous health benefits, especially on the heart, are entirely lacking in evidence or verging on the fraudulent. Independent reviews have found no evidence of benefit. Much coconut oil is heavily processed to remove impurities and natural chemicals, leaving little if any nutritional value. To keep the fat in solid form at room temperature but melt at body temperature, the coconut oil is mixed with other fats, inter-esterified and processed. Constantly reheating the oil can produce other chemicals labelled as 'potentially' carcinogenic, but without any of the reassuring data from long-term olive oil studies.[20] So while it is probably fine to use high-quality unprocessed coconut oil once in a while to liven up your Asian dishes, avoid it as a regular cooking oil. I am told it is excellent as a moisturiser or hair conditioner though, so your old supplies can still be put to good use.

Avocado oil is extracted from the flesh of the fruit rather than the stone, similar to EVOO in its extraction. Like olive oil, it is high in oleic acid and saturated fats with some similar characteristics, so may in theory be beneficial. It has a high smoke point and so can be fried, but is pricy at around £12 per litre.

More studies are needed, but it seems that cold-pressed avocado oil, also labelled unrefined virgin or extra virgin, could preserve a lot of the beneficial polyphenol compounds of the raw fruit, and so could be nearly as good as olive oil. However, the majority of avocado oil production uses heat or chemical solvents and bleaching resulting in a refined product with little to recommend it. Using more natural processes such as cold-pressed extraction results in a much lower yield, making this already expensive oil even less profitable.

Corn oil is cheap, common, and is usually highly refined and processed with a high smoke point (230°C), but very low stability at high temperatures because it has little saturated fat. It is heavily promoted in North America as healthy, because of enormous surpluses due to government subsidies to keep prices low. Recent advertising claims have said that it is 'healthier' than EVOO. This is based, first, on having more polyunsaturated than monounsaturated fats, and second on a randomised study of fifty volunteers comparing 4tsp daily of corn oil versus EVOO.[21] The authors found corn oil produced greater short-term changes in beneficial lipids by a few per cent. Strangely the authors didn't highlight the fact that corn oil increased blood pressure and heart rate, which is much more relevant, or the little detail that the study was sponsored by the corn industry.

Palm oil is used globally in most of the cheap UPFs produced today for its robust material properties and flexibility. It accounts for

40 per cent of oils used for food, animal feed and fuel, and demand is rising. But it lacks healthy fats, is not pleasant to cook with and is an environmental disaster causing devasting deforestation (50 per cent of Borneo), and in an ideal world should be avoided. Unfortunately, there is no real equivalent versatile fat that can be used in food processing, other than butter or lard which are arguably worse for the planet. Oil palm crops, for all the faults of palm oil, grow rapidly and take up much less land than equivalent crops (around 5 per cent of global oil-crop land) .

If, like most of us, you are not able to avoid UPFs, look out for 'sustainable palm oil' in your biscuits, which might be slightly better.

Ghee

Ghee (clarified butter without the milk) is a popular butter alternative in many parts of the globe, especially in Sri Lanka and southern India. It has a 20 per cent higher smoke point than butter (250°C) but with its high saturated fat content (over 60 per cent) it is naturally stable to oxidation. It will adversely alter blood fat levels compared to EVOO. Interestingly, butter (see page 303) has been compared in a 2018 trial with other oils in ninety people for four weeks and produces a worse blood lipid profile than EVOO or coconut oil.[22] This can't be simply explained by fat content, which is how many have so far simplistically graded fat for health risk. Whether this blood difference actually translates long term into more heart disease for butter consumption is unknown.

Nut oils

Most nut oils have a low smoke point and when used in cooking can really alter the taste and produce a range of unwanted aromas, so use them sparingly or mainly as a dressing. Peanut oil is the exception (as it is not really a nut), and can be used for frying where you want some nutty aromas. Sesame oil and flaxseed are more typical, with low smoke points of under 110°C and low saturated fat levels, making them less stable, so are best avoided for frying and used on salads instead. Flaxseed oil is a great plant source of omega-3 fatty acids, so is worth adding to your pantry, especially if you don't eat much fish. I prefer the milled seeds myself which are also better for your gut microbiome thanks to the fibre content. Walnut oil has been used in traditional Chinese medicine as a supplement and some studies in mice suggest it has powerful anti-inflammatory properties in the gut.[23] We don't know how well this translates in humans, but good-quality walnut oil does seem to have the highest level of polyphenols after olive oil (see table, page 444), so could be a good healthy alternative for dressings if you like the taste.

Argan oil is one of the most expensive oils you can buy unless you live in Morocco where it literally grows on trees. It is very labour intensive to cut the fruit and open the nut and dry roast and grind it, so traditionally the locals cut corners and allow their goats to feed on the trees, and they simply pick up the droppings. It is a mixture of several different fats, some similar to olive oil, and it also has high amounts of polyphenols. It is sold for hair and skin cosmetics and the drinking version costs around £100 per litre. It may be healthy, though we may not know for sure for another twenty years, and it is expensive to take the risk.

Hemp is no longer just used to make rope or soap. Seeds from a mild variety of the cannabis plant with a low level of THC are a new addition to health food shelves. It is low in saturated fat, so it goes off quickly, and compared to anything else except flaxseed, very high in omega-3 and six essential fatty acids. Its low smoke point makes it unsuitable for cooking, it is unstable and tastes grassy and nutty.

Condiments

Saucy stuff

Oils, sauces and condiments hold a special place on our plates, reminding us of home; from tomato ketchup to French aioli to Indian mango chutney. These culinary additions are not new; the Babylonians used oil and vinegar for dressing greens thousands of years ago.

Oils are liquid fats at room temperature, many made from distinctive seeds or spices. For millennia, we used natural oils made from animal fat (lard), seeds like sesame seeds, plants like olives (see page 399) or nuts, until margarine oils were invented a few decades ago. More recently, an American man named Caesar Cardini invented his eponymous salad, the key ingredient of which is its dressing. The French still look down disdainfully on English sauces, with Voltaire supposedly writing, 'In England, there are forty-two different religions and only two sauces,' and the French still regard mint sauce with lamb as revolting.

Many sauces and liquids are used to hide, mask, or accentuate flavour. Oils are used to season and cook food. As with spices, additional sauces have been used since the earliest times to improve food or extend its life. Over the centuries our palates have changed. In the West, early sauces were mainly used with meat, and often based on sweet fruits like figs or dates or with honey in the Middle Ages. The eighteenth-century French court cooks created much of modern 'haute cuisine' based on complex sauces, which has persisted today. As a broad generalisation, the more complex the cuisine and sauces of a country or region, the poorer the original quality of the meat centuries ago. Thus the British and American cuisines have very simple dishes and sauces because there was usually a ready supply of the best cuts of meat. When you compare national cuisines, this 'lazy cuisine' theory seems quite plausible, although genetics, religion (Catholic vs Protestant) and many other factors are likely to play a role in our choice of sauce.

Vinegars

As long as wine and alcohol were made and left too long, vinegars have existed, initially as a medicine and antiseptic, then for embalming and for cleaning, and finally as a condiment.

The word vinegar comes from the French *vin aigre* or sour wine. It can be made from any sugar-containing source that can be made into alcohol, such as white or red wine grapes, rice, malted grains and barley, various palms (such as nipa from the Philippines) and fruits such as apples. Microbes ferment the alcohol into acetic acid that increases the acidity to 4–8 per cent, ensuring that other non-acid loving bacteria can't survive and compete. In the process, the microbes also produce a range of other complex chemicals and flavours depending on the original plant that was used to generate the alcohol. A vinegar mother is often used to get a new batch started and is a mix of yeasts and bacteria that form a single blob as in kombucha. The vast majority of commercial vinegars are pasteurised with no living culture, as the fermentation process is often unstable and unpredictable. If you see a best-before date on the label, you can have a quiet laugh and ignore it, as vinegar should outlive you. Cheap clear vinegar is at the other extreme and is made from synthetic acetic acid plus water.

Cooks use vinegars to provide a balancing acidity in many dishes, particularly with fats, or to curdle milk. But it has tastes and aromas beyond the acidity, depending on the pungency of the acetic acid. The most famous wine vinegar is balsamic (from the Latin *balsamun* meaning restorative or curative) from Modena in Italy, made since Roman times using fermented, cooked and aged grape must. This is slowly caramelised, which concentrates the must, changing the colour and flavours. Real balsamic is made by adding cooked must to a wooden barrel, and blending it with the old cooler must already in it, initially for a year. Samples are then moved to refresh another barrel every year, as the temperature increases, keeping the balsamic must culture alive. This ageing and fermenting process continues for at least twelve years before the balsamic can be sold, sometimes for as long as twenty-five years as the samples rotate through the barrels. The result is a rich syrup with balanced complex flavours like the best vintage wines and the mother source is passed down through generations, often as a dowry. Unlike other foods in Italy, the use of the balsamic accreditation is not protected legally, leading to many imitators. The real ancient stuff is *Aceto Balsamico Tradizionale di Modena DOP*, but you are unlikely to ever see it, as production is tiny, just from sixty-six family producers in Modena, and sells for a minimum of £200 per litre.

But for the last twenty-five years millions of bottles of balsamic

vinegar from Modena have magically appeared everywhere at a surprisingly reasonable price. This stuff is made very differently, speeding
up the process using red wine vinegar with added wine must and sugar.
It is called balsamic vinegar of Modena (with an IGP label) found in
many supermarkets and may cost between £4 to £40 per litre, depending on how much time it spent in a wood barrel as opposed to a factory.
Many of these more expensive ones taste fine. To add to the confusion
there are a range of other certifications and labels according to ageing
and barrels. Outside Europe, the rules are even more lax and virtually
anything can be called balsamic from Modena. Further down the food
chain is plain 'balsamic vinegar', which doesn't claim to be from
Modena, a low-quality product made from industrial vinegar plus
caramelised sugar and variable grapes, and usually a sickly sugary taste.
Don't expect any major health benefits, though, as most microbes don't
survive, and any benefit will be from the quality of the grapes. As is
often the case, you get what you pay for.

Apple cider vinegar (ACV) is the new magic cure-all. A tablespoon
of the sour liquid each morning is the modern cod liver oil. The internet extols its twenty 'proven' benefits, including a daily tablespoon
for weight loss and energy. A pilot study kicked off the craze in 2004,
when twenty-one diabetic and pre-diabetic people took a drink of
ACV before a single carb meal and had promising improvements in
insulin and glucose responses.[24] Studies since have found up to 2kg
in weight loss over twelve weeks with reduced blood triglycerides in
groups taking 1–2tbsp before meals compared to control groups. The
results seem superficially impressive, but the evidence base is unsurprisingly littered with bias and small-scale human studies.[25]

If it does really work, it could be the microbes, the polyphenols or
the acetic acid itself. A few people (mainly rich celebs) believe unpasteurised ACV with live acetic acid bacteria is key. None of the human
studies used live vinegar, and the yeast will have died off leaving only
a few *acetobacter* microbes alive anyway, which grow naturally in our
guts. There have been several proposed ways ACV might be producing this effect; some suggest that the acetic acid could reduce the
speed at which food is emptied from the stomach. Others suggest it
may slow down the enzymes which break sugar down into glucose,

flattening glucose spikes. It may also make you feel fuller, meaning you eat less. It is still possible that a mix of the complex polyphenols with the vinegar could be beneficial, but with no big studies on the horizon don't waste your money on expensive versions – or the totally unhelpful ACV gummies. Any form of unsweetened good-quality acetic acid may also do the same, including the much cheaper red wine vinegar.

Table sauces

Tomato ketchup is one of the earliest processed foods and has existed since the seventeenth century. Ketchup scholars believe it may have originated in *kê-tsiap* (pronounced 'ki-chap'), a dark fermented fish sauce from China or Malaysia. English colonists in the early 1700s called it as 'catsup' and tried to replicate it at home, using oysters, mussels, mushrooms, walnuts, lemons, celery and even fruits like plums and peaches. The first tomato-based ketchup came much later when in 1812 James Mease, a Philadelphia scientist, is credited with inventing the recipe. The first mass-produced ketchup was made in 1837, followed by Henry John Heinz's version forty years later, which in its modified form is still the market leader in the UK and US. In the UK, Heinz, like others, has a 'clean label' of contents in order of concentration: tomatoes, vinegar, sugar, salt, herb extracts, spice and celery (to provide the nitrite preservatives). US versions have high-fructose corn syrup and are less worried about 'natural' flavourings.

Most brands have much more sugar than people realise (around 25 per cent), disguised by the vinegar and salt, and initially used to preserve shelf-life: a tablespoon of ketchup is the same as a teaspoon of pure sugar (4g) or half a Snickers bar, and many kids use much more. Low-sugar versions are available at the cost of many more added chemicals. But you can blend your own easily with some tomato paste, water, salt, vinegar, onion, mustard and ground clove – then add sugar to taste. The flow dynamics of ketchup are one of the scientific puzzles of our age: hitting the glass bottle or squeezing the plastic in the right places changes its viscosity and makes it more liquid, allowing it to flow out. The bottles are often coated with chemicals to help the flow, but these don't make it onto the label. After nearly two hundred years, ketchup may be on the way out as tastes change; sales have recently been overtaken by spicy salsa in the US and mayonnaise in the UK.

Mayonnaise is simply an emulsion of fresh eggs mixed with olive oil and vinegar or lemon. It probably originated from Mahon in the Mediterranean island of Menorca (*Salsa Mahonesa* in Spanish), as a simple and pure sauce which, by adding garlic, became aioli in many Mediterranean countries and made a delicious accompaniment to fish dishes. It is a common ingredient in many pre-prepared sandwiches, adding around 100 calories to each. The commercial market leader, Hellman's, was launched by German immigrants to New York around 1912 and is now made by the giant Unilever group.

Because of the egg content, mayo has always had an associated health risk of *salmonella* infections which thrive if the contents are not acidic enough. In 1976, a Las Palmas airline catering company got it badly wrong and *salmonella* infected over 2,000 travellers and killed six. This and other high-profile bad outbreaks added to the fear of the natural product, and cheaper, synthetic, mass-produced products with virtually no egg in them appeared on the market, with low-fat high-additive versions that never go off. A typical 'healthy' low-fat, low-calorie mayo will contain over twenty ingredients compared to the original three. Whether these ultra-processed mayonnaises are healthier than ketchup is unknown, but neither is likely to be good for your gut microbes.

Salad cream is a very British invention designed during World War One as a cheaper, watered down, brighter-yellow version of mayonnaise which is still popular today. At my school it was commonly served as a revolting 'sandwich spread' containing a few chopped unrecognisable vegetables. It is nearly 20 per cent sugar and has sunflower oil, mustard and a fistful of other chemicals to provide texture and colour. In short, it is best avoided.

Worcestershire sauce started life in 1837 in a pharmacy in Worcester run by chemists Mr Lea and Mr Perrins. Although the original product was supposedly based on a Bengali recipe, it has now evolved into a versatile, fermented mix of ingredients. The powerful umami flavours mean it is a great addition to intensify the taste of mush-rooms, lentils, or in a bloody Mary.

Brown sauce is a watery, more sugary version of Worcestershire sauce, and the vinegary peppery competitor to ketchup in the UK, Canada and Australasia. The HP sauce brand, named after the Houses of Parliament, whose restaurant was one of the first to serve it, is still the market leader. Brown sauce is made with a tomato base, blended with malt and spirit vinegar, plus a variety of items from the old empire including sugars, dates, cornflour, rye flour, salt, paprika, spices, and even tamarind and anchovies. There are no studies to suggest that these sauces with their high-salt and sometimes high-sugar content are good for us. Any polyphenol or fibre content from the fruit and vegetable ingredients is eradicated by the quantities of sugar, emulsifiers and other chemicals used to make them non-perishable.

Pickles and chutneys

Pickles and chutneys are found all over the world in different forms, many slowly fermented to bring out complex flavours of the vegetable and fruit ingredients. Some, like kosher dill pickles in vinegar, have relatively few additives and calories, while industrially manufactured brands contain whopping amounts of sugar. Branston pickle and shop-bought mango chutney contain 31g and 52g sugar respectively per 100g, making any beneficial live bacteria a biochemical impossibility. The only pickles worth eating are the true fermented types like sauerkraut, kimchi and more traditional preserves prepared using fresh herbs and spices and with minimal processing and added chemicals.

Ten tips on liquids, oils and condiments

1. There is no need to drink eight glasses of water a day if you are not thirsty.
2. Bottled water is no better than tap water in most high-income countries.

3. Soft drinks containing sugars or artificial sweeteners are virtually all unhealthy.
4. Coffee and green teas are fermented plant products that have real health benefits.
5. A cup of coffee contains more fibre than a glass of orange juice.
6. Alcohol is harmful for most people, except in very small amounts or as a single glass of red wine.
7. Extra virgin olive oil is the best oil for cooking and dressing food.
8. Most mass-produced condiments, including ketchup, mayonnaise and pickles, have no benefits and their extensive ingredients lists include excessive salt, sugar and additives.
9. Worcestershire sauce has powerful umami flavours and thus is great for accentuating ingredients when used in moderation. Tabasco is a fermented condiment, and is another good way to add flavour.
10. True fermented pickles like sauerkraut, kimchi and traditional preserves made with minimal processing are great for your gut.

33. Final word

My goal throughout this book, and in my recent work with ZOE, is to help empower people to make better food choices for their unique biology. Using my own lived experience plus the wealth of scientific evidence which continues to emerge on food, metabolism and the microbiome, I hope this book will be a good starting point for investing in your future health. There are other important factors – such as our environment, daily schedules and social context – which also play a huge role in our relationship with food. I have touched on some of these topics in this book, but there are plenty more to explore.

As I finish writing, the war in Ukraine, as well as being a major humanitarian and diplomatic emergency, has caused new challenges to our food environment: the ubiquitous sunflower oil is now a rarity and wheat is becoming scarce. Meanwhile, a sudden environmentally motivated ban on fertilisers and pesticides in Sri Lanka is leaving farmers with no crops resulting in food riots. Food prices have soared worldwide, and food insecurity and poverty are issues faced by even more families in the UK and globally.

At the same time, there have been some positive changes as I've written this book: the Covid-19 pandemic is slowly becoming a 'normal' part of our lives, travel is open again and vaccine science has made great progress. A long-overdue move towards including women and women's health in scientific studies is beginning to take place: the physiological impact of the menopause is now a well-reported scientific finding thanks to our diet study on over 20,000 women – the largest study on food and the menopause to date.[1] The use of the outdated calorie models to explain weight gain and obesity is becoming more and more distant to scientific practice, and the value of understanding the importance of quality and seasonality of food is gaining ground.

We know that the food choices we make on each of the roughly 20,000 days of our average lives impact our health, the planet's health and the health and livelihood of future generations. Moving away from ultra-processed foods wrapped in plastic is the simplest way to improve our health and help the environment. Later generations will have the tools and knowledge to safeguard their health from a younger age and be more informed about their own food choices. We must model this change for our own health and inspire those younger than us to do the same – the prospect of being a healthy and active 100-year-old is far more accessible than we thought even ten years ago, when metabolic disease and frailty seemed an inevitable part of ageing.

I hope this book has provided you with the tools to make better food choices. Whether you are shopping for yourself and your family, helping your clients improve their health, or teaching students or children, this collection of food facts should make your choices more diverse, informed and logical.

The immense power of food is in your hands. Here are twenty headline tips to remember as well as a number of useful tables and figures to help you rank and prioritise the foods in this book. Good luck!

Twenty tips to keep you and your microbes healthy

1. Sleep well and exercise regularly.
2. Avoid snacking and allow occasional long fasting intervals.
3. Try to eat up to thirty plant varieties a week, including nuts, seeds and spices.
4. Drink only moderate amounts of ideally high-polyphenol alcohol.
5. Eat fruit and vegetables high in polyphenols and fibre.
6. Eat less but higher-quality meat and fish.
7. Ignore calorie counts and seek out the higher nutritional quality of foods with the same calorific value.
8. Think about origins and ingredients – and how they affect your microbes.

9. Support small food producers and local shops instead of supermarkets.
10. Think about the environmental impact of your food choices.
11. Eat fungi regularly.
12. Don't use supplements unless you are ill or pregnant.
13. Always opt for real food when you have a choice.
14. If eating convenience foods, choose the least processed ones, with the fewest ingredients.
15. Don't follow blindly what someone else says is good for them – no one is average.
16. Understand that food is medicine and the right diet can be as effective as many drugs.
17. Eat something fermented every day and become an expert in fermenting.
18. Cook for yourself whenever you can.
19. Try to look at all food through a different lens.
20. Experiment on yourself and try something new.

PART THREE

Food Tables and Tips

34. Food Tables

Polyphenol, fibre and sugar content of fruits (per 80g serving

Fruit	Polyphenol (mg)	Fibre (g)	Sugar (g)
Acai berries	2560	3.4	1.8
Apple	161	1.9	8.0
Apricot	106	1.6	7.2
Avocado	122	5.6	0.6
Banana	124	3.0	9.6
Blackberry	456	4.0	3.9
Black chokeberry	1405	3.4	3.4
Black grapes	148	0.7	12.2
Black olives	94	3.4	0.0
Black raspberry	784	5.6	3.6
Blueberry	472	1.9	7.3
Cantaloupe	88	0.7	6.4
Cranberry	252	3.7	3.2
Fig	77	1.8	13.0
Goji berry	140	3.4	11.3
Gooseberry	376	2.0	0.0
Grapefruit	21	1.3	5.6
Green olives	129	3.4	0.0
Guava	101	4.0	7.2
Honeydew melon	48	0.6	6.4
Kiwi	144	1.5	7.2
Lemon	48	2.2	2.0

Fruit	Polyphenol (mg)	Fibre (g)	Sugar (g)
Lychee	23	1.0	12.0
Mango	116	2.1	11.2
Nectarine	44	1.2	6.2
Orange	223	1.4	7.2
Papaya	46	1.8	6.3
Passion fruit	46	8.0	8.8
Peach	223	1.2	6.8
Pear	86	2.5	8.0
Pineapple	118	1.2	8.0
Plum	328	1.3	8.0
Redcurrant	359	3.4	5.9
Red raspberry	124	5.6	3.5
Sour cherry	282	1.3	6.8
Star fruit	144	2.2	3.2
Strawberry	231	1.6	3.9
Sweet cherry	140	2.9	6.4
Tangerine	154	1.1	8.8
Watermelon	41	0.3	4.8
White grapes	97	0.7	12.2

Buy in season to maximise nutritional benefits and minimise harm to the environment. Alternatively, enjoy year-long tinned, dried, or frozen. Remember that while dried fruit alternatives have higher polyphenol content, their sugar content will also be higher so consume in smaller amounts.

Polyphenol values are calculated based on averages of currently available data. Exact values will change and evolve as new data emerges.

Source: Polyphenol Explorer and USDA Food Survey, figures correct January 2022.

Top 10 most frequently eaten fruits, ranked by average scores from all ZOE users

A ZOE score for an individual food is a composite score (from 0 to 100) based on personal blood responses to sugars, responses to fats, and the effect on personal gut health (microbes). These scores may not apply to you as no one is average. The bars in values show the wide range of personalised responses to some fruits, such as bananas, whereas raspberries were found to be universally good for the metabolisms of these participants.

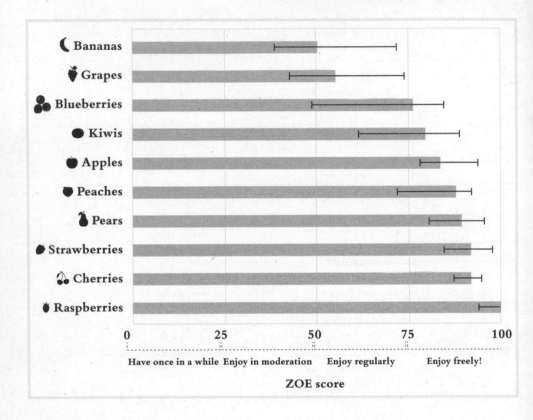

How frequently should we enjoy foods based on their score?

0–24 – 'Have once in a while'
There are no foods you can never eat. It's ok to eat these items but you should have them rarely or in small quantities.

25–49 – 'Enjoy in moderation'
There are healthier swaps for these foods but having them from time to time (2–3 times per week) in normal quantities is fine.

50–74 – 'Enjoy regularly'
You can eat these foods regularly (every other day). However, large quantities may have a negative impact.

75–100 – 'Enjoy freely!'
These foods are predicted to be the best for your metabolism. You can have these frequently.

The Rainbow Diet

This table shows my tips for vegetables and legumes categorised by colour to help you increase polyphenol diversity.

Red	Top tips
Beans (kidney, red, adzuki)	High in protein and beneficial polyphenols as well as fibre. Try to include beans in your meals every day.
Beetroot	Rich in fibre, vitamins and polyphenols including anthocyanin, with as little sugar as an apple. Eat raw when thinly sliced or cooked (but avoid boiling the nutrients to death).
Bell peppers	Higher in vitamin C than oranges. Eat raw in chopped salad for maximum vitamin C availability.
Chillies	Great for antioxidants and vitamin A. Add to curries and soups.
Radish	Slice into salads or sandwiches, ferment in kimchi, or roast.
Tomato	Cooked tomatoes are better than raw for their lycopene availability.
Orange	
Carrot	Best cooked for greater beta-carotene availability.
Pumpkin	A squash variety that is overshadowed by Halloween but is packed with fibre and vitamin A. Delicious in stews, soups or curries. Tap on the side to see if it's edible: the denser it is the tastier it'll be.
Sweet potato (and purple potatoes)	Great alternative to starchier white potatoes for a boost of polyphenols, ideally eaten with the skin on.
Squash	A nutritious power-packed vegetable; works well in stews, soups or curries.
Yellow/brown	
Cauliflower	Save the nutritious leaves, steam or briefly roast them, and serve with extra virgin olive oil (EVOO) and a spritz of lemon.
Chickpeas	Fantastic source of fibre and protein and shown to reduce blood glucose in trials. Best eaten whole in salads, soups and curries.
Corn	High in lutein and zeaxanthin, which may help maintain eye health (based on trials).
Garlic	Packed with prebiotic fibre inulin, which benefits the gut microbiome; excellent anti-inflammatory properties.

Mushrooms	Eat them every day for a great micronutrient boost, and a source of protein and vitamin D without the supplements.
Parsnips	Contains starch so they are energy-dense and contribute to fibre diversity.
Potato	Always leave the skin on. Contains more potassium than a banana and more fibre than an apple; high in vitamin C and a good source of iron.
Soybeans	A small snack of edamame gives you around 11 grams of protein and 8 grams of fibre. Enjoy in tofu form as a meat alternative.
Green	
Artichoke	High in the prebiotic fibre inulin to feed your gut microbiome. Delicious fresh but also when jarred or frozen.
Asparagus	Asparagus is one of the few exceptions to the polyphenol colour rule – green and white varieties have more polyphenols than purple asparagus.
Avocado	Excellent source of monounsaturated fats, fibre, vitamins and polyphenols.
Broad beans	Nourishing and versatile food frequently used in European and Middle Eastern cuisine but underused in the UK. A good source of fibre and protein and helps make meals more filling.
Broccoli	Try a range of broccoli varieties including purple. Can be eaten raw or cooked; contains iron as well as beneficial fibres.
Brussel sprouts	Roast them or steam them lightly to avoid the foul smell of boiled sprouts. A great seasonal vegetable packed with fibre.
Cabbage	Steam for less than 5 minutes to retain nutrients and avoid the rotten egg smell. Ferment to feed your gut.
Celery	When slowly braised it greatly enhances other flavours in tomatoes, olive oil and onions.
Cucumber	A good snack with hummus and counts as one of your plants, but otherwise nothing else special.
Iceberg lettuce	Its only good point is that it lasts for weeks in your refrigerator. My least favourite plant!
Lentils	High in protein, iron, fibre and nutrients, they are higher in iron gram-for-gram than steak or chicken. Cook from dried form to bring out their complex flavours.

Peas	Maintain structure well when frozen – keep a bag in the freezer to cheaply top up your meals.
Rocket and other leaves	The darker or redder the leaf the higher the polyphenols.
Spinach	Keep a bag of this leaf in your freezer for an affordable, nutritious boost to meals.
Blue/purple	
Aubergines (eggplant)	Salt or quickly boil then drain aubergine before baking, lightly frying in EVOO or adding to stews and curries for an excellent source of fibre, polyphenols and flavour.
Kale	Retains nutritional value relatively well when baked into chips with EVOO as a tasty snack as long as you don't overcook it.
Radicchio	Purple bitter leaf that's so full of polyphenols it can be overpowering when eaten raw in salad. Try grilled and add balsamic, or leave for an hour in a bowl of ice cold water to soften the bitterness.
Red cabbage	Switch to red cabbage which has three times the polyphenols of white. Great steamed, raw or fermented; adds colour and fibre to your plate.
Brown/black	
Black beans	High protein and polyphenol addition to salads, chillies and rice dishes.
Onions	Incredibly versatile vegetable; the darker the colour the higher in inulin and phytonutrients: red > yellow > white.
Peanuts and tree nuts	Eating these every day in their whole form has been shown to improve health. A handful of mixed nuts are high in polyphenols, high in fibre and help to regulate blood sugar responses. Generally, the whole nut is better than powdered, but introduce to babies in nut butter or powdered form.

Cereals, grains, pasta and bread

The following three tables show my personalised ZOE scores for cereals and grains, pasta and bread. These responses will vary by individual and can change over time. My personal score was calculated from my blood sugar response to carbohydrates, my blood fat response to fatty foods and whether that particular food is good or bad for my gut health. I've included my responses here to show just how varied our individual responses to carbohydrates can be.

My responses to cereals and grains, ranked from worst to best

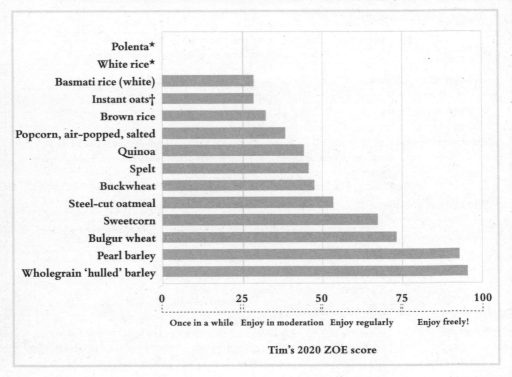

Tim's 2020 ZOE score

* My scores are 0 for polenta and white rice, showing they are foods I should only eat rarely.

† Instant oats have the same C:F ratio as rolled oats but the average ZOE score and GI index differ and individuals will have different responses to them, due to their different level of processing. This means they are the same on an ingredients list but will affect metabolism differently.

My responses to pasta, ranked from best to worst

Note that a low carbohydrate-to-fibre ratio is generally good, but individual responses will vary. Values will also vary by brand.

	Tim's 2020 ZOE score	Carb-to-fibre (C:F) ratio	Protein (percentage of total)
Chickpea pasta	59	4:1	20%
Whole-wheat pasta	49	8:1	6%
Whole-wheat couscous	45	6:1	5%
Fresh egg pasta	44	24:1	11%
Wholegrain spelt pasta	42	6:1	12%
Durum wheat pasta	41	18:1	14%
Buckwheat pasta	38	7:1	11%
Medium egg noodles	39	17:1	12%
Buckwheat noodles	35	12:1	13%
Dried egg pasta	34	22:1	15%
Rice noodles	34	16:1	3%
Semolina	32	23:1	5%
Couscous	22	18:1	6%
Potato gnocchi	21	12:1	5%
Instant noodles	16	21:1	2%

My responses to breads, ranked from best to worst

Note that values will vary depending on different recipes, brands and cooking techniques.

Bread type	Tim's 2020 ZOE score*	Carb-to-fibre (C:F) ratio*
Sourdough, rye	32	5:1 to 8:1
Sourdough, wholemeal	31	7:1 to 10:1
Loaf, rye, dark	30	3:1 to 8:1
Poppadoms	27	4:1 to 5:1
Chapati	26	7:1 to 9:1
Bagel, wholemeal	24	7:1 to 12:1
Sourdough, white	22	11:1 to 24:1
Supermarket loaf, seeded	20	7:1 to 12:1
Focaccia	14	13:1 to 20:1
Naan	9	16:1 to 19:1
Supermarket loaf, wholemeal	7	4:1 to 7:1
Supermarket loaf, white	4	17:1 to 22:1
Pitta, white	3	23:1 to 32:1
Bagel, white	0	16:1 to 19:1
Baguette	0	22:1 to 23:1
Ciabatta	0	12:1 to 23:1

Environmental impact of different sources of protein (per 100g of protein)

Note that these values will vary depending on a range of factors including the type of cheese, if animals are grass or grain fed, the energy source of growing modern proteins, and the location and scale of farming. For instance, lamb from New Zealand may have a lower carbon footprint than UK lamb, even if it's transported all the way to the UK.

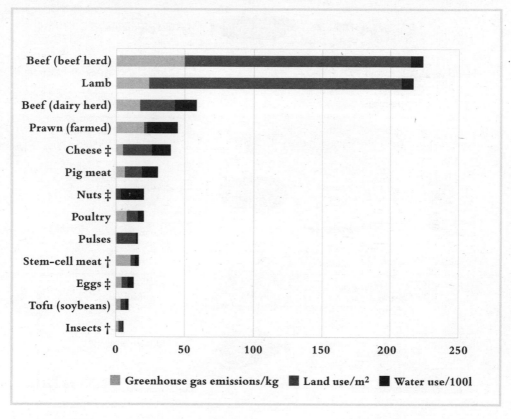

† Insects and stem-cell meat are approximates based on limited current data.

‡ Eggs, nuts and cheese are calculated per 50g of protein to better reflect realistic portion sizes.

Processed meats, ranked from worst to best

Low Quality		High Quality

SAUSAGE

Lowest-quality UK supermarket sausage*	Butcher's sausage
24 ingredients	4–10 ingredients
38% meat*	42–99% meat
Tim's ZOE score: 0	Tim's ZOE score: 31

BURGER

Lowest-quality UK supermarket burger	Highest-quality UK supermarket burger
17 ingredients	3 ingredients
62% meat	98% meat
Tim's ZOE score: 16	Tim's ZOE score: 37

HAM

Supermarket cooked ham	Prosciutto Cotto cooked ham
8 ingredients	2–5 ingredients
45–70% meat*	98% meat
Tim's ZOE score: 26	Tim's ZOE score: 33

SALAMI

Lowest-quality UK supermarket salami	Traditional Spanish chorizo
11 ingredients	5 ingredients
25–45% meat	95% meat
Tim's ZOE score: 0	Tim's ZOE score: 0

* Sausages must contain at least 42% pork to be legally called pork sausages in the UK, although to be classified as meat the pork can contain 30% fat and 25% connective tissue.

Omega-3 and mercury content of popular seafood

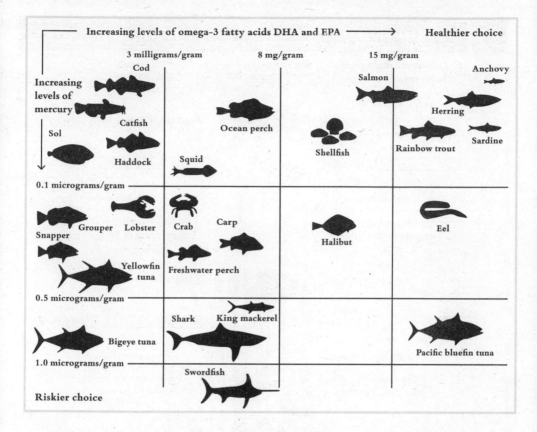

Bivalve shellfish such as mussels and clams are very sustainable.

How what we eat now compares to what we should eat for greater sustainability

The grey columns in this table show how much we typically eat from each food group in modern Western diets today. The dotted columns show how much food from each group we should consume to eat more sustainably.

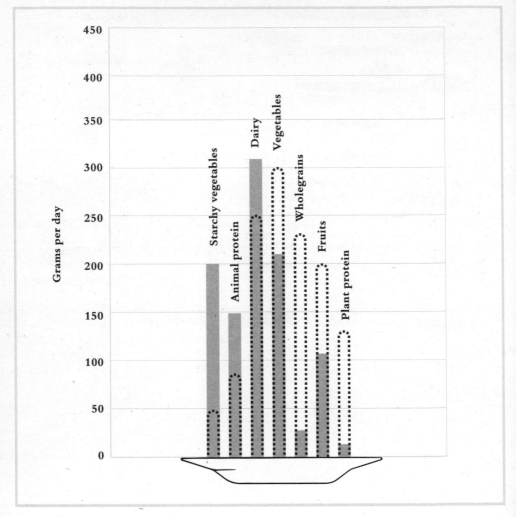

Sources: Our World in Data, 'Data Explorer: Environmental Impacts of Food': https://ourworldindata.org/environmental-impacts-of-food; R. E. Santo, 'Considering Plant-Based Meat Substitutes and Cell-Based Meats: A Public Health and Food Systems Perspective', *Frontiers in Sustainable Food Systems* (2020); 4:134; and C . Saunders, 'Food Miles, Carbon Footprinting and their potential impact on trade', *Australian Agricultural and Resource Economics Society* (2009).

Environmental impact of different types of milk (per 100ml glass)

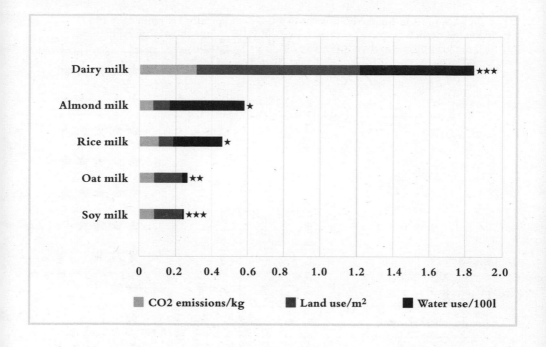

Stars show nutrient density from 1 star (least nutritious) to 3 stars (most nutritious) in terms of protein, fat and carbohydrate content per 100ml.

Fermented foods and dairy products, ranked by probiotic score and my personalised responses

Type	Tim's 2020 ZOE score	Probiotic score
Kimchi	92	★★★★★
Sauerkraut	91	★★★★★
Kombucha*	80	★★★★★
Kefir (milk)	76	★★★★★
Coconut kefir	70	★★★★★
Greek yogurt (full-fat)	78	★★★★
Blue cheese†	48	★★★
Water kefir	65	★★
Cheddar cheese†	56	★
Full-fat milk	58	☆
Semi-skimmed milk	50	☆
Butter	47	☆
Low-fat fruit-flavoured yogurt	41	☆
Skimmed milk	40	☆
Children's yogurt and fromage frais	24	☆
Full-fat cream	27	☆

5★★★★★ = Most probiotics   Empty star ☆ = No probiotics

* Based on my homemade kombucha. The higher the sugar content, the lower this score would be.

† Many of the probiotic strains in cheese are found in the rind, so it's good to eat the rind too (as long as not made of wax).

Microbial diversity of fermented drinks

Each shaded band indicates a different microbial strain. Absolute levels of microbes will differ in each batch of a fermented drink. Ensuring fermented drinks are live is the key to enjoying their health benefits and the greatest diversity and quantity of microbes.

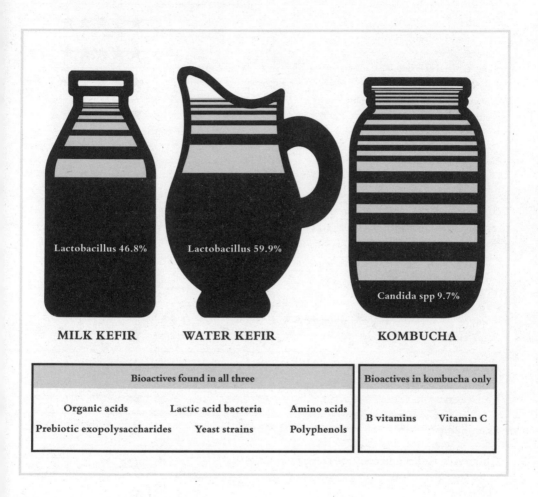

MILK KEFIR — Lactobacillus 46.8%

WATER KEFIR — Lactobacillus 59.9%

KOMBUCHA — Candida spp 9.7%

Bioactives found in all three			Bioactives in kombucha only	
Organic acids	Lactic acid bacteria	Amino acids	B vitamins	Vitamin C
Prebiotic exopolysaccharides	Yeast strains	Polyphenols		

Sources of calcium, ranked from highest to lowest

Food	Calcium per serving	Recommended daily intake (RDI)
Tofu (calcium set)	860mg in 126g (½ cup)	86%
Almonds (whole)	354mg in 143g (1 cup)	35%
Sardines	350mg in 92g (1 can)	35%
Cow's milk (whole)	350mg in 237ml (1 cup)	25%
Natural yogurt	300mg in 245g (1 cup)	30%
Amaranth	280mg in 132g (1 cup)	28%
Spring greens	266mg in 190g (1 cup)	26%
Dried figs	162mg in 1 dried fig	16%
White beans	130mg in 179g (1 cup)	13%
Poppy seeds	126mg in 9g (1 tbsp)	13%
Supermarket loaf, wholemeal	110mg in 10g (1 tbsp)	11%
Edamame	100mg in 155g (1 cup)	10%
Rhubarb	87mg in 240g (1 cup)	9%
San Pellegrino mineral water	40mg in 240ml (1 cup)	4%

My tips for using spices, seasoning and herbs every day

Spices	
Cardamom	Strong, sweet, pungent flavour and aroma, that can be bought as seeds, pods or ground.
Chilli peppers	Come in a variety of levels of sweetness and spice which we can be cautiously positive about: if eaten long term they may raise pain thresholds, maintain a healthy gut and reduce inflammation.
Cinnamon	Also contains eugenol (see cloves), comes in powder and stick form. Add to food for sweetness without adding sugar.
Cloves	Effective in treating gum pain and teething babies. Contains eugenol which is the active principle from clove extract, an anti-inflammatory and antimicrobial agent, but human studies are lacking. Delicious added sparingly to baked apples or mulled wine.
Cumin	A fragrant spice with great depth of flavour and over 100 chemicals and volatiles. Many claim it helps people slim down although the research is still evolving.
Ginger	Although there are plenty of unsubstantiated health claims, it can be helpful for nausea and possibly arthritis. Enjoy freshly grated or ground.
Kosher or sea salt	A purer form of table salt which comes in larger granules so is less concentrated than table salt – a good substitute for table salt when making kimchi if you're trying to lower your salt intake.
Mustard	Pungent seeds derived from the cabbage family, often used in curries.
Nutmeg	Pairs well with cinnamon and also contains eugenol (see cloves).
Paprika	Add near the end of cooking to avoid overcooking which diminishes colour and flavour. Made from dried and ground red peppers.
Pepper	Rich in protective antioxidants; whole peppercorns keep for years and are best ground onto food directly before eating.
Saffron	One of the most expensive substances on Earth by weight, but no proof yet of any health benefits.
Table salt	An essential nutrient that accentuates flavour but is hidden in large quantities in UPFs; usually comes in fine granules.

Turmeric (curcumin)	A balancing agent which is a great way to round off flavour to a dish. Add to anything orange (and edible) like sweet potatoes, carrots or eggs. There may be health benefits to eating turmeric daily.
Vanilla	Although it has potential antioxidant and antimicrobial effects, the vanilla bean extracted from orchids is best known for its unique aroma from the release of the chemical vanillin which most find relaxing. It can calm babies down nearly as well as breast milk.
Wasabi	Grate fresh to release many different chemical aromas; the strength is greatest after 5 minutes but after 20 minutes this overpowering aroma dissipates and it has a milder complexity.
Herbs	
Basil*	Rich nutrient profile with vitamins A, C and K, as well as anti-inflammatory polyphenols. Grow on your kitchen window sill and add liberally to pizza, pastas, salads and soups.
Coriander*	Similar health benefits to basil. For 1 in 5 of us it tastes like soap due to our genes.
Dill*	Pairs well with potatoes, pickles, fish, pickles and a wide range of vegetables.
Marjoram	Another versatile herb which can be added to almost everything Mediterranean or tomato-based.
Mint*	Very easy to grow at home – grows like a weed once it gets going! Add boiling water to make flavoursome tea or slice finely into salads, cocktails/mocktails, or to add to flavour your water.
Oregano	A bold, earthy flavour which is great sprinkled thinly sliced over salads, meats, poultry, fish and pasta. Use interchangeably with marjoram.
Parsley*	Similar health benefits to basil. Alternate curly with flat leaf variety for a change.
Rosemary	Hardy plant with lots of polyphenols, tastes great added to meat, beans and pulses.
Thyme	Similar to marjoram and oregano but with a slightly minty and lemony flavour.

*Best eaten fresh.

The spicy scoreboard

Ingredient	Scoville heat unit	
Pure capsaicin*	10,000,000	
US-graded police pepper spray	2,500,000–5,000,000	
Carolina Reaper	1,000,000–2,200,000	
Bhut jolokia (ghost pepper)	855,00–1,000,00	
Red Scandinavia habanero	350,000–580,000	
Habanero chile, Scotch bonnet	100,000–350,000	
Tabasco pepper	30,000–50,000	
Manzano pepper	12,000–30,000	
Serrano pepper	6,000–23,000	
Chipotle pepper, jalapeno	3,500–10,000	
Tabasco sauce	2,500–5,000	
Pasilla, poblano	1,000–2,500	
Paprika, pimiento, pepperoncini	100–900	
Bell pepper	0	

* This is a collector's item only and illegal to add to any food or sell as an ingredient due to the damage it can cause if ingested. If you're looking to challenge yourself with spice a Scotch bonnet will definitely be hot enough.

Smoke points of cooking fats, ranked by stability

Stability refers to the oxidation stability of the oil when heated to high temperatures, and how well it will retain its antioxidant properties. When considering which oil to use, both oxidative stability and polyphenol content play a part. Extra virgin olive oil contains the highest amount of antioxidants, and high oxidative stability, which is why I recommend choosing it for cooking, baking and frying, even at high temperatures.

Type	Smoke point	Oxidative stability	Polyphenols mg/100g
Coconut oil	175–200°C	★★★★★	0
Peanut oil	225–235°C	★★★★	0
Extra virgin olive oil	170–207°C	★★★★	60
Virgin olive oil	205–215°C	★★★★	35
Olive oil	195–245°C	★★★	20
Grapeseed oil	185–205°C	★★	2
Sunflower oil	220–240°C	★★	1
Ghee	245–255°C	★★	0
Rapeseed oil	190–230°C	★★	3
Walnut oil	160°C	★★	8
Avocado oil	270–300°C	★	6
Butter	150–175°C	★	0
Sesame oil	175–210°C	★	2
Flaxseed oil	107°C	★	5

Understanding ultra-processed foods

This table shows examples of foods in their minimally processed, processed and UPF forms. When choosing food, we should aim to have the majority of it in its whole form, sometimes in its processed form and very occasionally in its UPF form. Currently most of our calories come from the UPF form.

Minimally processed (whole food)	Processed	Ultra-processed food (UPF)
Corn on the cob	Tinned sweetcorn	Corn tortilla chips
Whole tomatoes	Tomato passata	Tomato-style pasta sauce
Whole peanuts	100% nut peanut butter	Chocolate peanut bars
Fresh strawberries	Strawberry jam	Strawberry fromage frais
Beef steak	100% minced beef	Frozen beef burgers
Green beans	Frozen green beans	Crunchy processed vegetable snacks
Stone-ground whole-wheat flour	Whole-wheat sourdough bread	Sliced bread loaf
Raw tuna (sashimi)	Tinned tuna	Tuna melt ready meal
Basmati rice	Parboiled basmati rice*	Rice puff breakfast cereal
Loose leaf green tea	Matcha tea latte	Commercial iced tea
Whole banana	Home-baked banana cake	Shop-bought banana cake
Whole unhomogenised milk	Live natural full-fat yogurt	Flavoured sugar-free low-fat yogurt
Whole orange	Freshly squeezed orange juice	Tropicana orange juice
Coffee bean	Espresso coffee	Mocha light caramel frappuccino
Whole skin-on baked potato	Potato fried in extra virgin olive oil (skin on)	Skinny potato fries
Steamed cod loin	Homemade fish goujons using breadcrumbs	Frozen fish fingers

* Parboiled rice is actually a good option when consuming rice as the resistant starch formed in the parboiling process leads to lower glucose load.

NOVA food classification

Classification	Definition	Examples
(1) unprocessed or minimally processed foods (MPF)	Comprising edible parts of plants, animals or fungi without any processes applied to them, or natural foods altered by minimal processing designed to preserve them and make them suitable for storage, or to make them safe, edible or more palatable.	Fresh fruit, vegetables, grains, legumes, meat and milk.
(2) processed culinary ingredients (PCI)	Substances extracted from group 1 or from nature used to cook and season MPF, not intended for consumption on their own.	Fats, oils, sugars and starches, salt.
(3) processed foods (PF)	Industrial products made by adding PCI to MPF.	Canned vegetables in brine, fruit in syrup, cheese, natural yogurt.
(4) ultra-processed foods (UPFs)	Formulations of ingredients, mostly of exclusive industrial use, that result from a series of industrial processes, many requiring sophisticated equipment and technology. Ingredients characteristic of UPFs include food substances of no or rare culinary use, including sugar, protein and oil derivatives, and cosmetic additives designed to make the final product look more palatable.	Sweet and savoury snacks, reconstituted meats, frozen pizza dishes and confectionery. High-fructose corn syrup, maltodextrin, protein isolates and hydrogenated oil. Colours, flavours, flavour enhancers, emulsifiers, thickeners and artificial sweeteners.

Source: Monteiro et al.

Glossary

Butyrate: a key healthy short chain fatty acid released when microbes digest fibre-rich foods which helps maintain a healthy intestinal barrier, key for good immune system function and reduced inflammation.

Caramelisation: the process by which slow, low-temperature cooking of sugars causes a change in appearance and flavour through a process which causes oxidisation of the food and the distinctive brown colour and rich, slightly nutty sweetness.

DNA: deoxyribonucleic acid is the building block of our genetic material; it is arranged as a double helix in chromosomes and contains roughly 20,000 genes in each cell of our bodies.

Endocrine Disrupting Chemicals (EDCs): chemicals found in plastics, fertilisers and some drugs that interact with human hormone pathways and contribute to infertility and other developmental issues in humans.

Epidemiology: the study of large groups or populations in order to discover the causes of disease.

Epigenetic: mechanisms by which chemical signals can switch genes on and off without altering the DNA structure. A normal process in babies and growth, which can be altered by diet and chemicals for up to several generations.

Esterification (inter-esterification): better for us than trans fats, new esterified fats are another way of turning liquid fats into solid or spreadable fats. We are not sure if they are any safer than hydrogenated fats and require processing methods.

Fat: a term with many different meanings; scientifically synonymous with lipids and not necessarily to be feared. Fats are normally solid at room temperature but oils which are liquid can be manipulated chemically.

Fermentation: a process involving microbes that break down food to produce chemicals that modify and preserve food to create alcohol in beer or wine, or lactic acid in milk products, sourdough bread or pickled cabbage.

Fibre: a general term for the complex, hard-to-digest parts of carbohydrates that reach the colon for our microbes to feed off. Crudely divided into soluble and insoluble fibres based on how they interact with water in our gut, which is not very helpful. They contain many different chemicals we understand little about, making fibre a very broad term that covers hundreds if not thousands of different chemical compositions and nutrients. High levels are found in fruit, legumes, other vegetables, whole grains and nuts. Artificial fibre is also available as additives.

FODMAP diet: often recommended as a treatment to those suffering with IBS (irritable bowel syndrome) symptoms, it excludes fermentable oligosaccharides, disaccharides, monosaccharides and polyols, found in many foods. It can lead to inadequate dietary intake as it is restrictive, and is not evidence-based for long-term intervention.

Free radicals: small chemicals released from cells as part of their normal function. If they accumulate they can be harmful to the body. Mopped up by antioxidants such as polyphenols.

Fructose: a carbohydrate sugar that makes up a percentage of table sugar and is much sweeter. Contained in most fruits and can be produced artificially from corn syrup and used in soft drinks.

Fungi: a large group (kingdom) of ancient organisms that include yeast, mould and mushrooms. Eating fungi confers many health benefits with few added calories.

Gene: a small group of chemicals on our DNA that tell the body to make a particular protein. We have about 20,000 in each of our cells. Estimates vary as our precise definition of genes changes.

Glycaemic Index (GI): a measure of the speed at which different foods produce an increase in glucose and then insulin in the blood. Low-GI foods are the basis of many diets. High-GI foods enable sugars to be released rapidly and cause rapid peaks in blood glucose and insulin (e.g. mashed potatoes) as opposed to low-GI, high-fibre foods like celery. An over-simplistic index, it is still unclear how important this mechanism is for influencing obesity and how it reflects our individuality.

Greenhouse gases (GHG): gases such as carbon dioxide and methane which absorb and emit infrared radiation and thus trap the world's heat leading to global warming.

Inflammation: the body's natural immune response to an injury or invasion by a foreign microbe, such as a painful swelling around a muddy scratch. Can also be brought on by chronic stress to the body which activates inflammatory pathways. Eating UPFs and insufficient fibre also causes inflammation after eating, known as postprandial inflammation. Obesity and type 2 diabetes and other diseases are linked to systemic low-grade inflammation.

Inflammatory Bowel Disease (IBD): a group of relatively rare diseases including Crohn's and ulceritive colitis are chronic, relapsing intestinal inflammation disorders with an unknown cause. Not to be confused with IBS, IBD can be diagnosed with endoscopy and samples taken from the colon. These diseases can be life-threatening if not treated correctly and have a significant impact on patients' lives.

Insulin: the hormone which, in response to blood glucose, controls how much sugar to store as glycogen in the liver and as fat in fat cells.

Insulin resistance: results when insulin doesn't rise as much after ingesting glucose, forcing the pancreas to produce more insulin so as to control glucose levels; leads to diabetes.

Intermittent fasting: reduced-calorie or no-calorie intake on 'fasting' days, either as the popular 5:2 diet or alternate-day fasting. Effective for weight loss due to reduced calorie consumption over the course of the week and sustainable in some people. Not to be confused with restricted-time eating, where there is no food consumed at all for an overnight fast of twelve to sixteen hours.

Inulin: not to be confused with insulin. A prebiotic fibre found in artichokes, leeks, onions, chicory and many other plants, now also a fashionable supplement. Fructose oligosaccharides (FOS) such as inulin are found naturally in these vegetables while galacto-oligosaccharides (GOS) are mostly synthesised from lactose. Neither is a magic bullet, we need a variety of fibre for maximum microbiome diversity and health.

Irritable Bowel Syndrome (IBS): a common, chronic intestinal condition with no obvious physical pathology. Results in pain, excessive wind, irregular bowel movements and a reduction in quality of life but is not usually life-threatening.

Kefir: a fermented milk drink that has several times the microbial composition of yogurt and is shown to have health benefits. Can also be made from water and sugar or fruit juice for vegans.

Keto diet: a diet designed to use ketone bodies for energy, based on at least 70 per cent of calories as fats. Found to help epilepsy in children, this is not to be confused with low-carb diets which are very effective to treat type 2 diabetes and have evidence supporting their efficacy.

Kimchi: a Korean dish of spicy fermented vegetables usually containing cabbage, garlic, radishes, onion and chillies with numerous health benefits.

Kombucha: a fermented tea drink that contains a wide range of healthy microbes with health benefits, and can produce small amounts of alcohol.

Leptin: a hormone released by the brain and closely related to body fat levels. Signals to our brains when we have consumed enough food.

Lipids: the scientific word for fats, but includes many other molecules, e.g. fatty acids. When combined with proteins lipids are called lipoproteins, which travel around the body and can be of different shapes and sizes.

Low-density lipoproteins (LDL): the less healthy form in which lipids are transported. They can get absorbed into blood vessels and lead to clogging of the arteries (atherosclerosis).

Low-fat products: this may just mean slightly less fat than normal, or that the fat has been replaced with sugars, starches or proteins like soy and a multitude of chemicals to make them palatable. Normally *not* the healthier option over the full-fat version.

Maillard reaction: the browning reaction or chemical process which takes place when we heat carbohydrates (reducing sugars) with proteins (amino acids) to over 140°C that gives browned food its distinctive flavour thanks to the extra flavours and aromas released from food.

Meal replacement powders: designed to help people who are overweight, obese or pre-diabetic lose weight rapidly. Contain added vitamins and minerals as well as target levels of macronutrients but are generally full of artificial colours, flavours, emulsifiers and artificial sweeteners, leading to their classification as UPFs.

Mediterranean diet (MD): a dietary pattern that is often misconstrued as meaning lots of pasta and pizza. This dietary pattern with legumes, nuts, whole grains, fruits, vegetables, cultured dairy, EVOO and occasional meat and fish has the most data to show it is beneficial for overall health. It is rich in unprocessed foods and is seasonal.

Meta-analysis: a technique for combining the results of different studies or trials to produce a single summary result. Provides better evidence than any single study, but can still be misleading if many of the studies are biased or missing data.

Metabolism: the way the body and all cells both use and expend energy. Can be modified by many factors, e.g. heat, exercise, illness, body weight and food composition.

Microbiome: the whole community of microbes as measured by genetics that may be in our guts or mouths or in the soil. Best considered as a novel organ in our bodies that acts as thousands of chemical factories that produce vitamins, and key signals for our immune systems, brain and metabolism.

Microbiota: the different biological species that make up a community of living microorganisms in our gut, on our skin and in our mouth. Used interchangeably with microbiome although measured differently.

Microplastics: extremely small pieces of plastic waste in the environment resulting from the breakdown of consumer products and industrial waste. Found primarily in water supplies and seafood, the effects of these microplastics on our health are still relatively unknown.

mTOR pathway: a nutrient-sensing pathway for cell growth in many tissues that has been implicated in obesity, ageing and cancer, as well as being essential for development and growth, affected by milk and certain drugs, like rapamycin.

Neurotransmitters: chemicals in the brain that allow nerve cells (neurons) to communicate and control mood (e.g. serotonin, dopamine), some of which are produced predominantly by gut microbes and modifiable by diet.

NOVA classification: used to identify foods according to their level of processing from minimally processed food (MPF) to ultra-processed food (UPF). Used in some enlightened countries to flag UPFs and in research to help analyse the association between types of food available to us and chronic disease.

Nutrients: chemicals found in food that have been identified for their clinically observed medical impact. These currently cover only a fraction of the potentially helpful chemicals found in our food and will be added to in the future.

Observational study: a type of epidemiological research that makes inferences by comparing risk factors (e.g. food) with outcomes like disease. Evidence is weak when solely cross-sectional but better when people are followed over long periods (prospective observational study, or cohort study). All observational studies can be biased by other factors which are hard to measure.

Oleic acid: a fatty acid (monounsaturated) that is one of the major components of olive oil.

Omega-3 fatty acid: a polyunsaturated fatty acid found in many oily fish and often used as a (much-hyped) health supplement for the heart and brain. It is an essential fatty acid that we can't make ourselves. There are three main types, DHA, EPA and ALA: ALA is an essential precursor to DHA and EPA and is found in plants, whilst DHA and EPA are mostly found in fatty fish and grass-fed animal products. Humans are not always efficient at converting ALA, so consuming DHA and EPA directly is thought to be helpful.

Omega-6 fatty acid: a similar polyunsaturated fatty acid found in many foods, e.g. soybean, palm oil, chicken, nuts and seeds, and an essential fatty acid. It has a bad (largely unfounded) reputation. Ratio of 3:6 fatty acids is often used as a marker of health which is still unproven.

Palm oil: made very cheaply from oil from palm tree plantations in the rain-forest and a main contributor to deforestation and endangerment of wildlife including orangutans. Used widely in UPFs and cheap foods as a low-cost, palatable fat with no health benefits.

Polyphenols: a group of many chemicals released from food after digestion by microbes, many of which are useful and healthy. Polyphenols include flavonoids and resveratrol, which have antioxidant properties. Contained in vegetables, fruits, nuts, tea, coffee, chocolate, beer and red wine.

Polyunsaturated fatty acids (PUFAs): a type of lipid that consists of long chain fatty acids with double bonds, that are part of many foods generally regarded as healthy.

Postbiotic: a term for the chemical products of microbes that have beneficial effects on the body (see SCFA). Are now being used as novel therapeutics producing, for example, gamma-aminobutyric acid.

Prebiotic: any food component that encourages healthy bacteria to flourish like a fertiliser. Found in all breast milk and plants. Bacteria often feed off prebiotics. Often contains inulin, which is found in high levels in Jerusalem and globe artichokes, celery, garlic, onions and chicory root.

PREDICT study: a series of large nutritional intervention studies funded by ZOE Ltd, involving thousands of normal volunteers eating identical meals, and measuring responses with glucose monitors, blood fat levels and measuring microbiome, aiming to personalise diets.

Probiotic: a term for foods and supplements that contain live organisms that are considered beneficial for health. This can be in cultured yogurts, kimchi, kombucha, and are best consumed in foods daily as opposed to supplements.

Resveratrol: a natural phenol found in blueberries, the skin of red grapes and raspberries. Has been falsely hypothesised as the reason why red wine may have beneficial health effects.

Saturated fat: a type of lipid that lacks hydrogen bonds and is contained in large amounts in oils like coconut and palm oil, dairy and meats. Previously thought to be harmful, but recent data is conflicting and depends on context.

Sequencing: a term for identifying all the key parts of DNA and genes in an organism. Usually the DNA is broken into millions of small pieces and reassembled (often referred to as 'shotgun'). Used to identify microbe species and disease genes in humans in great detail.

Short chain fatty acids (SCFA): postbiotic chemicals produced by our gut microbes as a by-product of phytonutrient digestion of fibres. An example is butyrate which helps maintain a healthy intestinal barrier, key for good immune system function and reduced inflammation.

Smoke point: the point at which a cooking fat or oil starts to burn with impurities which cause smoke. This varies between oils and is the point at which some claim oil can become dangerous or carcinogenic, though the thermal stability of a cooking fat is probably more important than its smoke point and saturated fat is generally more stable.

Sourdough bread: bread made using traditional fermentation methods which typically only needs a fermenting starter, flour and water to start.

Stem cell meat: a new way of growing real meat or fish protein in a laboratory for use in processed food. Likely to get progressively cheaper and become an ethical alternative to meat.

Sugar-sweetened beverages (SSB): drinks which have added sugar and have been linked to increased tooth decay, obesity and poor health outcomes. Can be in the form of fizzy drinks or fruit juices and concentrates.

Sugar: this term has different meanings: it is another common word for soluble carbohydrates; or refers to the white powder we eat called sucrose, which is a mix of glucose and fructose. The suffix '-ose' means that the chemical is a sugar (e.g. lactose).

The four Ks: fermented foods starting with K: Kombucha, Kimchi, Kefir and Krauts (specifically fermented sauerkraut).

Time-restricted eating (TRE): an approach to respect our body's and microbiome's circadian rhythm by eating within a certain time frame during the day, leaving twelve to eighteen hours of no food overnight – for example, dinner at 9pm and breakfast at 11am the next day. According to ongoing research, fourteen to sixteen hours' fasting is the sweet spot for improved metabolism and weight control that is feasible. Not to be confused with intermittent fasting 'diets', this approach focuses solely on timing and may be more sustainable long term.

TMAO: a gut microbiome-dependent metabolite of a chemical trimethylamine, mostly found in animal foods. Associated with worse heart health outcomes and strokes, it is an example of an unhelpful postbiotic, but is only produced in some people because of certain gut microbes.

Trans fats: also called hydrogenated fats, these are chemically transformed unsaturated fats that solidify and are easy to cook with, but hard to break down in the body. Common as dairy substitutes and in junk foods. Major cause of heart disease and cancer. Banned in some countries and slowly being phased out in others.

Ultra-processed food (UPF): UPFs are made from combining substances extracted from food such as fats and starches and reconstituted into food products with added colours, flavours and stabilisers. These make up more than half the calorie intake in the UK and the US without providing the beneficial phytonutrients, fibre and food matrix which we all need for a healthy life.

Umami: the fifth (savoury) taste sense that mimics meat. It comes from glutamate and is found in mushrooms. There is now a possible sixth sense called 'kokumi', meaning 'heartiness'.

Viruses: tiny microbes that outnumber bacteria five to one, and many feed off them (these devourers are called 'phages') to control their numbers. Most are harmless to us and live in our bodies and may have a health role.

Visceral fat: the internal fat that accumulates around your intestines and liver. Excess fat is associated with heart disease and diabetes. More harmful than fat on the exterior of the body.

Vitamins: molecules that are essential for the body's chemical reactions to work, which we can't produce ourselves. We get most from food, sunlight (vitamin D – though not a true vitamin) and our gut microbes.

Yeast: a member of the fungi kingdom that converts sugar into alcohol and carbon dioxide. Used in making bread and alcohol. May promote healthy gut microbes. Can happily live in our guts and is only rarely pathogenic, e.g. candida infections.

ZOE: a data-science company based in the US and UK that develops and sells home-testing kits and apps to personalise nutrition. Also developed a not-for-profit app to fight Covid-19 (joinzoe.com).

Acknowledgements

For a book like this, covering such a vast area, I needed plenty of help over the years. This is a huge team effort and my long-term and brilliant editor Bea Hemming of Jonathan Cape and my agent Sophie Lambert of Curtis Brown have been crucial to its success and evolution in its many forms and versions. A huge thanks to the talented scientist and nutritionist Federica Amati, assisted by medical student Lucy McCann, who helped get the book up to speed and put all the tables and figures together in the final year. Rose Davidson did an amazing job of pruning and copy-editing. Amrita Vijay and then Emily Leeming, who later became my gifted PhD student, helped start the project off. I was supported and protected as always by the ever-loyal Victoria Vazquez and Debbie Hart who protected my back, and lucky to be surrounded by many clever experts in nutrition and microbes, both in the personalised nutrition company ZOE Ltd (my co-founders George Hadjigeorgiou and Jonathan Wolf who read the whole draft) and King's College London.

My friend and colleague, nutritionist Sarah Berry who has been co-leading the PREDICT studies with me, has been an amazing font of knowledge, enthusiasm and new ideas. Nicola Segata from Trento is the brains behind all the latest breakthroughs in the microbiome and it has been an absolute pleasure working with him and his team. Spencer Hyman was a huge help with the chocolate chapters. Talking to real chefs was an inspiration and I was lucky to have had several memorable meals and discussions with Heston Blumenthal and latterly Jamie Oliver. I tried to get as many sources of information as possible and read more books, reviews and articles than I can mention or remember. Regular companions on my travels were Harold McGee's classic *Food and Cooking*, and some excellent regular podcasts such as BBC Radio 4 *The Food Programme*, BBC World Service *The Food Chain*, the US series *Gastropod*, and ZOE *Science and Nutrition*. A few of the other contributors who educated me or helped with my questions or fact-checked some chapters are listed below but the mistakes are all mine not theirs:

Haya Al Khatib; Lazlo Barabiasi; John Blundell; Lesley Bookbinder; Ruth Bowyer; Helen Browning; Richard Davies; Henry Dimbleby; Robyn Fitzgerald; Christopher Gardner; Amir Gehr; James Hoffman; George Hadjigeorgiou;

Deborah Hart; Nicky Hornzee; John the fishmonger; Caroline LeRoy; Laura McKenzie; Cristina Menni; Dariush Mozaffarian; Seb Ourselin; Bex Palmer; Bronwen Percival; Susana Puig; Maria Rodriguez; Dan Saladino; Luca Sirejol; Roz Smyth; Thomas Spector and his microbes; Claire Steves; Ana Valdes; Jessie Inshauspe; John Vincent; Matt Walker; Jonathan Wolf; Patrick Wyatt and the whole team at ZOE.

Notes

Introduction

1. J. Merino, 'Diet quality and risk and severity of COVID-19: a prospective cohort study', *Gut* (2021); 70:2096–2104
2. A. Afshin, 'Health effects of dietary risks in 195 countries, 1990–2017: a systematic analysis for the Global Burden of Disease Study 2017', *The Lancet* (2019); 393:1958–72
3. A. L. Barabási, 'The unmapped chemical complexity of our diet', *Nature Food* (2020); 1:33–37
4. H. Kolb, 'Health Effects of Coffee: Mechanism Unraveled?' *Nutrients* (2020); 12(6):1842
5. Genevieve Timmins, 'Urgent action needed to reduce harm of ultra-processed foods to British children', Imperial College London (14 June 2021)
6. https://joinzoe.com/our-science
7. H. R. Marston, 'A Commentary on Blue Zones: A Critical Review of Age-Friendly Environments in the 21st Century and Beyond', *International Journal of Environmental Research and Public Health* (2021); 18(2):837
8. S. Swaminathan, 'Associations of cereal grains intake with cardiovascular disease and mortality across 21 countries in Prospective Urban and Rural Epidemiology study: prospective cohort study', *BMJ* (2021); 372:m4948
9. S. B. Seidelmann, 'Dietary carbohydrate intake and mortality: a prospective cohort study and meta-analysis', *The Lancet Public Health* (2018); 3:e419–e428
10. J. Smylie, 'Our health counts: population-based measures of urban Inuit health determinants, health status, and health care access', *Canadian Journal of Public Health* (2018); 109(5–6):662–670
11. J. L. Heileson, 'Dietary saturated fat and health disease: a narrative review', *Nutrition Reviews* (2019); 78(6):474–485

1: What is the microbiome?

1. F. Amati, 'The gut microbiome, health and personalised nutrition', *Trends in Urology & Men's Health* (2022); 13(3):22–25

2. F. Asnicar, 'Blue poo: impact of gut transit time on the gut microbiome using a novel marker', *Gut (2021)*; 70(9):1665–1674

3. https://joinzoe.com/bluepoop

4. A. Reale, 'Tolerance of Lactobacillus casei, Lactobacillus paracasei and Lacto-bacillus rhamnosus strains to stress factors encountered in food processing and in the gastro-intestinal tract', *LWT-Food Science and Technology (2015)*; 60(2):721–728

5. M. O'Driscoll, 'Age-specific mortality and immunity patterns of SARS-CoV-2', *Nature* (2021); 590:140–145

6. R. J. Cox, 'Not just antibodies: B cells and T cells mediate immunity to COVID–19', *Nature Reviews Immunology (2020)*; 20:581–582

7. K. A. Lee, 'The gut microbiome: what the oncologist ought to know', *British Journal of Cancer* (2021); 125:1197–1209

2: Why do we love food?

1. E. Alder, 'A novel family of mammalian taste receptors', *Cell* (2021); 100(6): 693–702

2. C. Menni, 'Real–time tracking of self-reported symptoms to predict potential COVID-19', *Nature Medicine* (2020); 26:1037–1040

3. A. Gupta, 'Brain-gut-microbiome interactions in obesity and food addiction', *Nature Reviews Gastroenterology & Hepatology* (2020); 17(11):655–672

4. P. Rao, 'Addressing the sugar, salt, and fat issues the science of food way', *npj Science of Food* (2018); 2:12

3: What foods are really healthy?

1. P. Scheelbeek, 'Health impacts and environmental footprints of diets that meet the Eatwell Guide recommendations: analyses of multiple UK studies', *BMJ Open* (2020); 10:e037554

2. G. Grosso, 'Red orange: experimental models and epidemiological evidence of its benefits on human health', *Oxidative Medicine and Cellular Longevity* (2013); 2013:157240

3. E. Cameron, 'Supplemental ascorbate in the supportive treatment of cancer: Prolongation of survival times in terminal human cancer', *Proceedings of the National Academy of Sciences of the USA* (1976); 73(1):3685–3689

4. P. Louca, 'Modest effects of dietary supplements during the COVID-19 pandemic: insights from 445 850 users of the COVID-19 Symptom Study app', *BMJ Nutrition, Prevention & Health* (2021); 4:e000250

5. Brent Schrotenboer, 'Vitamin C by an IV and an FBI raid. How hope, rather than proof, sent the antioxidant's sales soaring during COVID-19', *USA Today* (21 July 2020)

6. M. Chakhtoura, 'Impact of vitamin D supplementation on falls and fractures – A critical appraisal of the quality of the evidence and an overview of the available guidelines', *Bone* (2020); 131:115112

7. K. Li, 'The good, the bad, and the ugly of calcium supplementation: a review of calcium intake on human health', *Clinical Interventions in Aging* (2018); 13: 2443–2452

8. P. Wyatt, 'Postprandial glycaemic dips predict appetite and energy intake in healthy individuals', *Nature Metabolism* (2021); 3:523–529

9. Y. Zhu, 'Increased number of chews during a fixed-amount meal suppresses postprandial appetite and modulates glycemic response in older males', *Physiology & Behaviour* (2014); 133:136–140

10. A. T. Goh, 'Increased oral processing and a slower eating rate increase glycaemic, insulin and satiety responses to a mixed meal tolerance test', *European Journal of Nutrition* (2021); 60(5):2719–2733

11. S. B. Barr, 'Postprandial energy expenditure in whole-food and processed-food meals: implications for daily energy expenditure', *Food & Nutrition Research* (2010); 54:10.3402

12. F. Asnicar, 'Microbiome connections with host metabolism and habitual diet from 1,098 deeply phenotypes individuals', *Nature Medicine* (2021); 27(2): 321–332

13. D. McDonald, 'American Gut: an Open Platform for Citizen Science Microbiome Research', *mSystems* (2018); 3(3):e00031–18

14. O. Mompeo, 'Consumption of Stilbenes and Flavonoids is Linked to Reduced Risk of Obesity Independently of Fibre Intake', *Nutrients* (2020); 12(6):1871

15. C. Menni, 'Gut microbiome diversity and high-fibre intake are related to lower long-term weight gain', *International Journal of Obesity* (2017); 41(7): 1099–1105

16. S. O. Fetissov, 'Role of the gut microbiota in host appetite control: bacterial growth to animal feeding behaviour', *Nature Reviews Endocrinology* (2017); 13: 11–25

4: What foods are unhealthy?

1. M. Mazidi, 'Meal-induced inflammation: postprandial insights from the Personalised REsponses to DIetary Composition Trial (PREDICT) study in 1000 participants', *The American Journal of Clinical Nutrition* (2021); 114(3):1028–1038

2. C. A. Monteiro, 'Ultra-processed foods: What are they and how to identify them', *Public Health Nutrition* (2019); 22(5):936–941

3. K. D. Hall, 'Ultra-processed diets cause excess calorie intake and weight gain: An inpatient randomized controlled trial of ad libitum food intake', *Cell Metabolism* (2019); 30(1):67–77

4. E. Leeming, 'Ultra-processed foods associated with atherogenic lipoproteins partially mediated by the gut microbiota', *in press* (2022)

5. https://joinzoe.com/post/what-is-predict

6. L. Wang, 'Trends in Consumption of Ultraprocessed Foods Among US Youths Aged 2–19 Years, 1999–2018', *JAMA* (2021); 326(6):519–530

7. S. Vandevijvere, 'Global trends in ultraprocessed food and drink product sales and their association with adult body mass index trajectories', *Obesity Reviews* (2019); 20(2):10–19

8. K. D. Hall, 'Ultra-Processed Diets Cause Excess Calorie Intake and Weight Gain: An Inpatient Randomized Controlled Trial of Ad Libitum Food Intake', *Cell Metabolism* (2019); 30(1):67–77

9. A. S. Livingston, 'Effect of reducing ultraprocessed food consumption on obesity among US children and adolescents aged 7–18 years: evidence from a simulation model', *BMJ Nutrition, Prevention & Health* (2021).

10. P. Song, 'Dietary Nitrates, Nitrites, and Nitrosamines Intake and the Risk of Gastric Cancer: A Meta-Analysis', *Nutrients* (2015); 7(12):9872–9895

11. A. Etemadi, 'Mortality from different causes associated with meat, heme iron, nitrates, and nitrites in the NIH-AARP Diet and Health Study: population based cohort study', *BMJ* (2017); 357:j1957

12. P. Qin, 'Sugar and artificially sweetened beverages and risk of obesity, type 2 diabetes mellitus, hypertension, and all-cause mortality: a dose-response meta-analysis of prospective cohort studies', *European Journal of Epidemiology,* (2020); 35(7):655–671

13. C. B. Ebbeling, 'Effects of Sugar-Sweetened, Artificially Sweetened, and Unsweetened Beverages on Cardiometabolic Risk Factors, Body Composition, and Sweet Taste Preference: A Randomized Controlled Trial', *Journal of the American Heart Association* (2020); 9(15):e015668

14. P. Wyatt, 'Postprandial glycaemic dips predict appetite and energy intake in healthy individuals', *Nature Metabolism* (2021); 3:523–529

5: Can foods 'boost' your immune system?

1. M. Roederer, 'The genetic architecture of the human immune system: a bioresource for autoimmunity and disease pathogenesis', *Cell* (2015); 161(2):387–403

2. P. Brodin, 'Variation in the human immune system is largely driven by non-heritable influences', *Cell* (2015); 160(0):37–47

3. K. A. Lee, 'Cross-cohort gut microbiome associations with immune checkpoint inhibitor response in advanced melanoma', *Nature Medicine* (2022); 28:535–544

4. V. L. Greto, 'Extensive weight loss reduces glycan age by altering IgG N-glycosylation', *International Journal of Obesity,* (2021); 45:1521–1531

5. K. F. Gey, 'On the antioxidant hypothesis with regard to arteriosclerosis', *Biblioteca nutria et dieta* (1986); (37):53–91

6. P.C.H. Hollman, 'The biological relevance of direct antioxidant effects of polyphenols for cardiovascular health in humans is not established', *The Journal of Nutrition* (2011); 141(5):989S–1009S

7. M. Maares, 'Zinc and immunity: An essential interrelation', *Archives of Biochemistry and Biophysics* (2016); 611:58–65

8. P. Louca, 'Modest effects of dietary supplements during the COVID-19 pandemic: insights from 445 850 users of the COVID-19 Symptom Study app', *BMJ Nutrition, Prevention & Health* (2021); 4:e000250

9. S. L. Klein, 'Sex differences in immune responses', *Nature Reviews Immunology* (2016); 16:626–638.

10. D. A. Jolliffe, 'Vitamin D supplementation to prevent acute respiratory infections: systematic reviews and meta-analysis of aggregate data from randomised controlled trials', *The Lancet Diabetes & Endocrinology* (2021); 9(5):276–292

11. J. B. Cannata-Andía, 'A single-oral bolus of 100,000 IU of cholecalciferol at hospital admission did not improve outcomes in the COVID-19 disease: the COVID-VIT-D-a randomised multicentre international clinical trial', *BMC Medicine* (2022); 20(1):83

12. Y. Wang, 'Probiotics for prevention and treatment of respiratory tract infections in children', *Medicine* (Baltimore) (2016); 95(31):e4509

13. V. Sencio, 'The lung-gut axis during viral respiratory infections: the impact of gut dysbiosis on secondary disease outcomes', *Mucosal Immunology* (2021); 14:296–304

14. J. Schluter, 'The gut microbiota is associated with immune cell dynamics in humans', *Nature* (2020); 588:303–307

15. C. Menni, 'High intake of vegetables is linked to lower white blood cell profile and the effect is mediated by the gut microbiome', *BMC Medicine* (2021); 19:37

16. A. R. Wolf, 'Bioremediation of a Common Product of Food Processing by a Human Gut Bacterium' *Cell Host & Microbe* (2019); 26(4);463–477

17. M. Siervo, 'Does dietary nitrate say NO to cardiovascular ageing? Current evidence and implications for research', *Proceedings of the Nutrition Society* (2018); 77(2):112–123

18. W. H. Tang, 'Intestinal Microbial Metabolism of Phosphatidylcholine', *The New England Journal of Medicine* (2013); 368:1575–1584

6: How can we choose better foods?

1. J.P.A. Ioannidis, 'The Challenge of Reforming Nutritional Epidemiologic Research', *JAMA* (2018); 320(10):969–970

2. Gary Lewis, 'I got a hoax academic paper about how UK politicians wipe their bums published', *The Conversation* (20 July 2018)

3. H. Jabeur, 'Extra-Virgin Olive Oil and Cheap Vegetable Oils: Distinction and Detection of Adulteration as Determined by GC and Chemometrics', *Food Analytical Methods* (2016); 9:712–723

4. Felicity Lawrence, 'Rotting meat at Irish factory "destined for burgers"', *The Guardian* (24 February 2014)

5. BBC News, 'Lamb curries and kebabs "often another meat"' (17 April 2014)

6. Mauricio Savarese, 'Meatpacking companies "bribed inspectors to keep rotten meat on the market", police say', *The Independent* (18 March 2017)

7. Stephen Leachy, 'Revealed: seafood fraud happening on a vast global scale', *The Guardian* (15 March 2021)

8. BBC News, 'Peanut curry death: Restaurant owner Mohammed Zaman jailed' (23 May 2016)

7: How does storing, processing and cooking alter food?

1. B. H. Bajka, 'The impact of replacing wheat flour with cellular legume powder on starch bioaccessibility, glycaemic response and bread roll quality: A double-blind randomised controlled trial in healthy participants', *Food Hydrocolloids* (2021); 114:106565

2. https://www.bbc.co.uk/programmes/articles/3LncBcDcCXKgtpFvrDZVnNQ/can-my-leftovers-be-healthier-than-the-original-meal

3. Shari Roan, 'Fake blueberries abound in food products', *Los Angeles Times* (20 Jan 2011)

4. J. S. Siracusa, 'Effects of bisphenol A and its analogs on reproductive health: A mini review', *Reproductive Toxicology* (2018); 79:96–123

5. https://www.mdpi.com/1660-4601/16/14/2521 K. Y. Kim, 'The Association between Bisphenol A Exposure and Obesity in Children – A Systematic Review with Meta-Analysis', *International Journal of Environmental Research and Public Health* (2019); 16(14):2521

6. M. A. Poiana, 'Assessing the effects of different pectins addition on color quality and antioxidant properties of blackberry jam', *Chemistry Central Journal* (2013); 7:121

7. R. Alkutbe, 'Nutrient Extraction Lowers Postprandial Glucose Response of Fruit in Adults with Obesity as well as Healthy Weight Adults', *Nutrients* (2020); 12(3):777

8. A. Bouzari, 'Vitamin Retention in Eight Fruits and Vegetables: A Comparison of Refrigerated and Frozen Storage', *Journal of Agricultural and Food Chemistry* (2015); 63(3):957–962

9. S. Yochpaz, 'Effect of Freezing and Thawing on Human Milk Macronutrients and Energy Composition: A Systematic Review and Meta-Analysis', *Breastfeeding Medicine* (2020); 15(9):559–562

10. L. Mutsokoti, 'Carotenoid transfer to oil during thermal processing of lower fat carrot and tomato particle based suspensions', *Food Research International* (2016); 86:64–73

11. M. Kuroda, 'Association between soup consumption and obesity: A systematic review and meta-analysis', *Physiology & Behavior* (2020); 225:113103

12. M. K. Virk-Baker, 'Dietary acrylamide and human cancer: a systematic review of literature' *Nutrition and Cancer* (2014); 66(5):774–90

13. Y. Du, 'Association Between Frequency of Eating Away-From-Home Meals and Risk of All-Cause and Cause-Specific Mortality', *Journal of the Academy of Nutrition and Dietetics* (2021); 121(9):1741–1749

8: What to eat to save the planet?

1. https://www.ipcc.ch/srcclhttps://www.ipcc.ch/srccl/

2. D. F. Pais, 'Reducing Meat Consumption to Mitigate Climate Change and Promote Health: but Is It Good for the Economy?', *Environmental Modeling & Assessment* (2020); 25:793–807

3. T. D. Searchinger, 'Assessing the efficiency of changes in land use for mitigating climate change', *Nature* (2018); 564:249–253

4. Craig Jones, 'Wonky Fruit and Veg: The Carbon Footprint of Food', *Carbon Footprint* (14 February 2018)

5. R. Geyer, 'Production, use, and fate of all plastics ever made', *Science Advances* (2017); 3(7):e1700782.

6. Oliver Franklin-Wallis, ' "Plastic recycling is a myth": what really happens to your rubbish?', *The Guardian* (17 Aug 2019)

7. C. G. Parks, 'Rheumatoid Arthritis in Agricultural Health Study Spouses: Associations with Pesticides and Other Farm Exposures', *Environmental Health Perspectives* (2016); 124(11)

8. https://efsa.onlinelibrary.wiley.com/doi/pdf/10.2903/j.efsa.2016.4611

9. Damian Carrington, 'Free school fruit contains multiple pesticides, UK food report shows', *The Guardian* (5 Sep 2017)

10. B. González-Alzaga, 'A systematic review of neurodevelopmental effects of prenatal and postnatal organophosphate pesticide exposure', *Toxicology Letters* (2014); 230(2):104–121

11. The Alliance for Natural Health USA, 'Glyphosate Levels in Breakfast Foods: What is safe?' (19 April 2016)

12. B. Gao, 'Sex-Specific Effects of Organophosphate Diazinon on the Gut Microbiome and Its Metabolic Functions', *Environmental Health Perspectives* (2017); 125(2):198–206

13. L. G. Smith, 'The greenhouse gas impacts of converting food production in England and Wales to organic methods', *Nature Communications* (2019); 10:4641

14. D. Średnicka-Tober, 'Effect of crop protection and fertilization regimes used in organic and conventional production systems on feed composition and physiological parameters in rats', *Journal of Agricultural and Food Chemistry* (2013); 6:61(5):1017–29

15. M. Barański, 'Higher antioxidant and lower cadmium concentrations and lower incidence of pesticide residues in organically grown crops: a systematic literature review and meta-analyses', *British Journal of Nutrition* 2014; 112(5):794–811

16. D. Średnicka-Tober, 'Composition differences between organic and conventional meat: a systematic literature review and meta-analysis', *British Journal of Nutrition* (2016); 115:994–1011

17. J. Baudry, 'Association of Frequency of Organic Food Consumption with Cancer Risk: Findings From the NutriNet-Santé Prospective Cohort Study', *JAMA Internal Medicine,* (2018); 178(12):1597–1606

18. K. E. Bradbury, 'Organic food consumption and the incidence of cancer in a large prospective study of women in the United Kingdom', *British Journal of Cancer* (2014); 110:2321–2326

19. J. W. Leff, 'Bacterial communities associated with surfaces of fresh fruits and vegetables', *PLoS One* (2013); 8(3):e69310

9: How are we all unique?

1. M. L. Pelchat,' Excretion and perception of a characteristic odor in urine after asparagus ingestion: a psychophysical and genetic study', *Chemical Senses* (2011); 36(1):9–17

2. M. Falchi, 'Low copy number of the salivary amylase gene predisposes to obesity', *Nature Genetics* (2014); 46(5):492–497

3. G. Rukh, 'Dietary starch intake modifies the relation between copy number variation in the salivary amylase gene and BMI', *The American Journal of Clinical Nutrition* (2017); 106(1):256–262.

4. Sharon Moalem, *The DNA Restart: Unlock your personal genetic code to eat for your genes, lose weight, and reverse aging*, Rodale Books (2016).

5. T. Pallister, 'Food Preference Patterns in a UK Twin Cohort', *Twin Research and Human Genetics* (2015); 18(6)793–805

6. S. Schrempft, 'Variation in the Heritability of Child Body Mass Index by Obesogenic Home Environment', *JAMA Pediatrics* (2018); 172(12):1153–1160

7. F. Asnicar, 'Microbiome connections with host metabolism and habitual diet from 1,098 deeply phenotyped individuals', *Nature Medicine* (2021); 27:321–332

8. https://joinzoe.com/learn/menopause-metabolism-study

9. https://joinzoe.com/

10. A. J. Johnson, 'Daily Sampling Reveals Personalization Diet-Microbiome Associations in Humans', *Cell Host & Microbe* (2019); 25(6):789–802

11. J. M. Santos, 'Pre and Post-Operative Alterations of the Gastrointestinal Microbiome Following Bariatric Surgery', *Cureus* (2021); 13(2):e13067

10. What is the future of food?

1. G. Brookes, 'Farm income and production impacts of using GM crop technology 1996–2015', *GM Crops Food* (2017); 8(3):156–193

2. A. Crimarco, 'A randomized crossover trial on the effect of plant-based compared with animal-based meat on trimethylamine-N-oxide and cardiovascular disease risk factors in generally healthy adults: Study With Appetizing Plantfood – Meat Eating Alternative Trial (SWAP-MEAT)', *The American Journal of Clinical Nutrition* (2020); 112(5):1188–1199

3. Zoe Williams, '3D-printed steak, anyone? I taste test this "game changing" meat mimic', *The Guardian* (16 Nov 2021)

4. Damian Carrington, 'Lab-grown meat firms attract sixfold increase in investment', *The Guardian* (11 May 2021)

5. Bloomberg, 'Maggot farmer to expand from Cape Town to California', *Engineering News* (31 Oct 2019)

6. C. Depommier, 'Supplementation with *Akkermansia muciniphila* in overweight and obese human volunteers: a proof-of-concept exploratory study', *Nature Medicine* (2019); 25:1096–1103

7. Alyx Gorman, 'Cooped up: is coronavirus lockdown a good time to start keeping chickens?', *The Guardian* (8 Apr 2020)

11. So, now what should I have for dinner?

1. Centres for Disease Control and Prevention, 'Childhood Obesity Facts', https://www.cdc.gov/obesity/data/childhood.html

2. https://joinzoe.com/our-science

3. M. Gibbs, 'Diurnal postprandial responses to low and high glycaemic index mixed meals', *Clinical Nutrition* (2014); 33(5):889–894

4. J. R. Lundgren, 'Healthy Weight Loss Maintenance with Exercise, Liraglutide, or Both Combined', *The New England Journal of Medicine* (2021); 384:1719–1730

5. R.I.M. Dunbar, 'Breaking Bread: the Functions of Social Eating', *Adaptive Human Behavior and Physiology* (2017); 3:198–211

12. Fruits

1. H. Du, 'Fresh fruit consumption and all-cause and cause-specific mortality: findings from the China Kadoorie Biobank', *International Journal of Epidemiology* (2017); 46(5):1444–1455

2. B. Baby, 'Antioxidant and anticancer properties of berries', *Critical Reviews in Food Science and Nutrition* (2017); 58(15):2491–2507.

3. A.D.M. Briggs, 'A statin a day keeps the doctor away: comparative proverb assessment modelling study', *BMJ* (2013); 347:f7267

4. I. Onakpoya, 'The effect of grapefruits (Citrus paradisi) on body weight and cardiovascular risk factors: A systematic review and meta-analysis of randomized clinical trials', *Critical Reviews in Food Science and Nutrition* (2019); 57(3):602–612

5. O. D. Rangel-Huerta, 'Normal or High Polyphenol Concentration in Orange Juice Affects Antioxidant Activity, Blood Pressure, and Body Weight in Obese or Overweight Adults', *Journal of Nutrition* (2015); 145(8):1808–1816

6. D. D. Wang, 'Fruit and Vegetable Intake and Mortality: Results From 2 Prospective Cohort Studies of US Men and Women and a Meta-Analysis of 26 Cohort Studies', *Circulation* (2021);143(17):1642–1654

7. E. E. Devore, 'Dietary intake of berries and flavonoids in relation to cognitive decline', *Annals of Neurology* (2012); 72(1):135–143

8. E. L. Boespflug, 'Enhanced neural activation with blueberry supplementation in mild cognitive impairment', *Nutritional Neuroscience* (2018); 21(4):297–305.

9. D. J. Lamport, 'Concord grape juice, cognitive function, and driving performance: a 12-week, placebo-controlled, randomized crossover trial in mothers of preteen children', *The American Journal of Clinical Nutrition* (2016); 103(3):775–83

10. A. R. Whyte, 'A Randomized, Double-Blinded, Placebo-Controlled Study to Compare the Safety and Efficacy of Low Dose Enhanced Wild Blueberry Powder and Wild Blueberry Extract (ThinkBlue™) in Maintenance of Episodic and Working Memory in Older Adults', *Nutrients* (2018); 10(6):660

11. S. Khalid, 'Effects of Acute Blueberry Flavonoids on Mood in Children and Young Adults', *Nutrients* (2017); 9(2):158

12. K. L. Barfoot, 'The effects of acute wild blueberry supplementation on the cognition of 7–10-year-old schoolchildren', *European Journal of Nutrition* (2019); 58(7):2911–2920

13. LS. Wang, 'A Phase Ib Study of the Effects of Black Raspberries on Rectal Polyps in Patients with Familial Adenomatous Polyposis', *Cancer Prevention Research* (2014); 7(7):666–74

14. C. Morimoto, 'Anti-obese action of raspberry ketone' *Life Sciences* (2005); 77(2):194–204

15. B. M. Cotton, 'Raspberry ketone fails to reduce adiposity beyond decreasing food intake in C57BL/6 mice fed a high-fat diet', *Food & Function* (2017); 8(4): 1512–1518

16. Michael Mosley, 'Why Dr Michael Mosley started the BBC Sleep Challenge', *BBC News* (3 May 2017)

17. G. Howatson, 'Effect of tart cherry juice (Prunus cerasus) on melatonin levels and enhanced sleep quality', *European Journal of Nutrition (2012)*; 51(8):909–16

18. K. M. Kaene, 'Effects of Montmorency tart cherry (Prunus Cerasus L.) consumption on vascular function in men with early hypertension', *The American Journal of Clinical Nutrition (2016)*; 103(6):1531–9

19. A. Luís, 'Can Cranberries Contribute to Reduce the Incidence of Urinary Tract Infections? A Systematic Review with Meta-Analysis and Trial Sequential Analysis of Clinical Trials', *The Journal of Urology* (2017); 198(3):614–621

20. M. Juthani-Mehta, 'Effect of Cranberry Capsules on Bacteriuria Plus Pyuria Among Older Women in Nursing Homes', *JAMA* (2016); 316(18):1879–1887

21. J. K. Udani, 'Effects of Açai (*Euterpe oleracea* Mart.) berry preparation on metabolic parameters in a healthy overweight population: A pilot study', *Nutrition Journal* (2011); 10:45

22. G. W. Cao, 'Observation of the effects of LAK/IL-2 therapy combining with Lycium barbarum polysaccharides in the treatment of 75 cancer patients', *Clinical Observations* (1994); 16(6):428–31

23. XF. Guo, 'The effects of Lycium barbarum L. (L. barbarum) on cardiometabolic risk factors: a meta-analysis of randomized controlled trials', *Food & Function* (2017); 8(5):1741–1748

24. M. Shirai, 'Oral L-citrulline and Transresveratrol Supplementation Improves Erectile Function in Men With Phosphodiesterase 5 Inhibitors: A Randomized, Double-Blind, Placebo-Controlled Crossover Pilot Study', *The Journal of Sexual Medicine* (2018); 6(4):291–296

25. A. Calvano, 'Dietary berries, insulin resistance and type 2 diabetes: an overview of human feeding trials', *Food & Function* (2019); 10:6227–6243

26. H. Du, 'Fresh fruit consumption in relation to incident diabetes and diabetic vascular complications: A 7-year prospective study of 0.5 million Chinese adults', *PLoS Medicine* (2017); 14(4):e1002279

13: Vegetables

1. B. Kulczyński. 'Antiradical capacity and polyphenol composition of asparagus spears varieties cultivated under different sunlight conditions', *Acta Scientarium Polonorum, Technologia Alimentaria* (2016); 15(3):267–279

2. K. Singh, 'Sulforaphane treatment of autism spectrum disorder (ASD)', *Proceedings of the National Academy of the Sciences of the USA* (2014); 111(43):15550–5

3. B. Christiansen, 'Ingestion of broccoli sprouts does not improve endothelial function in humans with hypertension', *PLoS One* (2010); 5(8):e12461

4. J. D. Clarke, 'Bioavailability and inter-conversion of sulforaphane and erucin in human subjects consuming broccoli sprouts or broccoli supplement in a cross-over study design', *Pharmacological Research* (2011); 64(5):456–463

5. World Health Organisation data: https://apps.who.int/gho/data/view.main.CTRY2450A

6. J. Y. Kim, 'Changes in Korean Adult Females Intestinal Microbiota Resulting from Kimchi Intake (longdom.org)', *Journal of Nutrition & Food Science* (2016); 6:2

7. E. K. Kim, 'Fermented kimchi reduces body weight and improves metabolic parameters in overweight and obese patients', *Nutrition Research* (2011); 31(6): 436–43

8. N. F. McMahon, 'The Effect of Dietary Nitrate Supplementation on Endurance Exercise Performance in Healthy Adults: A Systematic Review and Meta-Analysis', *Sports Medicine* (2017); 47(4):735–756

9. M. Siervo, 'Does dietary nitrate say NO to cardiovascular ageing? Current evidence and implications for research', *Proceedings of the Nutrition Society* (2018); 77(2):112–123

10. E. Lissiman, 'Garlic for the common cold', *Cochrane Database of Systemic Reviews* (2014); 2014(11):CD006206

11. K. Ried, 'Garlic Lowers Blood Pressure in Hypertensive Individuals, Regulates Serum Cholesterol, and Stimulates Immunity: An Updated Meta-analysis and Review', *Journal of Nutrition* (2016); 146(2):389S–396S

12. R. Arreola, 'Immunomodulation and anti-inflammatory effects of garlic compounds', *Journal of Immunology Research* (2015); 2015:401630

13. R. Llorach, 'Characterisation of polyphenols and antioxidant properties of five lettuce varieties and escarole', *Food Chemistry* (2008); 108(3):1028–38

14. S. C. Larsson, 'Potato consumption and risk of cardiovascular disease: 2 prospective cohort studies', *The American Journal of Clinical Nutrition* (2016); 104(5):1245–1252

15. D. Borch, 'Potatoes and risk of obesity, type 2 diabetes, and cardiovascular disease in apparently healthy adults: a systematic review of clinical intervention and observational studies', *The American Journal of Clinical Nutrition* (2016); 104(2):489–98

16. https://www.chipsandcrisps.com/world-records.html

17. Statista Research Department, 'Global snack food market – statistics & facts' (Sep 15 2021)

18. Anna Wiber, 'Public Health England launches healthy snacking campaign for children', *Baking Business* (1 March 2018)

19. H. M. Cheng, 'Lycopene and tomato and risk of cardiovascular diseases: A systematic review and meta-analysis of epidemiological evidence', *Critical Reviews in Food Science and Nutrition* (2019); 59(1):141–158

20. H. M. Cheng, 'Tomato and lycopene supplementation and cardiovascular risk factors: A systematic review and meta-analysis', *Atherosclerosis* (2017); 257: 100–108

21. F. Thies, 'Cardiovascular benefits of lycopene: fantasy or reality?', *Proceedings of the Nutrition Society* (2017); 76(2):122–129

22. K. Sahin, 'Lycopene Protects Against Spontaneous Ovarian Cancer Formation in Laying Hens', *Journal of Cancer Prevention* (2018); 23(1):25–36

23. J. L. Rowles, 'Processed and raw tomato consumption and risk of prostate cancer: a systematic review and dose–response meta-analysis', *Prostate Cancer Prostatic Diseases* (2018); 21:319–336

14: Legumes (aka pulses)

1. D. M. Winham, 'Perceptions of flatulence from bean consumption among adults in 3 feeding studies', *Nutrition Journal* (2011); 10:128

2. Rick Pendrous, 'Prim and proper beans', *Food manufacture* (5 Dec 2005)

3. P. Wang, 'Bacillus natto regulates gut microbiota and adipose tissue accumulation in a high-fat diet mouse model of obesity', *Journal of Functional Foods* (2020); 68:103923

4. M. D. van Die, 'Soy and soy isoflavones in prostate cancer: a systematic review and meta-analysis of randomized controlled trials', *BJU International* (2014); 113(5b):E119–30

5. J. Wu, 'Dietary Protein Sources and Incidence of Breast Cancer: A Dose-Response Meta-Analysis of Prospective Studies', *Nutrients* (2016); 8(11):730

6. G. Du Toit, 'Randomized Trial of Peanut Consumption in Infants at Risk for Peanut Allergy', *The New England Journal of Medicine* (2015); 372:803:813

7. D. M. Winham, 'Glycemic Response to Black Beans and Chickpeas as Part of a Rice Meal: A Randomized Cross-Over Trial', *Nutrients* (2017); 9(10):1095

8. M. Singh, 'Glycemic index of pulses and pulse-based products: a review', *Critical Reviews in Food Science and Nutrition* (2019); 61(9):1567–1588

9. C. E. O'Neil, 'Chickpeas and Hummus are associated with Better Nutrient Intake, Diet Quality, and Levels of Some Cardiovascular Risk Factors: National Health and Nutrition Examination Survey 2003–2010', *Journal of Nutrition & Food Sciences* (2014); 4:1

10. J. Erickson, 'Satiety Effects of Lentils in a Calorie Matched Fruit Smoothie', *Journal of Food Science* (2016); 81(11):H2866–H2871

11. A. L. Bonnema, 'The Effects of a Beef-Based Meal Compared to a Calorie Matched Bean-Based Meal on Appetite and Food Intake', *Journal of Food Science* (2015); 80(9):H2088–93

12. E. A. Magee, 'Contribution of dietary protein to sulfide production in the large intestine: an in vitro and a controlled feeding study in humans', *The American Journal of Clinical Nutrition* (2000); 72(6):1488–94

15: Cereals and grains

1. MR. Taskinen, 'Dietary Fructose and the Metabolic Syndrome', *Nutrients* (2019); 11(9):1987.

2. M. A. Cutulle, 'Several Pesticides Influence the Nutritional Content of Sweet Corn', *Journal of Agricultural and Food Chemistry* (2018); 66(12):3086–3092

3. Gaynor Selby, 'Global Breakfast Cereal Survey Reveals Major Differences Depending on Country', *Food Ingredients* (29 Nov 2016)

4. A.F.G. Cicero, 'A randomized Placebo-Controlled Clinical Trial to Evaluate the Medium-Term Effects of Oat Fibers on Human Health: The Beta-Glucan Effects on Lipid Profile, Glycemia and inTestinal Health (BELT) Study', *Nutrients* (2020); 12(3):686

5. T.M.S. Wolever, 'Increasing oat β-glucan viscosity in a breakfast meal slows gastric emptying and reduces glycemic and insulinemic responses but has no effect on appetite, food intake, or plasma ghrelin and PYY responses in healthy humans: a randomized, placebo-controlled, crossover trial' *The American Journal of Clinical Nutrition* (2020); 111(2):319–328

6. The Alliance for Natural Health USA, 'Glyphosate Levels in Breakfast Foods: What is safe?' (19 April 2016)

7. M. J. Davoren, 'Glyphosate-based herbicides and cancer risk: a post-IARC decision review of potential mechanisms, policy and avenues of research', *Carcinogenesis* (2018); 39(10):1207–1215

8. C. Shimizu, 'Association of Lifelong Intake of Barley Diet with Healthy Aging: Changes in Physical and Cognitive Functions and Intestinal Microbiome in Senescence-Accelerated Mouse-Prone 8 (SAMP8)', *Nutrients* (2019); 11(8):1770

9. D. Aune, 'Whole grain consumption and risk of cardiovascular disease, cancer, and all cause and cause specific mortality: systematic review and dose-response meta-analysis of prospective studies', *BMJ* (2016); 353:i2716

10. F. G. De Carvalho, 'Metabolic parameters of postmenopausal women after quinoa or corn flakes intake – a prospective and double-blind study', *International Journal of Food Sciences and Nutrition* (2014); 65(3):380–5

11. A. Arranz Otaegui, 'Archaeobotanical evidence reveals the origins of bread 14,400 years ago in northeastern Jordan', *PNAS* (2018); 115(31):7925–7930

12. Brendan Borrell, 'Stone Age sorghum found in African cave', *Nature* (17 Dec 2009)

13. M. P. Ostrowski, 'Mechanistic insights into consumption of the food additive xanthan gum by the human gut microbiota', *Nature Microbiology* (2022); 7:566–569

14. T. Bacchetti, 'The postprandial glucose response to some varieties of commercially available gluten-free pasta: a comparison between healthy and celiac subjects', *Food & Function* (2014); 5(11):3014–7

15. C. S. Johnston, 'Commercially available gluten-free pastas elevate postprandial glycemia in comparison to conventional wheat pasta in healthy adults: a double-blind randomized crossover trial', *Food & Function* (2017); 8(9):3139–3144

16. G. I. Skodje, 'Fructan, Rather Than Gluten, Induces Symptoms in Patients With Self-Reported Non-Celiac Gluten Sensitivity', *Gastroenterology* (2018); 154(3):529–539.e2

16: Rice

1. E. A. Hu, 'White rice consumption and risk of type 2 diabetes: meta-analysis and systematic review', *BMJ* (2012); 344:e1454

2. M. Dehghan, 'Associations of fats and carbohydrate intake with cardiovascular disease and mortality in 18 countries from five continents (PURE): a prospective cohort study', *The Lancet* (2017); 390(10107):2050–2062

3. J. Dias, 'Diabetes Risk and Control in Multi-ethnic US Immigrant Populations', *Current Diabetes Reports* (2020); 20:73

4. H. M. Boers, 'A systematic review of the influence of rice characteristics and processing methods on postprandial glycaemic and insulinemic responses', *British Journal of Nutrition* (2015); 114(7):1035–45

5. E. Kurtys, 'Anti-inflammatory effects of rice bran components', *Nutrition Reviews* (2018); 76(5): 372–379

6. Y. Fakhri, 'Concentrations of arsenic and lead in rice (Oryza sativa L.) in Iran: A systematic review and carcinogenic risk assessment', *Food and Chemical Toxicology* (2018); 113:267–277

7. L. W. Lu, 'Effect of Cold Storage and Reheating of Parboiled Rice on Postprandial Glycaemic Response, Satiety, Palatability and Chewed Particle Size Distribution', *Nutrients* (2017); 9(5):475

8. https://www.nhs.uk/common-health-questions/food-and-diet/can-reheating-rice-cause-food-poisoning/ (26 March 2020)

9. https://www.pbs.org/newshour/health/one-in-six-americans-gets-food-poisoning-every-year-cdc-finds PBS News Hour, '1 in 6 Americans get food poisoning every year, CDC finds' (15 Dec 2010)

17: Pasta

1. G. Punis, 'Association of pasta consumption with body mass index and waist-to-hip ratio: results from Moli-sani and INHES studies', *Nutrition & Diabetes* (2016); 6(7):e218

2. L.Chiavaroli, 'Effect of pasta in the context of low-glycaemic index dietary patterns on body weight and markers of adiposity: a systematic review and meta-analysis of randomised controlled trials in adults', *BMJ Open* (2018); 8:e019438

3. M. Vitale, 'Pasta Consumption and Connected Dietary Habits: Associations with Glucose Control, Adiposity Measures, and Cardiovascular Risk Factors in People with Type 2 Diabetes – TOSCA.IT Study', *Nutrients* (2019); 12(1):101

4. Y. Papanikolaou, 'Pasta Consumption Is Linked to Greater Nutrient Intakes and Improved Diet Quality in American Children and Adults, and Beneficial Weight-Related Outcomes Only in Adult Females', *Frontiers in Nutrition* (2020); 7:112

5. V. L. Fulgoni, 'Association of Pasta Consumption with Diet Quality and Nutrients of Public Health Concern in Adults: National Health and Nutrition Examination Survey 2009–2012', *Current Developments in Nutrition* (2017); 1(10):e001271

6. M. D. Russo, 'Nutritional Quality of Pasta Sold on the Italian Market: The Food Labelling of Italian Products (FLIP) Study', *Nutrients* (2021); 13(1):171

7. T. M. Robertson, 'The cumulative effects of chilling and reheating a carbohydrate-based meal on the postprandial glycaemic response: a pilot study', *European Journal of Clinical Nutrition* (2021); 75:570–572

8. Harold McGee, 'How much water does pasta really need?', *The New York Times* (24 Feb 2009)

9. A. Climini, 'Effect of cooking temperature on cooked pasta quality and sustainability', *Journal of the Science of Food and Agriculture* (2021); 101(12):4946–4958

18: Bread, pastries and biscuits

1. Vanessa Kimbell, *The Sourdough School: the ground-breaking guide to making gut-friendly bread*, Kyle Books (2018)

2. C. G. Rizzello, 'Sourdough Fermented Breads are More Digestible than Those Started with Baker's Yeast Alone: An In Vivo Challenge Dissecting Distinct Gastrointestinal Responses', *Nutrients* (2019); 11(12):2954.

3. James Cox, 'Year Old Sarnies: Pret a Manger "fresh" baguettes are up to a YEAR old after being frozen at a factory in France and shipped to UK', *The Sun* (9 Oct 2018)

4. M. Lindenmeier, 'Structural and functional characterization of pronyl-lysine, a novel protein modification in bread crust melanoidins showing in vitro antioxidative and phase I/II enzyme modulating activity', *Journal of Agricultural and Food Chemistry* (2002); 50(24):6997–7006

5. J.H.W. Brinch, 'The effect on mold formation when leaving the first slice in situ in white sliced bread', *Ugeskr Laeger* (2016); 12;178(50):V68834

6. L. Greco, 'Safety for patients with celiac disease of baked goods made of wheat flour hydrolyzed during food processing', *Clinical Gastroenterology and Hepatology* (2011); 9(1):24–9

7. The Global Sourdough Project: http://robdunnlab.com/projects/sourdough/

8. T. Korem, 'Bread Affects Clinical Parameters and Induces Gut Microbiome-Associated Personal Glycemic Responses', *Cell Metabolism* (2017); 25(6): 1243–1253

9. O. Prykhodko, 'Impact of Rye Kernel-Based Evening Meal on Microbiota Composition of Young Healthy Lean Volunteers With an Emphasis on Their Hormonal and Appetite Regulations, and Blood Levels of Brain-Derived Neurotrophic Factor', *Frontiers in Nutrition* (2018); 5:45

10. Nicole Sagener, 'Overwhelming majority of Germans contaminated by glyphosate', *Euractiv* (7 Mar 2016)

19: Fungi and Mushrooms

1. T. Spector, 'Should healthy people take vitamin D supplement in the winter months?', *BMJ* (2016); 355:i6183

2. I. K. Cheah, 'Administration of Pure Ergothioneine to Healthy Human Subjects: Uptake, Metabolism, and Effects on Biomarkers of Oxidative Damage and Inflammation', *Antioxidants & Redox Signaling* (2017); 26(5):193–206

3. S. Zhang, 'Mushroom Consumption and Incident Dementia in Elderly Japanese: The Ohsaki Cohort 2006 Study', *Journal of the American Geriatrics Society* (2017); 65(7):1462–1469

4. K. M. Jade Mattos-Shipley, 'The good, the bad and the tasty: The many roles of mushrooms', *Studies in Mycology* (2016); 85:125–157

5. R. B. Beelman, 'Is ergothioneine a "longevity vitamin" limited in the American diet?', *Journal of Nutritional Science* (2020); 9:e52

6. J. A. Jovanović, 'The Effects of Major Mushroom Bioactive Compounds on Mechanisms That Control Blood Glucose Level', *Journal of Fungi* (Basel) (2021); 7(1):58

7. N. L. Klupp, 'Ganoderma lucidum mushroom for the treatment of cardiovascular risk factors', *Cochrane Database of Systematic Reviews* (2015); 2:CD007259

8. D. Ba, 'Mushroom Consumption Is Associated with Low Risk of Cancer: A Systematic Review and Meta-Analysis of Observation Studies', *Current Developments in Nutrition* (2020); 12(5):1691–1704

9. D. Sharma, 'A Review on Phytochemistry and Pharmacology of Medicinal as well as Poisonous Mushrooms', *Mini-Reviews in Medicinal Chemistry* (2018); 18(13):1095–1109

10. J. Varshney, 'White button mushrooms increase microbial diversity and accelerate the resolution of Citrobacter rodentium infection in mice', *Journal of Nutrition* (2013); 143(4):526–32

11. C. J. Chang, 'Ganoderma lucidum reduces obesity in mice by modulating the composition of the gut microbiota', *Nature Communications* (2015); 6:7489

12. G. Guan, 'Dietary Chitosan Supplementation Increases Microbial Diversity and Attenuates the Severity of *Citrobacter rodentium* Infection in Mice', *Mediators of Inflammation* (2016); 2016:9236196

13. P. Rossi, 'B-glucans from Grifola frondosa and Ganoderma lucidum in breast cancer: an example of complementary and integrative medicine', *Oncotarget* (2018); 9(37):24837–24856

14. M. K. Panda, 'Promising Anti-cancer Therapeutics From Mushrooms: Current Findings and Future Perceptions', *Current Pharmaceutical Biotechnology* (2021); 22(9):1164–1191

15. X. Jin, 'Ganoderma lucidum (Reishi mushroom) for cancer treatment', *Cochrane Database of Systematic Reviews* (2016); 4(4):CD007731

16. S. Habtemariam, '*Trametes versicolor* (Synn. *Coriolus versicolor*) Polysaccharides in Cancer Therapy: Targets and Efficacy', *Biomedicines* (2020); 8(5):135

17. C. J. Torkelson, 'Phase 1 Clinical Trial of *Trametes versicolor* in Women with Breast Cancer', *International Scholarly Research Notices* (2012); 2012:251632

18. A. K. Panda, 'Traditional uses and medicinal potential of *Cordyceps sinensis* of Sikkim', *Journal of Ayurveda and Integrative Medicine* (2011); 2(1): 9–13

19. K. R. Hirsch, '*Cordyceps militaris* Improves Tolerance to High-Intensity Exercise After Acute and Chronic Supplementation', *Journal of Dietary Supplements* (2017); 14(1):42–53

20. R. R. Griffiths, 'Psilocybin occasioned mystical-type experiences: immediate and persisting dose-related effects', *Psychopharmacology* (2011); 218:649–665

21. A. K. Davis, 'Effects of Psilocybin-Assisted Therapy on Major Depressive Disorder: A Randomized Clinical Trial', *JAMA Psychiatry* (2021); 78(5):481–489

22. S. Ross, 'Rapid and sustained symptom reduction following psilocybin treatment for anxiety and depression in patients with life-threatening cancer: a randomized controlled trial', *Journal of Psychopharmacology* (2016); 30(12):1165–1180

23. G. I. Agin-Liebes, 'Long-term follow-up of psilocybin-assisted psychotherapy for psychiatric and existential distress in patients with life-threatening cancer', *Journal of Psychopharmacology* (2020); 34(2):155–166

24. R. L. Carhart-Harris, 'Psilocybin for treatment-resistant depression: fMRI-measured brain mechanisms', *Scientific Reports* 7 (2017); 7:13187
25. R. L. Carhart-Harris, 'Trial of silocybin versus Escitalopram for Depression', *The New England Journal of Medicine* (2021); 384:1402–1411

20. Meat

1. Henry Mance, *How to love animals in a human-shaped world* (Jonathan Cape, 2021)
2. L. A. MacFarlane, 'Gout: a review of nonmodifiable and modifiable risk factors', *Rheumatic Disease Clinics of North America* (2014); 40(4):581–604
3. S. Rohrmann, 'Meat consumption and mortality – results from the European Prospective Investigation into Cancer and Nutrition', *BMC Medicine* (2013); 11:63
4. A. Etemadi, 'Mortality from different causes associated with meat, heme iron, nitrates, and nitrites in the NIH-AARP Diet and Health Study: population based cohort study', *BMJ* (2017); 357:j1957
5. J. E. Lee, 'Meat intake and cause-specific mortality: a pooled analysis of Asian prospective cohort studies', *The American Journal of Clinical Nutrition* (2013); 1032–41
6. R. Iqbal, 'Associations of unprocessed and processed meat intake with mortality and cardiovascular disease in 21 countries [Prospective Urban Rural Epidemiology (PURE) Study]: a prospective cohort study', *The American Journal of Clinical Nutrition* (2021); 114(3):1049–1058
7. D. Zeraatkar, 'Red and Processed Meat Consumption and Risk for All-Cause Mortality and Cardiometabolic Outcomes: A Systematic Review and Meta-analysis of Cohort Studies', *Annals of Internal Medicine* (2019); 171(10):703–710
8. F. Petermann-Rocha, 'Vegetarians, fish, poultry, and meat-eaters: who has higher risk of cardiovascular disease incidence and mortality? A prospective study from UK Biobank', *European Heart Journal*, 42(12); 1136–1143
9. N. Bergeron, 'Effects of red meat, white meat, and nonmeat protein sources on atherogenic lipoprotein measures in the context of low compared with high saturated fat intake: a randomized controlled trial', *The American Journal of Clinical Nutrition* (2019); 110(1):24–33
10. H. Hamdallah, 'Conjugated Linoleic Acid (CLA) Effect on Body Weight and Body Composition in Women (Systematic Review and Meta-Analysis)', *Proceedings of the Nutrition Society* (2020); 70(OCE2):E262
11. E. Lanza, 'The polyp prevention trial continued follow-up study: no effect of a low-fat, high-fiber, high-fruit, and -vegetable diet on adenoma recurrence eight years after randomization', *Cancer Epidemiology, Biomarkers & Prevention* (2007); 16(9):1745–52

12. C. A. Thomson, 'Cancer Incidence and Mortality during the Intervention and Postintervention Periods of the Women's Health Initiative Dietary Modification Trial', *Cancer Epidemiology, Biomarkers & Prevention* (2014); 23(12): 2924–2935

13. W.H.W. Tang, 'The Gut Microbiome and Its Role in Cardiovascular Diseases', *Circulation* (2017); 135(11):1008–1010

14. Chris Mccullough, 'Alibaba: Artificial intelligence inside Chinese pig farms', *Pig Progess* (20 Feb 2018)

15. https://www.eggxyt.com/

16. D. R. Jones, 'Prevalence of coliforms, *Salmonella, Listeria*, and *Campylobacter* associated with eggs and the environment of conventional cage and free-range egg production', *Poultry Science* (2012); 91(5):1195–1202

17. Tim Spector, 'Is it safe to wash my hands, Doctor?', *The Conversation* (10 Oct 2016)

18. T. H. Jukes, 'Antibiotics in feeds', *Science* (1979); 204(4388):8

19. FDA, 'Steroid Hormone Implants Used for Growth in Food-Producing Animals': https://www.fda.gov/animal-veterinary/product-safety-information/steroid-hormone-implants-used-growth-food-producing-animals

20. K.M.C. Nogoy, 'Fatty Acid Composition of Grain- and Grass-Fed Beef and Their Nutritional Value and Health Implication', *Food Science of Animal Resources* (2022); 42(1):18–33

21. M. M. C. Sobral, 'Domestic Cooking of Muscle Foods: Impact on Composition of Nutrients and Contaminants', *Comprehensive Reviews in Food Science and Safety* (2018); 17(2):309–333

22. Consumer Reports: https://www.consumerreports.org/media-room/press-releases/2015/08/my-entry/

23. J.H.H. Wesley, 'Insects are a viable protein source for human consumption: from insect protein digestion to postprandial muscle protein synthesis in vivo in humans: a double-blind randomized trial', *The American Journal of Clinical Nutrition* (2021); 114(3):934–944

21: Processed meats

1. I. Ferrocino, 'RNA-Based Amplicon Sequencing Reveals Microbiota Development during Ripening of Artisanal versus Industrial Lard d'Arnad', *Applied and Environmental Microbiology* (2017); 83(16):e00983–17

2. G. Perrone, 'Penicillium salamii, a new species occurring during seasoning of dry-cured meat', *International Journal of Food Microbiology* (2015); 193;91–8

3. World Health Organization: https://www.who.int/news-room/fact-sheets/detail/hepatitis-e

4. V. Bouvard, 'International Agency for Research on Cancer Monograph Working Group. Carcinogenicity of consumption of red and processed meat', *The Lancet Oncology* (2015); 16(16):1599 600

5. S. Gallus, 'Meat consumption is not tobacco smoking', *International Journal of Cancer* (2016); 138:2539–2540

6. B. Chassaing, 'Dietary emulsifiers impact the mouse gut microbiota promoting colitis and metabolic syndrome', *Nature* (2015); 519(7541):92–6

7. E. Viennois, 'Dietary Emulsifier-Induced Low-Grade Inflammation Promotes Colon Carcinogenesis', *Cancer Research* (2017); 77(1):27–40

22. Fish

1. L. U. Sneddon, 'Evolution of nociception and pain: evidence from fish models', *Philosophical Transactions of the Royal Society B* (2019); 374:20190290

2. E. Sala, 'Protecting the global ocean for biodiversity, food and climate change', *Nature* (2021); 592:397–402

3. Jessica Sinclair Taylor, 'On the hook: Certification's failure to protect wild fish populations from the appetite of the Scottish salmon industry', feedback-global.org (2020)

4. Y. Hansa, 'Reconnaissance of 47 antibiotics and associated microbial risks in seafood sold in the United States', *Journal of Hazardous Materials* (2015); 282:10–17

5. M. J. Blaser, 'The theory of disappearing microbiota and the epidemics of chronic diseases', *Nature Reviews Immunology* (2017); 17(8):461–463

6. Y. Han, 'Fishmeal Application Induces Antibiotic Resistance Gene Propagation in Mariculture Sediment', *Environmental Science & Technology* (2017); 51(18):10850–10860

7. 'Scottish salmon sold by a range of supermarkets in the UK has sea lice up to 20 times acceptable limit', *The Independent* (29 Oct 2017)

8. R. E. Cooper, 'Omega-3 polyunsaturated fatty acid supplementation and cognition: A systematic review and meta-analysis', *Journal of Psychopharmacology* (2015); 29(7):753–63

9. J. Øyen, 'Fatty fish intake and cognitive function: FINS-KIDS, a randomized controlled trial in preschool children', *BMC Medicine* (2018); 16:41

10. J. E. Manson, 'Marine n-3 Fatty Acids and Prevention of Cardiovascular Disease and Cancer', *The New England Journal of Medicine* (2019); 380:23–32

11. D. Engeset, 'Fish consumption and mortality in the European Prospective Investigation into Cancer and Nutrition cohort', *European Journal of Epidemiology* (2015); 30(1):57–70

12. L. Schwingshackl, 'Food groups and risk of all-cause mortality: a systematic review and meta-analysis of prospective studies', *The American Journal of Clinical Nutrition* (2017); 105(6):1462–1473

13. T. Aung, 'Omega-3 Treatment Trialists' Collaboration. Associations of Omega-3 Fatty Acid Supplement Use With Cardiovascular Disease Risks: Meta-analysis of 10 Trials Involving 77 917 Individuals', *JAMA Cardiology* (2018); 3(3):225–234

14. M. Burckhardt, 'Omega-3 fatty acids for the treatment of dementia', *Cochrane Database of Systematic Reviews* (2016); 4(4):CD009002

15. N. K. Senftleber, 'Marine Oil Supplements for Arthritis Pain: A Systematic Review and Meta-Analysis of Randomized Trials', *Nutrients* (2017); 9(1):42

16. Paul Greenberg, *The Omega Principle: seafood and the quest for a long life and a healthier planet*, Penguin Books (2018)

17. Cochrane, 'New Cochrane health evidence challenges belief that omega 3 supplements reduce risk of heart disease, stroke or death', Cochrane.org (18 July 2018) https://www.cochrane.org/news/new-cochrane-health-evidence-challenges-belief-omega-3-supplements-reduce-risk-heart-disease

18. P. Middleton, 'Omega-3 fatty acid addition during pregnancy', *Cochrane Database of Systematic Reviews* (2018); 15(11):CB003402

19. C. Menni, 'Omega-3 fatty acids correlate with gut microbiome diversity and production of N-carbamylglutamate in middle aged and elderly women', *Scientific Reports* (2017); 7(1):11079

20. Oceana press release: https://usa.oceana.org/press-releases/1-5-seafood-samples-mislabeled-worldwide-finds-new-oceana-report/

21. Fox News, 'Study finds that 47 per cent of LA sushi is not the fish it claims to be' (13 Jan 2017)

22. Kashmira Gander, 'Fraudsters are dyeing cheap tuna pink and selling it on as fresh fish in £174M industry', *The Independent* (18 Jan 2017)

23. A. Planchart, 'Heavy Metal Exposure and Metabolic Syndrome: Evidence from Human and Model System Studies', *Current Environmental Health Reports* (2018); 5(1):110–124

24. J. McGuire, 'The 2014 FDA assessment of commercial fish: practical considerations for improved dietary guidance', *Nutrition Journal* (2016); 15(1):66

25. https://www.seafoodwatch.org/recommendations

23. Marine bugs and other seafood

1. L.G.A. Barboza, 'Microplastics in wild fish from North East Atlantic Ocean and its potential for causing neurotoxic effects, lipid oxidative damage, and human health risks associated with ingestion exposure', *Science of the Total Environment* (2020); 717:134623

2. T. S. Galloway, 'Marine microplastics spell big problems for future generations', *Proceedings of the National Academy of Sciences of the USA* (2016); 113(9): 2331–2333

3. N. Hirt, 'Immunotoxicity and intestinal effects of nano- and microplastics: a review of the literature', *Particle and Fibre Toxicology* (2020); 17(1):57

4. XiaoZhi Lim, 'Microplastics are everywhere — but are they harmful?', *Nature* (4 May 2021)

5. B. A. Froelich, 'Vibrio bacteria in raw oysters: managing risks to human health', *Philosophical Transactions of the Royal Society of London, Series B, Biological Sciences* (2016); 371(1689):20150209

6. A. Ludwig, 'Mislabeled and counterfeit sturgeon caviar from Bulgaria and Romania', *Journal of Applied Ichthyology* (2015); 31(4):587–591

7. E. M. Brown, 'Seaweed and human health', *Nutrition Reviews* (2014); 72(3): 205–216

8. Food and Agriculture Organization (FAO), 'The Global status of seaweed production, trade and utilization. Globefish Research Programme', Rome (2018);124

9. E. Abed, 'Impact of Spirulina on Nutritional Status, Haematological Profile and Anaemia Status in Malnourished Children in the Gaza Strip: Randomized Clinical Trial', *Maternal and Pediatric Nutrition* (2016); 2(2):110

10. E. Vardaka, 'Molecular diversity of bacteria in commercially available "Spirulina" food supplements', *Peer J* (2016); 4:e1610

24: Milk and cream

1. Hannah Clarke, 'Change in UK consumer preferences shows need for more cheese', *Agriculture and Horticulture Development Board* (6 Feb 2020)

2. R. G. Heine, 'Lactose intolerance and gastrointestinal cow's milk allergy in infants and children – common misconceptions revisited', *World Allergy Organizational Journal,* (2017); 10(1):41

3. H. A. Bischoff-Ferrari, 'Milk intake and risk of hip fracture in men and women: a meta-analysis of prospective cohort studies', *Journal of Bone and Mineral Research* (2011); 26(4):833–9

4. H.K.M. Bergholdt, 'Lactase persistence, milk intake, hip fracture and bone mineral density: a study of 97 811 Danish individuals and a meta-analysis', *Journal of Internal Medicine* (2018); 284(3):254–269

5. M. Dehghan, 'Prospective Urban Rural Epidemiology (PURE) study investigators. Association of dairy intake with cardiovascular disease and mortality in 21 countries from five continents (PURE): a prospective cohort study', *The Lancet* (2018); 392(10161):2288–2297

6. M. Salmon, 'The Cultural Significance of Breastfeeding and Infant Care in Early Modern England and America, Journal of Social History', *Journal of Social History* (1994); 28(2):247–269

25. Fermented Dairy (yogurt, kefir and fermented milk)

1. J. B. Moore, 'Evaluation of the nutrient content of yogurts: a comprehensive survey of yogurt products in the major UK supermarkets', *BMJ Open* (2018); 8(8):e021387

2. J. B. Moore, 'High levels of sugar in organic and children's yogurts – new survey', *The Conversation* (19 Sept 2018)

3. N. Zmora, 'Personalized Gut Mucosal Colonization Resistance to Empiric Probiotics is Associated with Unique Host and Microbiome Features', *Cell* (2018); 174(6):1388–1405.e21

4. L. Wu, 'Consumption of Yogurt and the Incident Risk of Cardiovascular Disease: A Meta-Analysis of Nine Cohort Studies', *Nutrients* (2017); 9(3):315

5. A. A. Dumas, 'A systematic review of the effect of yogurt consumption on chronic diseases risk markers in adults', *European Journal of Nutrition* (2017); 56(4):1375–1392

6. C. Sayon-Orea, 'Associations between Yogurt Consumption and Weight Gain and Risk of Obesity and Metabolic Syndrome: A Systematic Review', *Advances in Nutrition* (2017); 8(1):146S–154S

7. C. I. Le Roy, 'Yogurt consumption is associated with changes in the composition of the human gut microbiome and metabolome', *BMC Microbiology* (2022); 22:39

8. J. Zierer, 'The fecal metabolome as a functional readout of the gut microbiome', *Nature Genetics* (2018); 50(6):790–795

9. C. Menni, 'Omega-3 fatty acids correlate with gut microbiome diversity and production of N-carbamylglutamate in middle aged and elderly women', *Science Reports* (2017); 7(1):11079

10. P. Lauca, 'Modest effects of dietary supplements during the COVID-19 pandemic: insights from 445 850 users of the COVID-19 Symptom Study app' *BMJ Nutrition, Prevention & Health* (2021);4:e000250

11. The Cultured Coconut, 'How to Decipher Probiotics', *Nature's Finest Probiotic* (25 Jan 2021)

12. H. Demir, 'Comparison of traditional and commercial kefir microorganism compositions and inhibitory effects on certain pathogens', *International Journal of Food Properties* (2020); 23(1):375–386

13. D. A. Savaiano, 'Yogurt, cultured fermented milk, and health: a systematic review', *Nutrition Reviews* (2021); 79(5):599–614

26. Cheese

1. M. Alkhouli, 'Revisiting the "cheese reaction": more than just a hypertensive crisis?', *Journal of Clinical Psychopharmacology* (2014); 34(5):665–7

2. V. T. Martin, 'Diet and Headache: Part 1', *Headache* (2016); 56(9):1543–1552
3. Nick Squires, 'Italy's "Mozzarella King" arrested over "contaminated cheese"', *The Telegraph* (17 Jul 2012)
4. Jessica Haworth, 'One in four Italian mozzarella cheeses contain foreign milk products', *The Mirror* (21 Jan 2016)
5. Brittany Vonow, 'How takeaways are selling pizza topped with fake cheese', *The Sun* (4 Oct 2016)
6. S. Costard, 'Outbreak-Related Disease Burden Associated with Consumption of Unpasteurized Cow's Milk and Cheese', *Emerging Infectious Diseases* (2017); 23(6):957–964
7. P. Gosalvitr, 'Energy demand and carbon footprint of cheddar cheese with energy recovery from cheese whey', *Energy Procedia* (2019); 161:10–16

27. Diary alternatives

1. Clara Guibourg and Helen Briggs, 'Climate change: which vegan milk is best?', *BBC News* (22 Feb 2019)
2. I. Vitoria, 'The nutritional limitations of plant-based beverages in infancy and childhood', *Nutricion Hospitalaria* (2017); 34(5):1205–1214
3. S. C. Bath, 'A review of the iodine status of UK pregnant women and its implications for the offspring', *Environmental Geochemistry and Health* (2015); 37(4):619–29
4. M. A. van Rooijen, 'Palmitic Acid Versus Stearic Acid: Effects of Interesterification and Intakes on Cardiometabolic Risk Markers – A Systematic Review', *Nutrients* (2020); 12(3):615
5. Maga Flores-Trevino, 'The best vegan "cheese" taste tested 2022', *BBC Good Food* (April 2022)

28. Eggs

1. A. Missimer, 'Compared to an Oatmeal Breakfast, Two Eggs/Day Increased Plasma Carotenoids and Choline without Increasing Trimethyl Amine N-Oxide Concentrations', *Journal of the American College of Nutrition* (2018); 37(2):140–148
2. D. M. DiMarco, 'Intake of up to 3 Eggs per Day Is Associated with Changes in HDL Function and Increased Plasma Antioxidants in Healthy, Young Adults', *Journal of Nutrition* (2017); 147(3):323–329
3. J. Y. Shin, 'Egg consumption in relation to risk of cardiovascular disease and diabetes: a systematic review and meta-analysis', *The American Journal of Clinical Nutrition* (2013); 98(1):146–159
4. C. Qin, 'Association of egg consumption with cardiovascular disease in a cohort study of 0.5 million Chinese adults', *Heart* (2018); 104:1756–1763

5. N.R.W. Geiker, 'Egg consumption, cardiovascular disease and type 2 diabetes', *European Journal of Clinical Nutrition* (2017); 72(1):44–56

6. P. Evenepoel, 'Digestibility of Cooked and Raw Egg Protein in Humans as Assessed by Stable Isotope Techniques', *The Journal of Nutrition* (1998); 128(10): 1716–1722

7. https://assets.publishing.service.gov.uk/government/uploads/system/uploads/attachment_data/file/167972/Nutrient_analysis_of_eggs_Summary_Report.pdf

8. R. T. Wu, 'Opposing impacts on healthspan and longevity by limiting dietary selenium in telomere dysfunctional mice', *Aging Cell* (2017); 16(1):125–135

9. M. Hammershoj, 'Review: The effect of grass and herbs in organic egg production on egg fatty acid composition, egg yolk colour and sensory properties', *Livestock Science* (2016); 194:36–42

10. Tamar Haspel, 'Backyard eggs vs. store-bought: They taste the same', *The Washington Post* (2 June 2010)

11. James Kenji López-Alt, 'Do "Better" Eggs Really Taste Better?', *Serious Eats* (16 May 2019)

12. G. Secci, 'Quality of eggs from Lohmann Brown Classic laying hens fed black soldier fly meal as substitute for soya bean', *Animal* (2018); 12(10):2191–2197

13. T. Yamaguchi, 'Detection of antibiotics in chicken eggs obtained from supermarkets in Ho Chi Minh City, Vietnam', *Journal of Environmental Science and Health B* (2017); 52(6):430–433

14. The EAT-Lancet Report 'Commission Food in The Anthropocene: the EAT-Lancet Commission on Healthy Diets From Sustainable Food Systems' (2019)

15. Aditi Chattopadhyay, 'Fact Check: Plastic Eggs in Circulation in Indian Markets?', *The Logical Indian* (25 Aug 2020)

29: Sweet treats

1. B. Amoutzopoulos, 'Free and Added Sugar Consumption and Adherence to Guidelines: The UK National Diet and Nutrition Survey (2014/15–2015–16)', *Nutrients* (2020); 12(2):393

2. S. Ramne, 'Association between added sugar intake and mortality is nonlinear and dependent on sugar source in 2 Swedish population-based prospective cohorts', *The American Journal of Clinical Nutrition* (2019); 109(2):411–423

3. S. Berry, 'Human postprandial responses to food and potential for precision nutrition', *Nature Medicine* (2020); 26(6):964–973

4. H. Abuelgasim, 'Effectiveness of honey for symptomatic relief in upper respiratory tract infections: a systematic review and meta-analysis', *BMJ Evidence-Based Medicine* (2021); 26(2):57–64

5. Z. A. Asha'ari, 'Ingestion of honey improves the symptoms of allergic rhinitis: evidence from a randomized placebo-controlled trial in the East Coast of Peninsular Malaysia', *Annals of Saudi Medicine* (2013); 33(5):469–475

6. H. T. Tan, 'The antibacterial properties of Malaysian tualang honey against wound and enteric microorganisms in comparison to manuka honey', *BMC Complementary and Alternative Medicine* (2009); 9:34

7. US Immigration and Customs Enforcement, 'HIS Chicago seizes nearly 60 tons of honey illegally imported from China' (30 June 2016)

8. Cody Copeland, 'Honey is one of the most faked foods in the world, and the US government isn't doing much to fix it', *Insider* (26 Sep 2020)

9. European Parliament, Committee on the Environment, Public Health and Food Safety, 'Report on the food crisis, fraud in the food chain and the control thereof' (4 Dec 2013)

10. V. Bataille, 'The influence of genetics and environmental factors in the pathogenesis of acne: a twin study of acne in women', *Journal of Investigative Dermatology* (2002); 119(6):1317–22

11. S. Yuan, 'Chocolate Consumption and Risk of Coronary Heart Disease, Stroke, and Diabetes: A Meta-Analysis of Prospective Studies', *Nutrients* (2017); 9(7):688.

12. K. Ried, 'Effect of cocoa on blood pressure', *Cochrane Database of Systematic Reviews* (2017); (4): CD008893

13. Y. Lee, 'Effects of Dark Chocolate and Almonds on Cardiovascular Risk Factors in Overweight and Obese Individuals: A Randomized Controlled-Feeding Trial', *Journal of the American Heart Association* (2017); 6:e005162

14. C. Krittanawong, 'Association between chocolate consumption and risk of coronary artery disease: a systematic review and meta-analysis', *European Journal of Preventative Cardiology* (2020); 13:28(12):e33–e35

15. J. Morze, 'Chocolate and risk of chronic disease: a systematic review and dose-response meta-analysis', *European Journal of Nutrition* (2020); 59:389–397

16. A. Scholey, 'Effects of chocolate on cognitive function and mood: a systematic review', *Nutrition Reviews* (2013); 71(10):665–681

17. Ellie Kincaid, 'A much-hyped study about a diet that lets you eat chocolate daily was an elaborate hoax', *The Insider* (28 May 2015)

18. S. Xiang, 'Xylitol enhances synthesis of propionate in the colon via cross-feeding of gut microbiota', *Microbiome* (2021); 9(1):62

19. T. Uebanso, 'Effects of Consuming Xylitol on Gut Microbiota and Lipid Metabolism in Mice', *Nutrients* (2017); 9(7):756

20. A. Alsunni, 'Effects of Artificial Sweetener Consumption on Glucose Homeostasis and its Association with Type 2 Diabetes and Obesity', *International Journal of General Medicine* (2020); 13:775–785

21. M. Nasseripour, 'A systematic review and meta-analysis of the role of sugar-free chewing gum on Streptococcus mutans', *BMC Oral Health* (2021); 21(1):217

22. P. A. Nayak, 'The effect of xylitol on dental caries and oral flora', *Clinical, Cosmetic and Investigational Dentistry* (2014); 6:89–94

23. L. Bonifait, 'Probiotics for Oral Health: Myth of Reality?', *Professional Issues* (2009); 75(8):585–90

24. A. Thomas, 'Comparison of Antimicrobial Efficacy of Green Tea, Garlic with Lime, and Sodium Fluoride Mouth Rinses against *Streptococcus mutans, Lactobacilli* species, and *Candida albicans* in Children: A Randomized Double-blind Controlled Clinical Trial', *International Journal of Paediatric Dentistry* (2017); 10(3):234–239

25. R. Penninkilampi, 'The association between consistent licorice ingestion, hypertension and hypokalaemia: a systematic review and meta-analysis', *Journal of Human Hypertension* (2017); 31:699–707

26. BBC News, 'Man dies from eating more than a bag of liquorice a day', (24 Sept 2020)

27. M. C. Borges, 'Artificially Sweetened Beverages and the Response to the Global Obesity Crisis', *PLoS Medicine* (2017); 14(1): e1002195

28. A. G. Yunker, 'Obesity and Sex-Related Associations with Differential Effects of Sucralose vs Sucrose on Appetite and Reward Processing: A Randomized Crossover Trial', *JAMA Network Open* (Sept 2021); 4(9):e2126313

29. I. Laforest-Lapointe, 'Maternal consumption of artificially sweetened beverages during pregnancy is associated with infant gut microbiota and metabolic modifications and increased infant body mass index', *Gut Microbes* (2020); 13:1

30. A. C. Sylvetsky, 'Consumption of Diet Soda Sweetened with Sucralose and Acesulfame-Potassium Alters Inflammatory Transcriptome Pathways in Females with Overweight and Obesity', *Molecular Nutrition & Food Research* (2020); 64(11):e1901166

31. S. Becker, 'Effect of stevia on the gut microbiota and glucose tolerance in a murine model of diet-induced obesity', *FEMS Microbiology Ecology* (2020); 96(6):fiaa079

32. N. J. Buckland, 'Susceptibility to increased high energy dense sweet and savoury food intake in response to the COVID-19 lockdown: The role of craving control and acceptance coping strategies', *Appetite* (2021); 158:195917

30: Nuts and seeds

1. J. Sabaté, 'Does nut consumption protect against ischaemic heart disease?' *European Journal of Clinical Nutrition* (1993); 47 Suppl 1:S71–5

2. M. Guasch-Ferré, 'Nut Consumption and Risk of Cardiovascular Disease', *Journal of the American College of Cardiology* (2017); 70(20):2519–2532

3. X. Liu, 'Changes in nut consumption influence long-term weight change in US men and women', *BMJ Nutrition, Prevention & Health* (2019); 2(2):90–99

4. M. Guasch-Ferré, 'Frequency of nut consumption and mortality risk in the PREDIMED nutrition intervention trial', *BMC Medicine* (2013); 11:164

5. G. C. Chen, 'Nut consumption in relation to all-cause and cause-specific mortality: a meta-analysis 18 prospective studies', *Food & Function* (2017); 8(11):3893–3905

6. V. Y. Njike, 'Snacking, Satiety, and Weight: A Randomized, Controlled Trial', *The American Journal of Health Promotion* (2017); 31(4):296–301

7. A. Carughi, 'Pairing nuts and dried fruit for cardiometabolic health', *Nutrition Journal* (2015); 15:23

8. H. Li, 'Nut consumption and risk of metabolic syndrome and overweight/obesity: a meta-analysis of prospective cohort studies and randomized trials', *Nutrition & Metabolism* (2018); 15:46

9. D. J. Baer, 'Metabolizable Energy from Cashew Nuts is Less than that Predicted by Atwater Factors', *Nutrients* (2019); 11(1):33

10. V. Dikariyanto, 'The effects of whole almond snack consumption on fasting blood lipids and insulin sensitivity: a randomised controlled trial in adults', *Proceedings of the Nutrition Society* (2020); 79:OCE1,E5

11. H. D. Holscher, 'Walnut Consumption Alters the Gastrointestinal Microbiota, Microbially Derived Secondary Bile Acids, and Health Markers in Healthy Adults: A Randomized Controlled Trial', *Journal of Nutrition* (2018); 148(6): 861–867

12. A. M. Tindall, 'Walnuts and Vegetable Oils Containing Oleic Acid Differentially Affect the Gut Microbiota and Associations with Cardiovascular Risk Factors: Follow-up of a Randomized, Controlled, Feeding Trial in Adults at Risk for Cardiovascular Disease', *The Journal of Nutrition* (2020); 150(4):806–817

13. A. C. Creedon, 'Nuts and their Effect on Gut Microbiota, Gut Function and Symptoms in Adults: A Systematic Review and Meta-Analysis of Randomised Controlled Trials', *Nutrients* (2020); 12(8): 2347

14. H. D. Holscher, 'Almond Consumption and Processing Affects the Composition of the Gastrointestinal Microbiota of Healthy Adult Men and Women: A Randomized Controlled Trial', *Nutrients* (2018); 10(2):126

15. L. K. Brahe, 'Dietary modulation of the gut microbiota – a randomised controlled trial in obese postmenopausal women', *British Journal of Nutrition* (2015); 114(3):406–417

16. A. Calado, 'The Effect of Flaxseed in Breast Cancer: A Literature Review', *Frontiers in Nutrition* (2018); 5:4

17. S. L. Teoh, 'Clinical evidence on dietary supplementation with chia seed (Salvia hispanica L.): a systematic review and meta-analysis', *Nutrition Reviews* (2018); 76(4):219–242

31: Seasoning, herbs and spices

1. S. Alonso, 'Impact of the 2003 to 2018 Population Salt Intake Reduction Program in England', *Hypertension* (2021); 77:1086–1094

2. Laura Petrecca, 'Chinese takeout has so much salt it should carry a "health warning", UK advocacy group says', *USA Today* (March 2018)

3. A. J. Moran, 'Consumer underestimation of sodium in fast food restaurant meals: Results from a cross-sectional observational study', *Appetite* (2017); 113:155–161

4. F. Elijovich, 'A Scientific Statement From the American Heart Association', *Hypertension* (2016); 68(3):e7–e46

5. Y. W. Kong, 'Sodium and Its Role in Cardiovascular Disease – The Debate Continues', *Frontiers in Endocrinology* (2016); 7:164

6. N. A. Graudal, 'Effects of low sodium diet versus high sodium diet on blood pressure, renin, aldosterone, catecholamines, cholesterol, and triglyceride', *Cochrane Database of Systematic Reviews* (2017); 4(4):CD004022

7. K. R. Mahtani, 'Reduced Salt Intake for Heart Failure: A Systematic Review', *JAMA Internal Medicine* (2018); 178(12):1693–1700

8. I. Nikiforov, 'Salt Consumption and Myocardial Infarction: Is Limited Salt Intake Beneficial?', *Cureus* (2021); 13(2):e13072

9. A. Mente, 'Associations of urinary sodium excretion with cardiovascular events in individuals with and without hypertension: a pooled analysis of data from four studies', *The Lancet* (2016); 388(10043):465–75

10. A. Brand, 'Replacing salt with low-sodium salt substitutes (LSSS) for cardiovascular health in adults, children and pregnant women', *Cochrane Database of Systematic Reviews* (2022); 10;8(8):CD015207

11. C. Menni, 'Gut microbial diversity is associated with lower arterial stiffness in women', *European Heart Journal* (2018); 39(25):2390–2397

12. F. Asnicar, 'Microbiome connections with host metabolism and habitual diet from 1,098 deeply phenotypes individuals', *Nature Medicine* (2021); 27(2):321–332

13. N. Wilck, 'Salt-responsive gut commensal modulates *TH17* axis and disease', *Nature* (2017); 551:585–589

14. AM. Lewis-Mikhael, 'Effect of Lactobacillus plantarum containing probiotics on blood pressure: A systematic review and meta-analysis', *Pharmacological Research* (2020); 153:104663

15. J. Y. Dong, 'Effect of probiotic fermented milk on blood pressure: a meta-analysis of randomised controlled trials', *British Journal of Nutrition* (2013); 110(7):1188–94

16. A. Ricci, 'Homemade tomato sauce in the Mediterranean diet: a rich source of antioxidants', *Italian Journal of Food Science* (2018); 30:37

17. F. Mohseni, 'The effect of Cumin on anthropometric measurements: A systematic review of randomized controlled clinical trials', *Obesity Medicine* (2021); 23:100341

18. R. Zare, 'Effect of cumin powder on body composition and lipid profile in overweight and obese women', *Complementary Therapies in Clinical Practice* (2014); 20(4):297–301

19. K. Mansouri, 'Clinical effects of curcumin in enhancing cancer therapy: A systematic review', *BMC Cancer* (2020); 20:791

20. A. B. Kunnumakkara, 'Curcumin, the golden nutraceutical: multitargeting for multiple chronic diseases', *British Journal of Pharmacology* (2017); 174(11):1325–1348

21. K. Paultre, 'Therapeutic effects of turmeric or curcumin extract on pain and function for individuals with knee osteoarthritis: a systematic review', *BMJ Open Sport & Exercise Medicine* (2021);7:e000935

22. Q. X. Ng, 'Clinical Use of Curcumin in Depression: A Meta-Analysis', *Journal of the American Medical Directors Association* (2017); 18(6):503–508

23. L. T. Marton, 'The Effects of Curcumin on Diabetes Mellitus: A Systematic Review', *Frontiers in Endocrinology* (Lausanne) (2021); 12:669448

24. J. Rubert, 'Saffron authentication based on liquid chromatography high resolution tandem mass spectrometry and multivariate data analysis', *Food Chemistry* (2016); 204:201–209

25. V. E. Attari, 'A systematic review of the anti-obesity and weight lowering effect of ginger (Zingiber officinale Roscoe) and its mechanisms of action', *Phytotherapy Research* (2018); 32(4):577–585

26. G. Bolognesi, 'Movardol® (N-acetylglucosamine, Boswellia serrata, ginger) supplementation in the management of knee osteoarthritis: preliminary results from a 6-month registry study', *European Review for Medical and Pharmacological Sciences* (2016); 20(24):5198–5204

27. A. Bameshki, 'Effect of oral ginger on prevention of nausea and vomiting after laparoscopic cholecystectomy: a double-blind, randomized, placebo-controlled trial', *Electronic Physician* (2018); 10(2):6354–6362

28. A. Alqareer, 'The effect of clove and benzocaine versus placebo as topical anesthetics', *Journal of Dentistry* (2006); 34(10):747–50

29. T. Pallister, 'Food Preference Patterns in a UK Twin Cohort', *Twin Research and Human Genetics* (2015); 18(6):793–805

30. M. Chopan, 'The Association of Hot Red Chili Pepper Consumption and Mortality: A Large Population-Based Cohort Study', *PLoS ONE* (2017); 12(1): e0169876

31. J. Lv, 'Consumption of spicy foods and total and cause specific mortality: population based cohort study', *BMJ* (2015); 351:h3942

32. Y.-H. Chen, 'High Spicy Food Intake and Risk of Cancer: A Meta-analysis of Case–control Studies', *Chinese Medical Journal (English)* (2017); 130(18):2241–2250

33. W. Shen, 'Anti-obesity Effect of Capsaicin in Mice Fed with High-Fat Diet is Associated with an Increase in Population of the Gut Bacterium *Akkermansia muciniphila*', *Frontiers in Microbiology* (2017); 8:272

34. J. Zheng, 'Dietary capsaicin and its anti-obesity potency: from mechanism to clinical implications', *Bioscience Reports* (2017); 37(3):BSR20170286
35. J. D. Mainland, 'The Missense of Smell: Functional Variability in the Human Odorant Receptor Repertoire', *Nature Neuroscience* (2014); 17(1):114–120
36. W.W.T. Khine, 'A single serving of mixed spices alters gut microflora composition: a dose–response randomised trial', *Scientific Reports* (2021); 11:11264

32. Liquids, oils and condiments

1. P. Zuchinali, 'Effect of caffeine on ventricular arrhythmia: a systematic review and meta-analysis of experimental and clinical studies', *Europace* (2016); 18(2):257–66
2. P. Zuchinali P, 'Short-term Effects of High-Dose Caffeine on Cardiac Arrhythmias in Patients With Heart Failure: A Randomized Clinical Trial', *JAMA Internal Medicine* (2016); 176(12):1752–1759
3. R. Poole, 'Coffee consumption and health: umbrella review of meta-analyses of multiple health outcomes', *BMJ* (2017); 359
4. M. J. Gunter, 'Coffee Drinking and Mortality in 10 European Countries', *Annals of Internal Medicine* (2017); 167(4):236–247
5. J. Simon, 'Light to moderate coffee consumption is associated with lower risk of death: a UK Biobank study', *European Journal of Preventive Cardiology* (2022); 29(6):982–991
6. G. Grosso, 'Coffee, Caffeine, and Health Outcomes: An Umbrella Review', *Annual Review of Nutrition* (2017); 37:131–156
7. O. I. Brown, 'Coffee reduces the risk of death after acute myocardial infarction: a meta-analysis', *Coronary Artery Disease* (2016); 27(7):566–72
8. NHS The Eatwell Guide: https://www.nhs.uk/live-well/eat-well/food-guidelines-and-food-labels/the-eatwell-guide/
9. Kate Taylor, 'Bottled water just surpassed a major milestone – thanks to the "marketing trick of the century"', *Insider* (9 Mar 2017)
10. Magnus Jern, 'What's healthier – bottled, filtered or tap water?', *Tapp Water* (26 Apr 2022)
11. A. Iranpour, 'A Review of Alcohol-Related Harms: A Recent Update', *Addiction & Health* (2019); 11(2)
12. A. M. Wood, 'Risk thresholds for alcohol consumption: combined analysis of individual-participant data for 599 912 current drinkers in 83 prospective studies', *The Lancet* (2018); 391(10129):1513–1523.
13. R. Estruch, 'Primary Prevention of Cardiovascular Disease with a Mediterranean Diet Supplemented with Extra-Virgin Olive Oil or Nuts', *The New England Journal of Medicine* (2018); 378:e34

14. G. Fiorito, 'DNA methylation-based biomarkers of aging were slowed down in a two-year diet and physical activity intervention trial: the DAMA study', *Aging Cell* (2021); 20(10):e13439

15. K. Sarapis, 'Extra virgin olive oil high in polyphenols improves antioxidant status in adults: a double-blind, randomized, controlled, cross-over study (OLIVAUS)', *European Journal of Nutrition* (2022); 61:1073–1086

16. V. Meslier, 'Mediterranean diet intervention in overweight and obese subjects lowers plasma cholesterol and causes changes in the gut microbiome and metabolome independently of energy intake', *Gut* (2020); 69:1258–1268

17. CBS News, 'Don't fall victim to olive oil fraud' (3 Jan 2016)

18. B. de Roos, 'The nutritional and cardiovascular health benefits of rapeseed oil-fed farmed salmon in humans are not decreased compared with those of traditionally farmed salmon: a randomized controlled trial', *European Journal of Nutrition* (2021); 60(4):2063–2075

19. R. Hoffman, 'Can rapeseed oil replace olive oil as part of a Mediterranean-style diet?', *British Journal of Nutrition* (2014); 112:1882–1895

20. S. Srivastava, 'Genotoxic and carcinogenic risks associated with the dietary consumption of repeatedly heated coconut oil', *British Journal of Nutrition* (2010); 104(9):1343–52

21. K. C. Maki, 'Corn oil intake favorably impacts lipoprotein cholesterol, apolipoprotein and lipoprotein particle levels compared with extra-virgin olive oil', *European Journal of Clinical Nutrition* (2017); 71(1):33–38

22. K.-T. Khaw, 'Randomised trial of coconut oil, olive oil or butter on blood lipids and other cardiovascular risk factors in healthy men and women', *BMJ Open* (2018); 8:e020167

23. F. Miao, 'The protective effect of walnut oil on lipopolysaccharide-induced acute intestinal injury in mice', *Food Science & Nutrition* (2021); 9(2):711–718

24. C. S. Johnston, 'Vinegar Improves Insulin Sensitivity to a High-Carbohydrate Meal in Subjects With Insulin Resistance or Type 2 Diabetes', *Diabetes Care* (2004); 27(1):281–282

25. T. L. Launholt, 'Safety and side effects of apple vinegar intake and its effect on metabolic parameters and body weight: a systematic review', *European Journal of Nutrition* (2020); 59:2273–2289

33. Final word

1. K.M. Bermingham, 'Menopause is a key factor influencing postprandial metabolism, metabolic health and lifestyle: The ZOE PREDICT study', *American Society for Nutrition* 2022 (abstract)

Index